LEONARDO'S LEGACY

The Science and Philosophy of Diet and Cancer
Through the Ages

Colin E. Champ, M.D.

CDR Health & Nutrition Publishing
Durham, NC

For information about special discounts for bulk purchases or to book
an event with the author contact
admin@colinchamp.com

ISBN-13: 978-1-7352862-0-4

"Neither need you tell me," said Candide, "that we must take care of our garden."

"You are in the right," said Pangloss; "for when man was put into the garden of Eden, it was with an intent to dress it; and this proves that man was not born to be idle…"

"Excellently observed," answered Candide; "but let us cultivate our garden."

Candide by Voltaire, 1759

For Juli and Aurelia

Table of Contents

INTRODUCTION

T he following book is a culmination of questions and topics on cancer, diet, and lifestyle habits brought forth to me by my cancer patients over the past 15 years. An attempt to answer these questions leads us down a long and winding path throughout the history of diet and cancer research with unexpected detours to address philosophy and religion – which have had an immense impact on the relationship between diet and cancer – all in the context of my great-grandfather's emigration from Italy to the United Stated during the turn of the 20th century, which parallels these points. The latter hopefully helps you to persevere through the thicker scientific discussions. They are, however, vital to the discussion and could not be removed or simplified any further. A "takeaway" section is included at the start of each chapter to highlight some of these points.

Yes, the science within has been kept dense at times. Publishers disagreed with this approach and felt it would be more appropriate to write an "Idiots Guide to Diet and Cancer" or "Top Ten Ways to Prevent Cancer with your Diet" and warned that I should keep it "simple and stupid" to sell more books. I felt this advice was rather offensive to my readers. While they may be correct in terms of book sales, that strategy would defeat the purpose of this work. The questions posed by my patients are not simple ones, nor are the answers. This book was not written for income potential. What publishers and marketing agents do not understand is that the quest to answer these questions is more rewarding than book sales, and perhaps it is best to keep the two apart to some degree.

If you are interested in diving head first to the difficult answers that accompany these questions, then you may find this book enjoyable and informative. If you are looking for an "Idiot's Guide to Diet and Cancer," you will certainly be disappointed with this book and the realization that cancer and diet are far too complicated topics to lend to such a discussion. A deeper dive is not only required, but it will likely leave us asking more questions than were answered. The hope is that this book will serve as a springboard in seeking knowledge while conveying tangible, evidence-based actions we can take to help combat cancer.

We need to view science and food differently. Both require dedication. There are no easy answers, and as long as we refuse to dig deeper and instead attempt to distill it down to simple, yet perhaps lucrative, yes and no answers, we will remain lost along the journey.

Diet and Cancer Studies

DR. C. MORESCHI: 1909
Beziehungen Zwischen Ernahrung und Tumorwachstum

Sarcoma growth was slowed by calorie restriction in mice.

ROUS: 1911
Proceedings of the Society of Exeripental Biology and Medicine

Underfed mice experienced decreased rates of tumor growth.

VAN ALSTYNE AND BEEBE: 1913
Journal of Medical Research
Carbohydrate restriction left mice more resistant to tumor growth inthe largest mouse study to this day.

ROUS: 1914
Journal of Experiential Medicine

Only 41% of mice on a calorically restricted diet experienced tumor implantation and growth versus 81% eating ad libitum.

KEYS: 1944
Military Archives
The
Minnesota Starvation Study took 36 individuals and calorically restricted them for 14 months, tracking physical and psychological distress.

TANNENBAUM: 1947
Annals of the NY Academy of Science

An array of studies revealed decreased tumor incidence, implantation and growth with calorie restriction. Particularly, carbohydrate restriction had a greater effect.

Doll and Armstrong: 1975
International Journal of Cancer

Assessed 32 countries to evaluate links between dietary habits and cancer. Some relationships were identified but difficult to control for GNP and western lifestyles.

WILLETT: 1987, 1992, 1999
NEJM, JAMA
The diets of 90,000 nurses were assessed to link breast cancer and dietary fat. No link was reported, but reducing fat and increasing carbohydrates was linked to increased risk of breast cancer.

PART I

THE ABSTRACT

1

JOURNEYS: PHYSICAL, EMOTIONAL & SCIENTIFIC

"La cucina di un popolo è la sola esatta testimonianza della sua civiltà."

Translation: "The cuisine of a country is the only exact attestation of its civilization."

- Eugène Briffault, 19th century food critic

Takeaways:

Leonardo Pesce, the story's protagonist, is introduced. Through his chronicled journey from Italy to the United States in the late 1800s, the stage is set to explore the tradeoffs that are made in society. The dichotomy of the promised land of America, with its glitz, glam, temptation, and assured prosperity to all-comers in exchange for Old World traditions and cultural practices will be further revealed in the context of diet, health, and well-being.

The sun's rays began to trickle in through the bedroom ceiling skylight, creating a warm rectangular glow cutting its way onto and across the black and white carpeting. I stared at the beautiful light – mesmerized, speechless, unable to move. The light brightened and the realization set in that I was experiencing a hypnopompic hallucination – a vivid dreamlike episode one encounters while awakening. I gradually exited my slumber and entered into consciousness; birds chirped in the background, creating the familiar soundtrack of serenity that signaled it was Saturday morning. Awaking naturally – without an alarm and instead relying on the sun's rays to gently nudge my brain back to consciousness – was my favorite weekend tradition. Today was a strange exception: this morning's rousting was rooted partly in dream but mostly in reality. A slightly muted chatter echoed up the stairs, emanating from the kitchen below. While this was not an uncommon weekend occurrence in my house, I was wide awake already, so decided to put on some shorts and head downstairs to investigate.

My grandmother Rose had leaned a picture on the edge of the glass kitchen table, tilting it upwards to catch my mother's eye. The same rays of sunshine that poked through my bedroom window now illuminated the kitchen, casting an eerily angelic silhouette onto the wall behind my mother. The sun's glow threw me off for a moment, and as I squinted and rubbed my eyes, I gathered my senses and noticed that Rose was distraught in tears over the man in the picture. He had a kind, familiar look to him, but my sleep-addled, sun-spotted brain was still tuning in to reality.

"Who is that in the picture?" I asked.

"That's your great Great-Grandfather Leonardo," my mother replied, answering for my now sobbing grandmother.

Earlier in the day, Rose found the old picture in her basement during some delayed spring cleaning. It was tucked away in some dusty file boxes stuffed with yellowing papers and bills, untouched for decades. The well-preserved black-and-white portrait measured over a foot tall. The man in the picture was standing in what appeared to be a small grocery store, wearing a grocery apron but appearing as though he was out of place, or just in costume. The corners of his mouth bent upwards while the corners of his eyes jutted downwards, projecting an air of cleverly subtle emotional restraint about him. He was leaning against the counter of the store, and his face radiated a comfortable natural visage even though he was clearly posing for the camera.

The year was 2001 and I was home from college for the summer, electing to spend my time working on artificial organ design at the University of Pittsburgh. Summer was halfway over, and I had spent my days slaving away at my biomedical engineering internship and nights nostalgically relaxing and then comfortably sleeping in my childhood bedroom. The internship work was intense but still I was quite content: I had my nights and weekends free to play in several basketball summer leagues, and even in the busy daylight hours I had ample time not only to be woken up naturally by the sun every day, but also to have that same sun bathe me as I sat poolside two to three times during the week. Today, my plan was more of the same: I would work in the lab in the morning, then head to the pool in the afternoon, and then there would be a basketball game or two waiting for me after a hearty dinner.

On this day, however, I was abruptly shaken from my daily routine and sent into a time machine by Grandma Rose's basement discovery. The man in the photo was Leonardo Pesce, affectionately known on this side of the Atlantic Ocean as Lawrence. Leonardo was born in San Lorenzo, a small town on the southwest coast of Italy perched high in the mountains overlooking the Mediterranean Sea. San Lorenzo is located in Calabria, the southernmost province in Italy – only 800 km from the North African coast – that makes up the "wedge" of the Italian boot. Nondescript towns like San Lorenzo, Condofuri, Bagaladi, Roccaforte del Greco, Melito di Porto Salvo, and Montebello Ionico are stuffed into this wedge like cramped toes. A trip throughout the mountainous areas of Calabria reveals a landscape similar to any general topography map: an assortment of brown and grey blotches with occasional smudges of green, intermixed with small stone-grey towns, surrounded by the sweeping turquoise of the sea. San Lorenzo was perhaps the most famous of these towns due to its history during the battle for Italian Independence in the late 1800s. Giuseppe Garibaldi, the controversial albeit successful French-born military leader of the 19th century and erstwhile Italian national hero, fought for his adopted country's independence from Austrian forces. Since before the time of Napoleon, France and Austria had nonchalantly traded territorial ownership in the yet-to-be-formed country of Italy. After a skirmish in a nearby town led to several fatalities among his men, Garibaldi was wounded and captured by Austrian commanders in San Lorenzo.

The village of San Lorenzo hovers high in the mountainside, clinging to the cliffs and floating along the edge of the mountainous terrain like cumulus clouds. The barely navigable terrain on which the town sits is sharply cut by rocks, steep cliffs and valleys, every so often interrupted by the presence of a hardy, weathered tree or two. As opposed to the Mediterranean paradise that most outsiders envision when contemplating southern Italy, many areas of Calabria more closely resemble a rocky desert; a much smaller minority of the land is tillable for subsistence farming. The abundance of rocks produces frequent landslides and creates unsafe surface conditions for travel. Poverty in the region is endemic, and the locals are mostly confined to a life of hardy agriculture, traditional artisanal work, and raising livestock. In other words, life was not easy; the Calabrese toiled with their hands, and they had few alternatives for eking out a living.

In his early years, Leonardo was no exception to the rule of life in Calabria. He was born to Lorenzo and Catterina Pesce in 1869; they lived like a typical Southern Italian family at the time, growing their own vegetables, slaughtering their own animals, and making their own wine, cheese, and soppressata. One soothing daily comfort to the difficult back-breaking life high in the Calabrian mountains was the view: the Pesces were privy to a spectacular panoramic of the Tyrrhenian, Ionian, and Mediterranean Seas – natural beauty that stood in stark contrast to the daily grind of their typical Mediterranean lives. On a clear day, one could even spot the famed shores of Sicily from the southwest lookout points of the province.

The pathways of life and work in young Leonardo's San Lorenzo seemed to veer sharply in opposing directions. Realities of daily life stood in stark contrast to the beautiful rolling hillsides, breathtaking views of the sea, and collegial village community day-to-day atmosphere. Life was hard, the work was backbreaking, and simply traveling around town required the scaling of steep hills on unstable pebbled trails that would leave the most fit of individuals out of breath.

Family life was important in 19th-century Calabria. The villagers produced wine and cheese, shared goods with their neighbors, socialized often and late into the night, and ate prolonged meals that more often resembled social gatherings than dinners. And oddly enough, many inhabitants of small Italian towns similar to San Lorenzo have experienced remarkable health and longevity. To this day, towns like Acciaroli and Pioppi tucked away farther north along the coast are teeming with centenarians at rates that can only be imagined within the United States and other developed countries.

The local sheep had called the Calabrian mountains home for many generations before their human companions arrived, and the Pesce family made their living serving as shepherds. Young Leonardo would follow his flock daily as it grazed on the trace amounts of grass and plants poking out between the rocky landscape. Using the flock's milk for cheese, its wool for clothing, and eventually its meat for sustenance, the Pesce family depended on their sheep to provide nourishment and a source of income. Leonardo, however, would find the most difficulty with the ultimate role of the shepherd, which would eventually cause a rift between his upbringing and family trade. When it was time to slaughter any one of the sheep, young Leonardo, the gentle soul, would scurry away from his parents to shield himself from the inevitable yet unbearable end to the life of any member of his beloved flock. He could not even bear the thought of butchering his sheep let alone perform the task himself... or even watch others do it, for that matter. This role conflict marked a crossroads that would change the direction of his life forever.

Only in his early twenties, Leonardo made the monumental decision to leave his parents and homeland, never to see either again. In 1897, he would officially sign his declaration of citizenship, renouncing his allegiance and fealty to the King of Italy. The United States – a faraway land of opportunity – advertised a life that might remove the hardship that he faced with each passing day in the rugged mountains. Much like Garibaldi's capture and hasty departure from Calabria, Leonardo suddenly and unexpectedly departed from his birthplace, unaware of what the future might hold but willing to take the risk. With nothing more than a head full of dreams and a trunk full of clothes, he set sail for a promising up-and-coming metropolis in this new land of opportunity, the land of ostensible riches and wealth, the land of endless job prospects: Pittsburgh, Pennsylvania. It would hardly be the promised land he envisioned, but the small Steel City suburb of McKees Rocks would welcome him and at the very least provide him an opportunity to avoid the slaughtering of sheep.

Leonardo was not alone in his decision to brave the long and grueling ocean voyage from Calabria to America, and many of his Southern Italian compatriots also ended up in Pennsylvania. Pittsburgh and the surrounding areas may have flourished culturally and economically from this century-long Italian exodus, but the toll on the motherland was steep: Leonardo's hometown of San Lorenzo, along with several other neighboring towns along the rocky coast, has stood nearly uninhabited since the first half of the twentieth century.

2

KILLING YOUR DARLINGS: A MATTER OF FAT

"You must kill your darlings."

- William Faulkner

Takeaways:

Contemporary research by some of the most renowned dietary researchers has led to the modern-day vilification of fat. While various studies and research protocols were conducted through the better part of the 20th century, even some of the brightest minds in science could not look beyond their hypotheses to see what was in plain sight regarding dietary and nutrition habits, eating patterns, and risk of cancer.

In the healthcare setting and oncology clinic, patients tend to have a similar set of questions revolving around what foods they should eat, what types and how much alcohol they can drink, and whether or not intimacy is safe while they are undergoing treatment. Those questions are asked and answers revealed.

This book is not a lengthy accounting of the history of dietary recommendations. Nor is it another tired addition to the mountainous pile of books claiming to readers that there is some magical path to health and that unless they starve themselves, go vegan, count calories, eat raw vegetables, avoid all animal products, or engage in other miserable activities, they can expect to be doomed to a lifetime of poor health. Neither is this book a scare tactic warning people "how not to die." (Yes, that book exists.) And I can assure you that this work will not be the further promulgation of dietary and lifestyle recommendations backed by little data yet claiming to improve your health or reduce your risk of cancer, especially when such recommendations have not been examined in the context of other parallel healthy lifestyle changes.

And finally, this book will not be an exoneration of fat, the macronutrient that has been so heavily chastised over the past half-century that you may be wondering if it provides any health benefits at all or was simply implanted within our diet by the Creator as a temptation and cruel joke. That being said, dietary fat has been so strongly entwined within the world of dietary recommendations that no adequate discussion may take place with at least providing some background on how it became America's most wanted dietary criminal, especially when it comes to cancer (and more specifically, breast cancer).

The stark contrast between a) the condemnation of fat and many other current aspects of health, lifestyle, and dietary dogma and b) the familial upbringings and cultural backgrounds of so many of us is what this book is about. And as you will see, it is a long, winding, and at times shocking tale – a story that practically writes itself. Dietary fat has been the most vilified of all food substances over the last fifty years. From heart disease to obesity to cancer, fatty foods have borne the brunt of criticism and blame for the current demise of our health, ushering in the rise of the anti-fat crusaders and anti-lipid evangelicals. Fat was relentlessly and systematically pulled from our grocery store shelves and replaced with imposters, often low-fat versions of the foods our parents and grandparents enjoyed. Around the midpoint of the twentieth century, the lipid and cholesterol hypothesis ushered in the creation of the Food Pyramid and Standard American Diet (SAD), with the base of the pyramid endorsing a hearty – and wholly unnecessary – six to eleven servings of grain, pasta, cereal, and bread. Shortly afterwards, the anti-fat sentiment picked up momentum and began its virulent spread throughout the medical field. Fatty foods quickly gained a reputation as the responsible party for nearly every malady large and small, from clogged arteries to acne.[1] Scientific studies filled tabloids, magazines, and news segments, implicating the thick, gooey substance as the grease that collected within our arteries, developed into arterial congestion and eventual complete obstruction, culminating in the incarceration of arterial blood and subsequent shutdown of our entire health system.[2] The detrimental health effects of any substance or activity are rarely viewed in isolation, and it was only a matter of time before the pervasive blame of fatty foods for health issues spread to the cancer world.

For decades the "evidence" was accumulating, and fat had no exonerating witnesses nor alibis. Most scientific studies, known as epidemiologic studies, took a bird's-eye view of a group of individuals by surveying their dietary habits at random times. Scientists running these studies would then perform a series of complicated statistical calculations to analyze whether a relationship extended between fatty foods and heart disease. The results of these studies further reinforced the preconceived notions about dietary fat, cholesterol, and saturated fat. Medical and government sources were convinced by these studies to strongly advise the American public to avoid all fatty foods. Eventually, public opinion shifted considerably, and Americans were told to replace foods heavy in saturated fats with foods cooked in lighter vegetable oils. Traditional diets were abandoned, and tiny Italian grandmothers like the one sobbing over Leonardo's picture at the dinner table threw out their cooking lard and began steaming their vegetables. The taste of steamed Brussels sprouts was so repulsive that she and others eventually abandoned many vegetables, replacing them with more palatable foods that were touted as heart healthy such as bread and whole grains.

Before we get into the precise mechanisms of how fat and breast cancer may be connected, the history behind their association provides some insights into why this message, regardless of any general accuracy or specific flaws, was so pervasive prior to the turn of the 21st century. One of the first major scientific discussions on the association between dietary fat and breast cancer took place in a massive worldwide population study that remains one of the most comprehensive to date. Prior to this study, no work had undertaken such a sweeping examination of the connections between different lifestyle habits and cancer. Furthermore, the researchers involved in the study had recently obtained scientific celebrity status. These factors combined to produce a powder keg of a study, ready to explode and send shockwaves throughout the scientific world.

Englishman Richard Doll was born in Middlesex in 1912. Some thirty years later – and after a failed attempt at studying mathematics at Cambridge University – Doll decided to enroll in King's College in London with the goal of following in his physician father's footsteps. Doll excelled in his medical studies and served in the Royal Army Medical Corps during World War II; by the mid-nineteenth century, he found himself enthralled with medical research, specifically regarding studies that aimed to associate daily and occupational exposures with medical issues ranging from peptic ulcers to cancer. A budding epidemiologist, Doll in 1957 became one of the first medical scientists to independently confirm that irradiation could cause leukemia.[3] Several years before this breakthrough, Doll joined forces with Austin Bradford Hill, another pioneer in the field of epidemiology and statistics. Doll, a smoker, had surmised that lung cancer was caused by car fumes or tarmac, the new (at the time) tar-like material used in road pavement. He and Hill set out to prove that lung cancer was associated with these occupational exposures. After surveying 20 hospitals throughout London, they found that lung cancer was indeed associated with an occupational exposure; unfortunately for Doll, that exposure was to tobacco smoke. They had found that individuals who smoked cigarettes were experiencing lung cancer at such an alarming rate that it could only be concluded that smoking caused cancer.[4] According to their findings, lung cancer risk reached as high as 3000% in heavy smokers. With a twist of irony, they confirmed their hypothesis in a study of over 40,000 British physicians, cementing a link not only between lung cancer and smoking, but also between premature death and a slew of other health issues. Horrified with his findings, Doll immediately stopped his smoking habit, replacing it with a work ethic few had seen before within the field of medical research. He would even publish long-term data for the smoking study five decades later in the *British Medical Journal*.[5] Doll died in 2005 at age 92; his popularity spread quickly throughout the scientific field on the heels of his multiple ground-breaking achievements.

Back in 1975, Doll attempted another career-defining research project with colleague Bruce Armstrong: he sought to analyze the lifestyle and dietary habits of 32 countries to assess for links between cancer deaths and overall mortality. Spanning multiple fields of study and utilizing intense statistical methods, Doll and Armstrong established several important links, including those between meat consumption and colon cancer, fish consumption in Asia and stomach cancer, coffee consumption and kidney cancer, and dietary fat consumption and cancer of the breast and uterus.[6]

However, unlike with the earlier reports of the incontrovertible link between smoking and lung cancer, Doll and Armstrong sternly cautioned restraint this time around. While their study did reveal that different behaviors and foods were associated with several types of cancer, they also strongly emphasized the term "associated." In their words, the findings from this study may "reflect some other variable correlated with economic development" and "the quality of the cancer incidence data is significantly affected by economic factors, particularly as controlling for any of the food consumption variables can reduce the correlation." To paraphrase, more affluent and westernized groups were experiencing higher rates of cancer, a trend that continues to this day for many cancers. In reflecting upon the results of their study, however, Doll and Armstrong advocated that coffee, for instance, may have been associated with kidney cancer, but coffee does not necessarily cause kidney cancer. Those individuals were at higher risk of kidney cancer due to one or more of their Western behaviors and tendencies to drink more coffee in parallel. Furthermore, as Doll and Armstrong had realized, individuals who drank more coffee were usually living in more developed countries and societies and thus engaging in a wider array of unhealthy behaviors. Coffee could have been related to cancer, but it may have been a distant fifth cousin.

To underscore this point, the increase in the gross national product of a country may be a better predictor of cancer than any food its citizens were regularly eating or behaviors they were repetitively undertaking, unhealthy or not. Armstrong and Doll further cautioned that the strong relationship between breast cancer and obesity made further calculations difficult – overweight women had generally worse health and a higher risk of breast cancer, both of which could conflate the available data. Finally, Armstrong and Doll warned of the inherent dangers of controlling for food consumption, along with the possibility of discovering associations that were merely coincidentally impacted by an unknown factor.

Their warnings went largely ignored as numerous questions surfaced regarding these relationships, from fears of coffee to the connection between dietary fat and breast cancer. The fifth cousins were now husband and wife, and while further studies were warranted, Doll's burgeoning reputation unwittingly seemed to hurl their data beyond its limitations, launching the perception that dietary fat caused breast cancer. This perception catapulted far across the pond, landing squarely on Longwood Avenue in Boston, Massachusetts. Several decades later at the Channing Laboratory with the Department of Medicine at Harvard University, Dr. Walter Willett followed Doll and Armstrong's lead as he set out to explore the link, if any, between fatty foods and breast cancer. However, this time around, Willett had at his disposal modern and well-organized data along with his subjects' diet journals known as food frequency questionnaires. Willett and his colleagues at Harvard created the 61-question survey in an attempt to quantify the diet of study subjects instead of piecing it together with calculated guesswork, like Doll and Armstrong.

Breast cancer, the most common non-skin cancer in women, affects one out of every eight women in the United States. Any implication that a specific food within our diet could affect rates of this goliath combined with the now famous Doll's association between dietary fat and cancer provided a natural impetus for further investigation in a more modern setting. However, instead of traveling the world over combing for data, Willett could simply use a massive database of Americans. Doll had already made his mark on the global scientific community throughout the world with respect to lung cancer, and now Willett – the Fredrick John Stare Professor of Epidemiology and Nutrition and Chair of the Department of Nutrition at Harvard School of Public Health – was ready to make his own.

A tenured Professor of Medicine at Harvard Medical School, Willett, and his team at Harvard spent countless hours evaluating the diets of nearly 90,000 female nurses with ages ranging from 34-59. These women, with no documented history of cancer, would periodically check in with medical personnel to fill out dietary questionnaires, adding to Willett's massive databank. Reminiscent of the high school days with standardized tests, participants found themselves filling in bubbles with "Number 2" pencils. The results were collected, analyzed, and then used to estimate the amount of total fat, saturated fat, linoleic acid (polyunsaturated fat), and cholesterol within the diets of these women. These diets were then compared with rates of heart attacks, cancer, and other medical issues to unearth any potential associations. Rudimentary in nature, food frequency questionnaires were a revolutionary tool during the days before the internet and desktop computer.

Willett's team of experts tediously rifled through the results, reconstructed the participants' diets, and then like their predecessors Armstrong, Doll, and Hill, patiently waited to observe correlative relationships. With their focus on fat, Willett's team compiled a more extreme subsample of women – 173 in total – who either consumed the most dietary fat at 44% of their diet, or the least at 32% of their diet. All women within the overall study were meticulously followed, and by four years 601 of them had been diagnosed with breast cancer.[7]

By 1987, these women had been followed long enough to generate the first accurate reports on any relationships between their diets and breast cancer. The medical world eagerly awaited the groundbreaking results. However, this excitement would quickly dissipate, as the scientists' comparison between the highest and lowest fat consumers revealed no difference in rates of breast cancer. Willett's group did warn that these findings were based on a limited period of follow-up, and perhaps if these women were assessed further down the road, associations might surface.

But, why was the study hailed as negative? Why was follow-up not an issue in Doll and Armstrong's earlier study? The groups' conclusions, which attempt to answer these questions, provide more insight into the unsuccessful attempt to link fat and cancer. The easy answer could have simply been that there was no tangible link between dietary fat and cancer. The authors attempted to ignore this dull and scientifically unsatisfying conclusion, and instead claimed that their results "do not exclude a possible influence of fat intake before adulthood or at levels lower than 30 percent of calories." In what could best be described as "doubling down" scientifically, the authors chose to hypothesize that the amount of dietary fat consumed by all women in the study was simply too high to reveal any benefit for the lowest fat consumers. This thought process was not unreasonable; if a moderate reduction in fat is unlikely to reduce the risk of breast cancer, perhaps a significant reduction in fat will be successful. In their words, "a moderate reduction in fat intake by adult women is unlikely to result in a substantial reduction in incidence of breast cancer."

This utterly confusing final conclusion illustrates that one negative study was certainly insufficient to negate the potential association between fat and breast cancer. Hatched in Doll and Armstrong's study, this dubious view still remained alive and well. Furthermore, many within the research community began to wonder whether the scientific question being asked was no longer, "Is fat associated with breast cancer?" but rather "How much fat is associated with breast cancer?" as supported in Willett's conclusion. Other possible explanations surfaced as well; perhaps many of the women were not honestly completing their questionnaires? In the phenomenon known as response bias, self-reporting participants are often found to respond to answers in a manner that supports a biased view of oneself. A type of response bias known as social desirability bias leads individuals to incorrectly, and perhaps even dishonestly, respond that they avoid certain foods considered unhealthy and instead turn to healthier choices. Other respondents may unknowingly over-emphasize good behaviors while underreporting bad ones. This bias typically leads to subtle influencing of response data within the dietary questionnaires, producing inaccurate data.[8] (While reading this, you might be thinking that you would never allow this to happen. If so, then take note – you have just fallen victim to this same social desirability bias.)

The other possible explanation, of course, was that there simply was no connection between dietary fat and breast cancer. The emotional environment during the time, however, would prevent such an explanation. Doll had recently achieved stardom within the scientific community for his work linking tobacco smoking, a social habit, with lung cancer. Next up on the docket was to link common foods and cancer, with the scientific steam engine aimed directly at fat, barreling down the tracks and picking up significant momentum. Doll's latest study threw additional kindle into the engine boiler, and the prevailing viewpoint was that other connections would surface if researchers dug deep enough. Doll's warnings about any conclusions from his data fell by the wayside – when a notable rock star scientist like Doll presented data, the scientific world followed blindly and molded it to validate their preexisting conclusions. After all, he was a highly credible source, and many of their careers were at stake.

An additional hypothesis, perhaps unthinkable at the time, was that the medical community was focusing our interrogation on the wrong suspect. In a strange twist of events, the actual results of the study more closely corroborated this hypothesis. According to the findings, the risks of breast cancer based on each type of fat were as follows: 1) Total fat consumption was associated with an 18% *reduced* risk of breast cancer; 2) Saturated fat consumption was associated with a 16% *reduced* risk of breast cancer; 3) Linoleic acid consumption was associated with a 12% *reduced* risk of breast cancer; 4) Dietary cholesterol was associated with a 9% *reduced* risk of breast cancer.

Each category of fat consumption assessed by the surveying group was associated with a reduced risk of breast cancer, the opposite of their hypothesis. A shocking finding at first glance, these relationships were actually only trends; none were statistically significant enough to be consistent with, or opposing, Willett's conclusions. For instance, the 18% reduced risk of breast cancer in those women eating more total fat was a substantial value, and while quite close to significance, it still may have been landed upon by chance. Furthermore, as the results segued from total fat to saturated fat, linoleic acid, and finally cholesterol, the findings were even less significant. Regardless, the more fat these women consumed, the *lower* risk they had of being diagnosed with breast cancer in each category, a finding that was difficult to reconcile with the groups' stated conclusions. Willett and his team were justified in describing no link between dietary fat and breast cancer, but their conclusion could just as easily have read that there was indeed a potential link – an inverse one. Nevertheless, the massive undertaking and its "groundbreaking" results were awarded publication in the *New England Journal of Medicine*, the oldest continuously published medical journal in the world and by far the most prestigious. Despite the publication, Willett and his group were unable to unearth their dietary diamond in the rough. The biased undertones were acceptable at first, as they were based on Doll and Armstrong's initial findings and, in theory, were attempting to prove the earlier duo's link between dietary fat and breast cancer. However, the lack of connection between dietary fat and breast cancer was glaring, not to mention hardly unique to their study: a smaller, less known study published two years prior had found no association between dietary fat and breast cancer.[9] Willett's group's work hinted at the exact opposite of their preconceived notions, and so it became a launching point for further studies assessing the connection between diet and cancer, which up to that point was an underexplored area within the medical world. Other colleagues followed their lead, and less than a decade later six additional studies emerged assessing the link between dietary fat and breast cancer. Willett and his group combined all six, yielding dietary data on over 337,000 women with 4980 cases of breast cancer. Confirming their initial findings, they found no link between dietary fat and the risk of breast cancer.[10]

⁘

Years later after my encounter with Leonardo at the kitchen table during that warm summer morning, I sat in my office and my mind began to wander.

When it began to meander – a relatively common occurrence – it would most often traverse through time, hopping from one standout memory to another. These memories often involved sports – the crucial basketball shots I made (and mostly missed) over the course of my career – or unforgettable details from the numerous academic classrooms where I spent much of my life. Perhaps somewhat strangely, my wandering thoughts often included food, which was without exaggeration a critical element and key focus of my childhood and adult life. Raised in a household of Italians, I spent nearly every Sunday watching my grandmother work her culinary magic, adding immeasurable pinches of ingredients with a composed fluidity that would without fail culminate in a masterful, delicious work of art. These marvelous cooking sessions were followed by countless hours of a multi-course meal. Similar to Grandma Rose's recipes, the dinner table was an intricate blending of ingredients: food, wine, laughing, socializing, and even relaxation. Our dinner table was more than a place for physical nourishment, it was a sounding board for all members of the family.

These childhood and adolescent Sundays at the dinner table had left an indelible impression on me, so much so that my medical career and adult persona gradually became an extension of these meals, with a constant dedication to food, its role in our lives, and its physical and psychological benefits. And at this particular moment as I sat in my office, my thoughts once again began to sink deeper and deeper into my past. Much like the hypnopompic hallucination I had the morning of Grandma Rose's discovery, I had – or at least I thought I had – an uncanny ability to delve deep into my own thoughts while simultaneously engaging in a completely unrelated work or leisure activity.

And just then, I was suddenly snapped out of my own mind, and my thoughts were abruptly ushered into a topic that would prove much more interesting.

"Can I drink alcohol, Doc?"

Paul Cooper stared at me intently as he waited for my response. The top of his crisp-white dress shirt pulled further open as he leaned forward with his elbows resting on his knees. His dark grey wool suit caught the white sleeves of his shirt and dragged them upwards, exposing the same silver Omega Seamaster worn by Daniel Craig in *Casino Royale*. Moments before, he sat with his left foot crossed over his right knee, revealing his impossibly shiny black Ferragamo loafers in which I remember being able to see my reflection.

I liked Mr. Cooper from the start, and with him sporting my dream watch from my favorite James Bond movie, I liked him even more now. I had pegged him as a whiskey drinker – probably a Bourbon guy. We spent that first half of the consultation discussing his family, his remarkably successful company, and how he spent his time on the weekends. At this precise moment of the consultation, however, he was ready to get down to brass tacks. It was the hundredth time I had been asked this specific question by a patient, and my response was well-prepared and well-rehearsed by now. I began to wonder whether I would make a better bartender than a physician, and it suddenly dawned on me just how similar the two professions are. To paraphrase the great French philosopher Voltaire, medicine is the art of amusing or entertaining the patient while the body heals itself. Oftentimes, we medical professionals need to provide more forms of entertainment to deliver the mix between preparing patients for what lies ahead, while attempting to avoid the inevitable evoking of large amounts of fear.

I had just finished reviewing with Paul every painstakingly precise detail of the radiation plan he would be receiving as part of his non-small cell lung cancer treatment. He had several lymph nodes tucked around the heart in an area known as the mediastinum, which disqualified him from a surgical resection. This disqualification meant that Paul would be venturing to my office every Monday through Friday for the next six weeks – he would now have a second "office job" of receiving radiation therapy. He would also be given a weekly chemotherapy regimen known as carbotaxol; while this treatment is generally better tolerated by most healthy patients, the sheer number of exposures can wear down even the strongest of wills. He could also expect fatigue, decreased blood cell counts, and an uncomfortable feeling when swallowing, referred to medically as esophagitis. Simply put, Mr. Cooper was going to get a sunburn along his esophagus as we pushed radiation to attack the lymph nodes nearby, which was a potential concern for someone I assumed to be a whiskey drinker.

After I finished reciting to Paul the laundry list of possible side effects from his upcoming treatment, he without hesitation asked if he would be able to continue working during treatment, if his hair would fall out, and if he was any risk to his children. Once we reviewed the basics – our review of the side effects resembling the dropdown screen after a prescription drug commercial – we got into the important stuff: his nightly cocktail. He shared his confidence in my ability to treat him for this potentially lethal disease but woefully exposed my lack of knowledge as a bartender.

"Is just a glass of wine with dinner OK?", he asked.

I responded, "I had you pegged as a Bourbon guy."

"Maybe in my younger days," he chuckled. "Give me a nice glass of red and I am good for the night."

Discussing wine with patients is one of my favorite and most frequently touched-upon conversation points during office visits. Radiation oncologists engage in a variety of conversations with patience broaching many topics, far too many concerning the specter of impending death. A nightly glass of red wine was much more than a serving of fermented red liquid; it held social, cultural, and even emotional importance for many of my patients, transcendent significance that I would never have predicted prior to my on-the-job medical training. We often underestimate the cultural importance of both alcohol and wine in other non-American cultures, and the cultural importance many patients held for red wine was remarkably close to that of my Sunday dinners in many respects.

After the alcohol question, the question "Can I have sex?" was almost equally as common, and of course much more awkwardly presented at times. I once had a patient's daughter leave the room after her father asked me this, half laughing and half horrified. Her mother was present, and she walked out before I could answer. That being said, "What should I eat?" was by far the most common question that I have encountered, with it being asked at least a dozen times over the course of my average workday.

Not long ago, I was a young student studying engineering at MIT in Boston, MA and then medicine at Thomas Jefferson University in Philadelphia, PA. It amused me to no end that just a handful of years later, in the first year of my otherwise quite humbling radiation oncology residency stint, I now had individuals twice my age and ten times more successful than me asking my permission to engage in normal behaviors such as eating, drinking, going to the bathroom, and having sex. What made it weirder was that I was advising on many subjects that were seen as taboo vices in my Catholic upbringing.

The first two questions were easy to answer. Alcohol was likely harmless in small amounts, provided it was not interacting with a treated area. In Mr. Cooper's case, he would find himself out of luck after about three to four weeks of treatment. Radiation therapy works by bombarding an area with free radicals via ionizing radiation. These free radicals cause damage to the underlying DNA of both normal cells and cancer cells. The major difference that is exploited with treatment is the tendency of normal cells to repair this damage. The cancer cells, on the other hand, have the primary goal of multiplying rapidly. This rapid growth leads to the prototypical palpable lump of tumor that often portends breast cancer. This tendency to rapidly multiply leaves cancer cells less willing to repair the DNA damage, and after enough treatments and accumulated damage the cancer cells die off. However, over time DNA damage in those normal cells can accumulate, leading to the laundry list of side effects I had discussed with Paul Cooper.

In Mr. Cooper's case, the damage from the daily bombardment of free radicals will eventually cause irritation to his esophagus and its surface over which his food and drink pass. As pouring alcohol on a sunburn is never a good idea, he would likely find himself turning to a differently nightly habit of the nonalcoholic variety. For other patients, such as women receiving radiation therapy for breast cancer, a glass of wine a night does not seem to cause any problems. In fact, a scientific study – from the Campania region of Southern Italy, no less – has revealed that women who enjoy one glass of red wine per day experience less skin toxicity from radiation treatment.[11] This study, much like Willett's initial work, was simply reviewing medical records to discover an association. This one happened to provide a valuable tidbit of information that permitted many women to continue one of their favorite nightly activities. Of course, the study may have been at least somewhat biased, as it took place in one of the largest wine-producing (and consuming) countries in the world. However, I continue to withhold any criticism, as it is not often that physicians can quote the benefits of red wine to our patients.

In fact, since Italians comprised a large amount of our patient population in the vicinity of Thomas Jefferson, this study was a fan favorite. It was particularly enjoyed by those patients who would make and bring in their own wine – and there were many. The Southern Philadelphia Italians even held a yearly contest called Vendemmia, where local families would enter their homemade wine in a competition for local bragging rights. The Vendemmia Foundation is a non-profit organization that is "dedicated to preserving Italian culture and fostering pride in their South Philadelphia community." Clearly, my patients and their community at-large loved their wine.

Sex was no different than alcohol. In contrast to red wine, the medical field lacks a specific study to support the health benefit of sex during cancer treatment; however, patients are generally told to proceed as desired, while avoiding pregnancy of course. If radiation treatment is directly interfering with the pelvic areas, then caution would be advised, and we would have an entirely different conversation with the patient (though this often does little to stop most motivated patients). The potential benefits of continuing these behaviors were obvious even without a study – physical exercise and emotional bonding during perhaps the most stressful time in one's life.

For the third and perhaps most important question, a good answer was surprisingly absent from available medical literature. My views have been pieced together over many years by available studies, personal anecdotal experience and self-experimentation, and decades of being raised in a family that valued nutrition and traditional foods. Unlike dietary dogma's darlings that seemed to play out in the aforementioned studies, my own beliefs incorporated more traditional cultural foods, and some of these generally forbidden foods hung from the ceilings of the grocery store that Leonardo Pesce would eventually build from the ground up in McKees Rocks, PA to serve the local population during the Great Depression.

With each passing conversation I had with my patients about what they should eat during treatment and after, it seemed that their interest in food was mounting. Over time, discussing food with patients – and eventually exercise, sleep, and most aspects of a healthy lifestyle – began to dominate our visits. During many of these conversations, I found that patients had few places to turn to for nutrition and food recommendations. Dieticians often read them the typical mantras of the time, which – based on studies like Doll and Armstrong's pioneering work – would often advise they avoid fat. More often, patients were left with vague recommendations, like follow a "plant-based" diet, count calories, exercise more and eat less, avoid processed foods, or my favorite: eat what your grandfather and his grandfather ate. Some of this advice was certainly reasonable, but still it lacked tangible recommendations, which were a necessity for most patients. The most beneficial aspect of the advice – or lack thereof – is that it provided me insights into the field of oncology's lack of attention to one of the three most common questions.

Regarding the final question of what to eat, little did they know that Leonardo's family saved him the fattiest part of the meat during those Sunday dinners and, perhaps most egregious, had generations-old family recipes for homemade cheese and cured meats. Leonardo was not alone in his small shop outside of Pittsburgh in the early 1900s, as only steps from my office at Thomas Jefferson University Hospital in Philadelphia, Rocky Balboa took his famous run along 9ᵗʰ Street, just south of Center City. With no filming permits or street closures needed, Balboa dashed through the Italian Market, inching closer to the hospital. In one of the most famous scenes of *Rocky*, he effortlessly caught an orange that was tossed by an Italian market vendor who, supposedly, had no idea they were even filming the movie.

In other words, the foods that Rocky, Leonardo, and many of my Italian patients were making at home and eating were the same foods many of their physicians were snubbing. A disconnect was forming between traditional cultural foods and the perceived notion of those foods that our grandparents and their grandparents ate. I began to inquire where my patients were gathering their dietary recommendations, especially since they were unlikely to be receiving them from their physicians. The disconnect between dietary recommendations, the lack of tangible food endorsements, and Willett's long and winding scientific journey illustrated some of the major issues of teaching nutrition and specific dietary recommendations at medical school – nobody was quite sure what to teach when it came to specifics. (The startling lack of basic diet and nutrition education in American medical schools was and continues to be a much larger issue that thankfully is undergoing attempts at reformative correction.) To the surprise of no one, most patients were turning to the internet and Google searches for their answers.

On the surface, the realization was quite damning: we were treating patients with heavy doses of ionizing radiation and chemotherapy for weeks to months at a time, yet we were unable to provide an answer to one of their three most common questions. Furthermore, many of their cancers were related to unhealthy dietary habits and obesity, further illustrating the necessity for lifestyle guidance. Since our patients were turning to the internet for their nutrition questions out of necessity, we decided to follow their lead and evaluate the online recommendations of the National Cancer Center

27

Network. The top universities within the cancer world are part of this network, and they provide online treatment recommendations and guidelines for the practicing oncologist. Surely, they were providing patients with adequate answers.

Only they were not. Only four university and hospital sites provided any dietary recommendations, and another four outsourced these to other websites. The paucity of recommendations was surely concerning, yet it paled in comparison to the concern over inconsistency of information. In total, eight sources, including the outsourced websites, supplied drastically conflicting recommendations for patients to follow during and after cancer treatment. In other words, depending on which website patients visited they were instructed to eat an entirely different diet, ranging from a heavy carbohydrate diet to one high in both fat and calories. Many cautioned against weight loss, which has traditionally been associated with worse outcomes after cancer treatment, and nudged patients to consume calorie-packed foods. Others endorsed a low-fat diet, which at the time was considered heart healthy. In corroboration of the vague nature of these website recommendations, we doctors had often heard from many hospital wards that the nutritional endorsements given by their cancer doctors were equally contradictory.

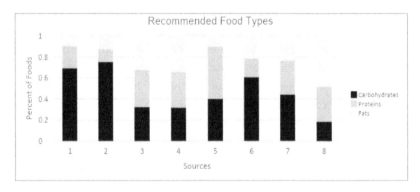

Figure 1: Four NCCN institution websites and four external outsourced websites supplied dietary recommendations for patients during and after cancer treatment.

The contradictory advice further complicated an already unacceptable aspect of our patient care: we physicians were providing few dietary recommendations, when we did, they were often intangible, and the sources providing those recommendations online were incredibly inconsistent. Judging these findings as nothing less than an astounding failure on our end, we quickly compiled our research data on this sore subject into a 23-page manuscript detailing our findings. With our anticipation running high, I submitted our work to one of the major oncology journals, hopeful for them to share in our enthusiasm and disseminate our findings among their readership. We titled the scientific paper *Dietary recommendations during and after cancer treatment: Consistently inconsistent?*

My enthusiasm was not shared by the medical field, as the work was met with disapproval and dismissal, and they quickly rejected the paper. Other journals seemed equally unimpressed and heaped upon us more rejections, which in turn led me to provide my fellow trainees a sampling of expletive-laden tirades directed towards the editors-in-chief of the journals (shouted only behind closed doors, of course). After the paper was rejected, and rejected, and rejected, my enthusiasm began to morph into mild despair. Time and again I received one of two general responses from the reviewers: 1) we do not have any data showing an effect of diet on cancer treatment or outcomes; and/or 2) diet is unlikely to play any part in cancer care; therefore this article is irrelevant for this journal."

Patients may have been interested, but it seemed that the medical field had other priorities.

⁘

While Willett and his team's initial biases were obvious, they could easily be forgiven. Like others at the time, the researchers were merely following the path laid down by a knighted researcher whose work implicated, or at least associated, dietary fat as a potential accomplice in the cause of breast cancer. Furthermore, data was only as reliable as the methods of accumulating that data, and the often-used food frequency questionnaires in these studies have repeatedly been shown to be quite inaccurate. Legitimate doubts and concerns should indeed accompany a scientific survey dependent on subjects' ability to accurately recall their meals over several days, weeks, and years. Furthermore, the risk of reporting bias was always looming; individuals would tend to underreport, lie about, or at best massage the truth when reporting how many "forbidden" foods they consume, in veiled attempts to minimize how much they misbehave.[8] For instance, in Willett's data, women reported that they were consuming an average of 1,500 calories per day, an impossibly small number. However, these women were consistently told they should eat less calories, and unintended reporting bias may have led them to lessen this number. The multitude of issues has led many researchers to abandon the use of these questionnaires.[12] Such issues provided difficulties for groups like Willett's, and while hard to overcome, many researchers did persevere to provide valuable insights into the connections between diet and cancer. Housing individuals and monitoring their food consumption is cost-prohibitive, but with newer technologies and personal devices, increasing surveying and measurement accuracy may soon become a reality.

However, these technologies were decades away from Willett and his group of researchers. Furthermore, Willett's group's work resulted in not one, but two studies – with the latter being a comprehensive analysis of several studies – contradicting their preconceived notions about fat. Yet these notions proved difficult to slay, even in the face of repeated mortal blows inflicted by the results of their own studies. Resisting any visible signs of injury, the biases instead grew stronger and began to spread further. These issues are not unique to medical researchers; American novelist William Faulkner famously advised his fellow writers, a group also prone to obsession with their own ideas, to "kill their darlings." Oftentimes, with careers and tenure on the line, medical researchers personify their hypotheses, creating difficulty in "killing" their theories and finding acceptance when they fail to succeed.

In fact, the conclusions of the original study seemed to be a thinly disguised hypothesis formed by the group. It is unclear if this came about before the initial study or during their synthesis of the results, but Willett attempted to test this theory by following the group of nurses for a bit longer. His second study had expanded the follow-up for eight years after the end of the first; as suggested in their initial publication, perhaps longer follow-up or a more extreme lowering of fat would unearth the link between dietary fat and cancer that was buried in the data. Indeed, Willett achieved both in his updated study, which he published in 1992.[13] This time around, his findings, which ended up in the *Journal of the American Medical Association*, were no different. Publication in *JAMA,* an esteemed but less prestigious journal than the *NEJM*, further signaled the beginning of the decline of the theory that dietary fat was associated with breast cancer.

In this new edition of the study, they began to expand their reach by including an analysis of the interaction between dietary fiber and cancer. While fat was finding itself the dietary whipping boy of the 1980s, fiber had reached stardom as the poster child of a healthy diet. The potential miracle compound found in many foods was felt to regulate our bowels, slow the digestion of food, and leave those who ate it more satiated after a meal, which could decrease the propensity of its consumers to overeat.[14] If true, several of the factors – and particularly the last – could lower the risk of cancer. Furthermore, several studies had linked dietary fiber with lower serum cholesterol levels and lower rates of heart disease. While findings were inconsistent, scientists and physicians studying disease rates in Africa during the mid-twentieth century had hypothesized that dietary fiber was at least partially responsible for a lower risk of cancer. Studies published by members of the British Royal Army Medical Corps stationed in Africa during World War II described an astonishing dearth of the westernized diseases that were abundant in their homeland of England. The theories gained substantial momentum when Denis Burkitt, the famous Irish surgeon and discoverer of a pediatric cancer that holds his name (Burkitt lymphoma), theorized to Richard Doll that colorectal cancer and other malignancies were exceedingly rare in Africa. Burkitt surmised this was due in large part to the amount of fiber in the diet of the continent's inhabitants. Burkitt even wrote an international bestseller on his theory, *"Don't Forget Fibre in your Diet."*

Yet, in a similar vein to the initial observation study of Doll and Armstrong, Willett's findings here did not substantiate the observation studies of Denis Burkitt. Dietary fiber did not appear to be a protector against breast cancer, just as dietary fat did not appear to be a catalyst for it. By this point, some individuals, like the reviewer of our original dietary recommendation paper, had begun to question whether any link between food and cancer existed. Around the same time, mounting public fears of the artificial sweetener aspartame and its role in cancer had now provoked scientists to study the potential association. These studies had exonerated the chemical, which further promoted the mindset that foods and food chemicals may be unrelated to cancer in humans.

31

Returning to the Willett team's third report, the group avoided scientific "doubling down" this time around, but they did provide a peculiar conclusion in the write-up. Around this time, some studies – similar to Doll's initial population study years ago – had suggested an association between meat, fat, and colon cancer. In Willett's paper on breast cancer, the authors concluded that while there was no association between dietary fat and breast cancer, the "positive association between intake of animal fat and risk of colon cancer observed in many studies provides ample reason to limit this source of energy."

While the conclusions of their initial study may have been harmless enough, the strange interweaving of colon cancer risk and their straw-man approach had begun to raise eyebrows within the scientific community. Two studies had now failed to provide a relationship between fat and breast cancer, and in response, the group still recommended avoiding fat by tangentially referring to an association between dietary fat and colon cancer. This non-sequitur further fueled the belief that bias was beginning to get the best of the researchers in what appeared to be no longer a theory, but rather a strong belief that dietary fat caused cancer. The groups' darlings had not been killed, but instead had withstood three fatal blows and continued to run amok, fueled – and perhaps shielded – by biased opinion. These conclusions also provided insight into just how far the darlings expanded beyond Willett's group: the fact that this comment shockingly made it through the peer review process as a primary conclusion of the study, and even more shockingly was published by a prestigious journal, further illustrated how deep the anti-fat sentiment had permeated into the medical world.

Seven years later, Willett and his group further responded to any lingering doubts about both their academic perseverance and personal determination to promote the importance of implanting nutrition and epidemiology within the medical world. After almost a decade and a half of following up, they published a final analysis of their group of nurses.[15] By then, they had succeeded in solving both issues voiced in their first report: they had achieved their long-term follow up and had finally accumulated enough data from women whose diet was less than 20% fat. (By the end of the twentieth century, nearly all these women had been subject to decades of aggressive low-fat dietary advice, and it finally began to take hold.) Yet despite the extended follow-up and the more extreme fat restrictions, their findings continued to be in stark contrast to their hypothesis. The researchers once again reported no benefit in reducing breast cancer risk by avoiding the consumption of fatty foods. However, buried deeper within the results were findings consistent with those of the initial study, as a higher fat consumption again trended with a lower risk of breast cancer.

However, in his third and final analysis of their data, Willett again decided to expand the reach of his research. This time, he would again assess fiber, but also include an analysis of dietary fat versus carbohydrate consumption. This strategy would take into consideration the premise that a diet rarely includes one macronutrient in isolation, and viewing them as such may be a major limiting factor of their prior work. Furthermore, when people decrease one dietary macronutrient, they most often increase another one. While the inclusion of fiber revealed no association with breast cancer, replacing dietary carbohydrates with fats and subsequently increasing fatty food consumption by 5% *lowered* the risk of breast cancer by 4%. Unlike the past trends of fat consumption and a lower risk of breast cancer, this analysis revealed a statistically significant reduction in the number of breast cancer cases in those women who swapped out carbohydrates for fatty foods. While the numbers were small, the findings were a major blow to dietary recommendations at the time and to fiber, the poster child of dietary recommendations over the past three decades. Subset analysis within the study also revealed a statistically significant increase in breast cancer in women who ate less dietary fat, ending their trilogy of reports with results that were the most impactful in finally dealing the death blow to their initial hypothesis. That being said, the undertones of deep-rooted biases still lingered: they reported that they "found no evidence that lower intake of total fat or specific major types of fat was associated with a decreased risk of breast cancer."

Since this publication, multiple population studies have supported the belief that dietary fat is associated with both an increased and decreased risk of breast cancer, while other studies still support the view that fatty foods are unrelated to breast cancer. Food studies vary so widely in their methods and interpretations that a recent analysis of all foods used as ingredients in the *Boston Cooking School Cookbook* concluded that there is scientific evidence to support that nearly all foods can cause or prevent cancer.[16] Pick your view, and there is likely a study to support it. In Willett's case, his own work supported the villain of his hypothesis.

Willett's data, along with several other studies, seemed to float under the radar while anti-fat recommendations permeated throughout the cancer world and society at large. Prior to Sir Richard Doll's death in 2005, he left us with several warnings that were formed from his concern over the implications of his original findings. At the end of his decades-old analysis of the environmental influences associated with cancer incidence, he provided Willett and the medical world with advice that could surely be perceived as modesty over his findings; others viewed it as an omen of what was to come in the dietary world:

"Given the many weaknesses of this method in terms of the quality of the data, allowances for latent periods and the uncertainty as to whether the most relevant environmental variables have even been included in the correlation matrices, it is clear that these and other correlations should be taken only as suggestions for further research and not as evidence of causation or as bases for preventive action."

Doll strongly believed that these correlations should be taken only as suggestions for further research and studies, or in other words a starting point or hypothesis with a clean slate to be equally proven or disproven. Since Willett's initial comprehensive study, numerous other studies have attempted to link dietary fat and breast cancer. Studies remain negative, and to Willett's credit, he has been vocal about the lack of data that implicated dietary fat as a cause of breast cancer, going as far as to state publicly that "support for a major relationship between fat intake and breast cancer risk has weakened considerably as the findings from large prospective studies have become available."[17] At the National Cancer Institute's Cancer Prevention Symposium in 2012, Willett boldly stated that "there was never any strong evidence for this idea, but it was repeated so often that it became dogma in the 1980s and 1990s ... The hypothesis that the percentage of calories from fat in the diet is an important determinant of cancer risk, at least during midlife and later, is not supported by the data."

Willett has even commented that a low-fat, high-carbohydrate diet may increase the risk of breast cancer for a portion of women.[18] While few researchers are able to follow the advice of William Faulkner, Willett succeeded. He had finally killed his darlings.

3

STRONG-ARMING STUDIES

"There are three kinds of lies: lies, damned lies, and statistics."

- Popularly (and erroneously) attributed to Mark Twain

Takeaways:

A variety of animal, population, and epidemiologic studies are explored, including Doll and Hill's groundbreaking finding that smoking and lung cancer are strongly related. This ushered in a wave of new research endeavors hypothesizing the link between foods and different cancers, with the research community vying to find the next trailblazing link. The overall theme is that not only does correlation not equal causation – as evidenced through the various studies and observations – but it may lead us down the wrong path for decades.

Over a decade before Doll and Armstrong published their seminal study, Abraham Kaplan, a philosopher and behavioral scientist, discussed in his book *The Conduct of Inquiry* what he called the "law of the instrument." Wrote Kaplan: "Give a small boy a hammer, and he will find that everything he encounters needs pounding." When Doll, who was widely celebrated for his impact on the health of future generations, connected fat with cancer and began expanding the reach of epidemiologic studies, the dietary wing of Big Medicine was given its hammer. Doll's omen seemed all but forgotten as the medical research community, acting like the small boy with his new toy, hammered on the implications of dietary fat and its relationship with cancer, providing the public with what seemed like a purposeful dismissal of the countless other aspects of a healthy diet. The connections between coffee and fish to cancer were placed on the backburner as an afterthought, only to slowly resurface years later during the heyday of the media's infatuation with dietary studies. But in the meantime, fat was the nail, and the burgeoning field of epidemiology was ready to pounce on it with their hammer, blaming it for everything from obesity to clogged arteries and eventually cancer as well. So, was fat's indictment justified, or had the jury wrongfully accused it based on inadequate evidence? Or perhaps, fat might indeed be guilty, but the punitive sentencing was simply too harsh?

The sheer number of foods, nutrients, vitamins, minerals, spices, and medicinal compounds that comprise a balanced diet – not to mention their interactions with each other – leaves a reliable and isolated analysis of any one of these dietary elements as a difficult, if not impossible, task. Factor in the sheer complexity of cancer initiation and progression, and the ability to predict which exact foods can cause or prevent cancer for a wide population of individuals is nearly impossible. Further confounding this process of epidemiologic examination is that a physical or biological mechanism is required to explain the relationship, otherwise it may simply be coincidence without concrete evidence.

Figuring out which foods may lead to obesity and heart disease is problematic in nature. The former remains controversial, while the latter has led to the lipid hypothesis, another provocative theory that permeated throughout the medical field. Regardless of the current debate surrounding the lipid hypothesis – that cholesterol and fat accumulate within our arteries, slowing blood flow, and eventually leading to total arterial incarceration – its simplistic view is reasonable on the surface. Fats are thicker than liquids at room temperature, and much like the blocked drain pipe removed from our malfunctioning sink, they can accumulate and eventually stop the natural flow within. In other words, there was a physical mechanism to describe how this theory might be reasonable. Ignoring that our bodies are 98.6 degrees and significantly higher than room temperature, the initial mechanism was at least conceptually feasible. Or, take carbohydrates for instance; they raise our blood sugar after we eat them, prompting the pancreas to secrete the hormone insulin, which then pulls sugar from our blood and into our cells to lower blood sugar – a simple cause and effect. If we abuse this process by overeating carbohydrates for decades, our pancreas eventually exhausts its ability to make insulin and becomes fatigued, our blood sugar rises, and we are stricken with Type II diabetes. In keeping with this theory, Type I diabetes is when the pancreas is unable to make insulin due to more innate issues, but the end result is similar. Both processes are considerably more complicated than these simple descriptions, but from a mechanistic point of view, they offer a sensible basis to construct a theory – even to those same old Italian women throwing away their lard in hopes of protecting their arteries. (For the record, the lipid hypothesis is significantly more complicated than this, and we now know that we first need inflammation and subsequent damage to the walls of the arteries for the Band-Aid-like cholesterol to coat it, so we may have been wrongfully blaming the police officer for the crime for decades. Science, especially medical science, always strives to get us closer to the correct answer, but it should always be expected that with every scientific discovery, we can expect several flaws to be lurking within.)

The higher caloric content of fat theoretically linked it to obesity, and cholesterol accumulation theoretically linked fat to atherosclerosis. On the other hand, a tenable mechanism by which fat was inherently harmful when it came to cancer remained elusive. Many believed that fat, which densely contains nine calories as opposed to the "thinner" four calories for protein and carbohydrates, simply led to higher rates of obesity. Individuals with obesity – the state of having too much adipose tissue throughout the body and within the abdomen, encompassing and strangling vital organs – are at a significantly higher risk of many health issues, including a higher risk of cancer due to higher rates of cancer-promoting inflammation, hormones, and blood sugar.[1]

Beyond the hypothesis that fat within the diet was innately linked to fat within the body, scientists were puzzled for decades at the inability to link dietary fat to cancer. It was as though the suspect stood directly in front of them staring them in the eyes, but they somehow lacked the evidence to prosecute. As we will touch upon later, fat within the diet and fat stored within the body are vastly different entities, and these differences were beginning to exert influence on the bulk of studies being conducted within the research world. Fat may have been associated with a higher risk of cancer – along with affluence and many other nonmedical health indicators – but data proving that dietary fat caused breast cancer were few and far between. We needed more proof, and epidemiologic studies were not providing it.

What we needed were human studies to test this hypothesis – studies that provided different diets to two or more groups of similar individuals. Such studies are complicated, expensive, and long-winded, and ideally possess subject observation periods spanning not months or years but decades.

Perhaps most importantly in this era of modern research, the limited immediate economic benefits to any individual or company for financially supporting these studies often leaves them unfunded or underfunded, and potential researchers are most often left with nothing more than a good idea. Furthermore, studies seeking to analyze harmful chemicals and carcinogens – the agents that cause cancer – through the intentional exposure of participants to these substances are obviously unethical and, while they have occurred in the past, should and will hopefully never occur again. The moral burden that limits these studies in humans is less problematic when it comes to animal studies; not surprisingly, the last decade has provided us with a plethora of mouse studies evaluating the cancer promoting and preventing properties of different foods. Humans and mice share 99% of the same genes, and while phenotypically mice are a far cry from humans, these studies are the closest we may come to directly analyzing the carcinogenic interactions of varying chemicals and food.

·❖·

In 1909, three decades before Willett was even a twinkle in his father's eye, Dr. C. Moreschi changed the course of nutritional scientific research forever when he published the small study *Beziehungen Zwischen Ernahrung und Tumorwachstum.*[2] Translated from German, the title reads *Relationships Between Diet and Tumor Growth*. Moreschi, who had faded into scientific oblivion during the twentieth century, has only recently – with the rise of the Information Age and the internet – become recognized for his scientific efforts. His pioneering work on the effects of diet and cancer growth performed from his small laboratory in Europe set the wheels in motion for events of the next century. Moreschi was focusing his efforts on sarcomas, the soft tissue tumors that grow almost superficially, emanating out of the fibrous tissues of tendons and muscles and tracking along the bones and muscles of our extremities. The locations of these lesions allow them to be more easily observed, measured, and studied than other cancer sites such as lung or even breast cancer.

Moreschi's experiment included 36 mice in total, and he separated them into four groups. He supplied the first group with the least amount of daily food, considerably underfeeding them in what might have seemed like cruel and unusual punishment at the time. The other groups were supplied with successively greater amounts of food by Moreschi, with the fourth group being able to eat as much as they pleased, known as *ad libitum* feeding, or Latin for "at one's pleasure." While the latter would be viewed by an outsider as the most humanely treated of the mouse groups, the same cannot be said when considering cancer's approach. Tumors did not grow similarly across the four groups, as would be expected if diet played little role in cancer growth, providing a future rebuttal to the dismissive reviewers of my manuscript on diet and cancer. Instead, the tumors grew in proportion to the amount of food the mice were fed, with the mice eating to their pleasure experiencing the worst fates by means of the largest cancerous growths. Those so-called "tortured" mice of the first group were actually spared the rapid tumor growth observed in the other three groups that had been fattening themselves up before their unknowing demise. They appeared to be feeding not only their appetites, but also their implanted cancer cells, which grew in proportion to their food consumption. In an unexpected twist of fate, the mice who were starved of food experienced the slowest tumor growth.

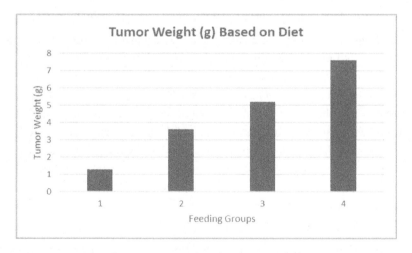

Figure 2: In Moreschi's experiment, as rats were fed more, their tumors grew larger. Group 1 ate 1 g/day, Group 2 ate 1.5 g/day, Group 3 ate 2 g/day, and Group 4 ate until they were full.

As is the case with any groundbreaking experiment that challenges the status quo, Moreschi was criticized for his crude methods. He decreased all three macronutrients, carbohydrates, protein, and fat, in the same proportions, and many felt that the tumors, along with the mice, were simply unable to grow due to malnutrition. Shortly thereafter, Moreschi faded into scientific obscurity following this experiment, but decades later he may have gotten the last laugh.

Intrigued by Moreschi's work, Francis Peyton Rous began performing his own dietary experiments with mice. Rous, a pathologist and virologist, was experimenting with viruses at the Rockefeller Institute for Medical Research in New York at around the same time Moreschi was running his experiments across the Atlantic Ocean. In 1911, only two years after Moreschi's initial pioneering experiment, Rous observed in his studies that a virus could transfer sarcomas – the same sarcomas that Moreschi was inhibiting by underfeeding mice – from one bird to another. This discovery was eventually named the Rous Sarcoma Virus, and Rous' findings earned him a Nobel Prize in Physiology or Medicine in 1966 (after being originally nominated 40 years earlier in 1926). A newcomer to the field, Rous' results were vehemently contested, following the trend of reluctance to accept new ideas within the field of cancer research, especially in nutritional science.

Rous became accustomed to dealing with controversy, and following in Moreschi's footsteps became the modus operandi for the Nobel Laureate as he turned his attention to studying the impact of diet on cancer growth. He even sought to further Moreschi's studies by attempting to prevent cancer with dietary changes; Moreschi had only succeeded in slowing its growth. Rous began harvesting tumors on mice and then transplanting them to other mice whose diets were manipulated. Like Moreschi, he would calorically restrict the mice to varying degrees, but taking his studies a step further he also exposed these mice as well as the normally fed mice to varying carcinogenic chemicals. This method would allow Rous to test whether diet alone could prevent tumor development in mice.

Rous' second research focus would prove to be another first for the medical field. Shortly after completing his Nobel Prize-worthy work, he followed with several groundbreaking studies revealing that different diets can potentially slow the growth of tumors, and more importantly that the dietary changes could provide mice with the ability to prevent cancer before it struck. For instance, simply decreasing the amount of food each mouse was fed would reduce their risk of successful implantation and growth of the foreign-grown tumors. Rous's findings were staggering – he was able to successfully transplant a tumor that would become embedded and grow within 83% of mice eating an unrestricted *ad libitum* diet, while only 41% of those mice on a restricted diet experienced tumor growth.[3,4] Mice that ate less were also resistant to cancer after Rous exposed them to a carcinogenic chemical, further revealing the preventative potential of dietary restriction. However, even during Rous' series of successful studies, he would report on the stubborn nature of cancer, as some tumors were impervious to even the most extreme dietary changes. Much like in humans, it appeared that some cancers were destined to occur.

Colleagues of Rous and Moreschi shared their enthusiasm of the link between diet and cancer. Dr. Albert Tannenbaum, who served as president of the American Association for Cancer Research, dedicated perhaps the most time and effort to furthering studies on the connection between diet and cancer prevention. His peers teased him about his incessant weighing of the mice to ensure precision measurement, the amount of food the mice were consuming, and the proportion of macronutrients being allotted. Despite all the teasing, Tannenbaum stayed the course, with the goal of effectively eliminating the common criticisms of Moreschi's study. When I sat down to discuss these studies with one of his colleagues, Dr. Renato Baserga, he smiled when I mentioned Tannenbaum. "Oh yes, Albert and his mice. He was always running to weigh them. He was quite particular." Unsurprisingly given the sentiment regarding diet research at the time, Tannenbaum also seemed to all but disappear into oblivion, leaving behind only his now invaluable research papers.

Tannenbaum's meticulous nature would prove vital for future researchers, as he would provide the largest and perhaps most significant studies on the effects of dietary manipulation and cancer prevention to this day. His studies no longer assessed crude states like underfeeding, but rather referred to the more precise scientific term: caloric restriction. This term, created to imply more specificity, would unfortunately create confusion within the field of nutrition and cancer for nearly a century.

Years before Tannenbaum began withholding food from mice, and decades before Walter Willett attempted to connect fat with breast cancer, dietary fat had received a scathing indictment via several rudimentary animal studies. Tar, a major carcinogen in tobacco products, produces skin cancer when applied to the surface of mice. When fat was first applied to the skin of mice, the tar-painted mice experienced higher rates of skin cancer. Scientists eventually attempted the same experiment, instead feeding the fat to the mice, and it seemed to cause a similar increase in skin cancer rates – along with producing a fatty coating on the skin of mice overconsuming butter – leading to the dubious hypothesis that fat within the diet increased fat within the skin, and thus ultimately enhanced carcinogen-induced skin cancers.[5] This series of earlier studies, along with those of Moreschi, Rous, and Tannenbaum, prompted the medical establishment to place hitman targets on both calories and fat, with the latter meriting more focus. As Doll had influenced Willett and his colleagues, so too did Tannenbaum's work lead to dozens of follow-up studies with the goal of narrowing down the mechanisms by which fat consumption might increase the risk of cancer, or even outright cause it.

Tannenbaum performed hundreds of experiments in mice; like Rous, his work focused on methods to prevent cancer by testing mice that were exposed to carcinogenic chemicals. He also began experimenting with genetically altered mice that were naturally prone to develop cancer. Both of these test groups represented a model of predetermined cancer in mice, enabling Tannenbaum to assess whether any activity could alter their fate by lowering or raising their cancer occurrence rate. Furthermore, this was the first crude prototypical experiment to model the mice after humans, since we also have plenty of genetic alterations and daily exposures to carcinogens that could predispose us to a cancer diagnosis. As fat possesses more than double the calories of protein and carbohydrates, and Moreschi and Rous had already shown that high-calorie diets could aid in cancer induction and growth, the prevailing expected outcome was that dietary fat would lead to higher rates of cancer growth. The same concerns from Moreschi's original study were adopted by later scientists; even if calories consumed were proportional to both mouse weight and tumor growth, was this not a potential mechanism to stunt tumor growth, or perhaps conversely to cause its growth to accelerate? Indeed, Tannenbaum and his colleagues found that supplying mice with extra fat led them to consume more calories and experience higher rates of cancer.

Predating Willett and the group at Harvard by almost 40 years, Tannenbaum and his contemporaries started to discover the exact opposite of their expected results in a handful of their studies. By 1945, some of his meticulous data strangely began to point to something inherently detrimental about dietary carbohydrates. As Tannenbaum described in one of his paramount studies: "*It appears that mice receiving the diet restricted in carbohydrate only developed fewer tumors, and at a later mean time of appearance.*"[6] Tannenbaum, like his predecessors, found that calorie restriction would increase the ability to prevent cancer, but those mice with diets restricted in carbohydrates often experienced even lower rates of cancer.

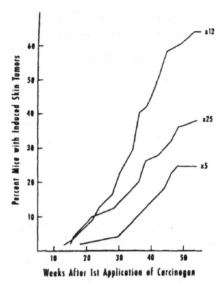

Fig. 1.—Cumulative curves of formation of induced skin tumors, illustrating effect of composition of diet on inhibition caused by caloric restriction. x12, *ad libitum* control; x5, restricted in carbohydrate only; x25, restricted in all components.

Figure 3: As mice went from an ad libitum diet (x12) to a calorie restriction diet (x25), rates of skin tumors dropped. Mice with only carbohydrates restricted (x5) experienced the lowest incidence of cancer.

It appeared that some unexpected inherent biologic property of dietary carbohydrates may have fueled cancer initiation and growth, and restricting carbohydrates in the diets of study mice might reduce the risk of cancer and delay its presentation. Yet, Tannenbaum's findings were not unique; decades before his results, several similar studies were completely overlooked by the

43

medical research world. Perhaps the most famous of these forgotten studies was performed in 1913, around the same time Peyton Rous was conducting his groundbreaking Nobel Prize-winning experiments. This separate study remains the largest mouse study to date, and it sought to assess the effects of diet on cancer growth in 303 mice.[7] Silas Palmer Beebe, an early pioneer in the cancer research world, teamed up with Eleanor Van Ness Van Alstyne of the Huntington Fund for Cancer Research at Cornell University to complete the study. Similar to Tannenbaum's work, the duo's data strongly implicated an unknown factor that was inherently favorable for cancer growth when carbohydrates were consumed in the diet. Their conclusions were somewhat bolder than Tannenbaum's, though the overall theme was similar:

"There seems to be no reasonable ground for doubt in view of these experiments that a lack of carbohydrate in the diet produces such an influence upon the rats as to make them more resistant to tumor growth."

"When the diet includes carbohydrate, the tumors grow luxuriantly. When the diet does not include carbohydrate, the animals show a marked resistance."

After their presentation to the American Association for Cancer Research – where Tannenbaum would serve as president over 40 years later – Van Alstyne and Beebe published their data, and almost immediately the report was fervently challenged. In a strange turn of events, Beebe was expelled from Cornell University two years later for apparently attempting to profit from an ineffective cancer treatment called autolysin.[8] His work in research continued, albeit in a different direction as he focused his subsequent studies on the thyroid gland.

In 1947, Tannenbaum presented his work to the prestigious New York Academy of Science. His groundbreaking findings revealed a consistent and considerable decrease in cancer rates – lung cancer, skin cancer, breast cancer, leukemia, and Moreschi's sarcomas – via a simple reduction in calories consumed. Furthermore, his underfed mice also experienced greater longevity and a healthier appearance. Over the decades, Tannenbaum's work has since been referenced thousands of times by modern doctors and nutritionists, yet back then only in a single editorial was there a brief comment about one small but potentially massive component of his work. In a 1945 editorial on earlier work by Tannenbaum in an issue of the *Journal of the American Medical Association* titled *"Cancer and Calorie Restriction,"* the carbohydrate conundrum was only briefly mentioned, as it repeatedly referred to the remarkable effect of calorie restriction as the major finding of his work.[9]

Tannenbaum's findings, knowingly or not, were paying homage to Van Alstyne and Beebe's earlier study. While Tannenbaum's coinage of the term calorie restriction defined his work for the future generation of researchers, a close examination reveals that the largest anti-cancer benefit was seen when dietary carbohydrates were restricted. Tannenbaum would provide summary graphs from his multiple studies, with the work illustrating the effect of underfeeding by carbohydrate withdrawal and its tendency to produce the largest decrease in cancer incidence. Tannenbaum even placed a "C" above them for "carbohydrates" for easy visualization, yet these findings remained understated throughout his text.

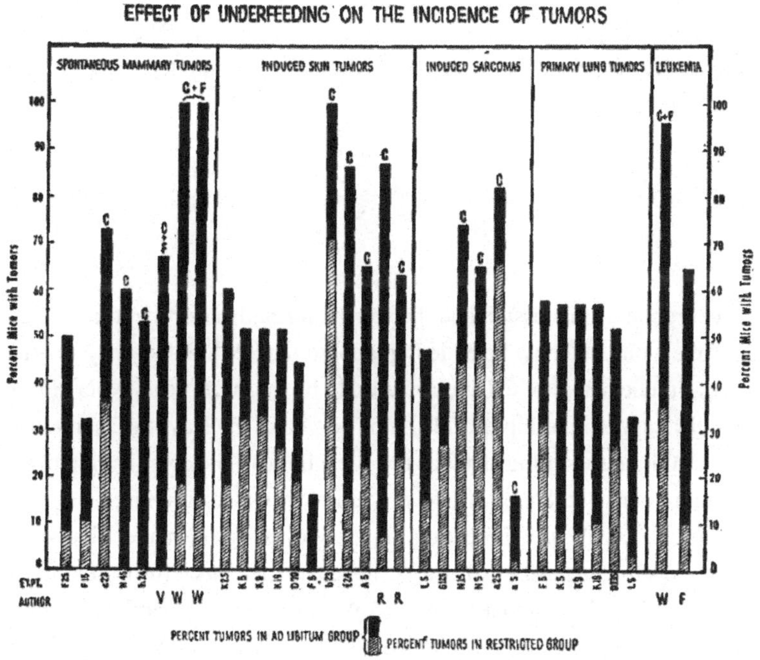

Figure 4: Tannenbaum linked the association between high carbohydrate and high calorie diets almost a century ago.

While much of Tannenbaum's data would implicate carbohydrates, Tannenbaum's meticulous approach would eventually unearth a phenomenon that would plague the dietary world for decades to come. Even with the first dietary study, Rous and his colleagues were feeding their mice a mixture of oatmeal, cornmeal, rye, flour, milk, and sugar. Such diets often consisted almost entirely of carbohydrate ingredients, with little protein and fat. As the findings of Willett's final study suggested, the macronutrient composition of the diets plays an important role in its impact on health. If these mice were being fed an almost entirely carbohydrate diet, it is difficult to tell if calorie restriction was indeed restricting calories or simply providing less carbohydrates and thus less of the mysterious factor that stimulated cancer growth in the earlier mouse studies. Furthermore, Tannenbaum's experiments suggested that increasing dietary fat while consuming a similar diet rich in carbohydrates – a diet resembling that of the Standard American Diet – may be the perfect storm for cancer development. Over time, scientists began to ask whether the general restriction of calories was responsible for aiding in cancer prevention, or if it was simply reducing the dosage level of an unhealthy, cancer-promoting diet. Almost a century later, the question remains unresolved.

❖

A surgeon by profession and the son of an English merchant, James Lind must have wondered how he ended up aboard the HMS Salisbury just off the coast of France being tossed about violently by the angry seas. After entering his medical apprenticeship in 1731, Lind served in the Navy as a surgeon-in-training, ultimately sailing as far as the West Indies. The combination of poor ventilation, constant dampness, severe food and water rationing, and lack of personal space onboard these floating cesspools surely made Lind further question his life decisions. Instead, he channeled his efforts to improve hygienic conditions aboard ships by promoting general cleanliness, ventilation, and fumigation of corridors below deck at a time when cholera, typhus, and dysentery were common epidemics ravaging passengers. His efforts to distill seawater provided passengers with a clean drinking source, a proven successful metric for decreasing rates of dysentery and other water-borne illnesses.

However, a rampant condition aboard Britain's navy vessels continued to stymie Lind and other physicians. It had been known for nearly a century that sailors were commonly plagued by an ailment known as scurvy, yet no treatment was in sight. A typical barrage of symptoms would strike a scurvy victim, starting with fatigue, weakness, and soreness within the arms and legs, and eventually progress to bleeding, nonhealing wounds, and finally, death. Lind was often quoted as declaring that scurvy was killing more sailors than opposing armies. The cause of this dreadful disease had remained elusive, and Lind and others surmised it came from the rotting of food within the body, a process known as putrefaction. The natural cure, Lind hypothesized, was to increase acids within the body to help accelerate the breakdown of the rotting organic matter.

The hypothesis of curing scurvy with acids was not unique to Lind. Over a century before, John Woodall, the surgeon for the East India Company, had recommended fresh foods and citrus fruits for similar symptoms. Prior to this, Portuguese explorers were consuming citrus fruits as a scurvy remedy in the early 1500s. Unlike his predecessors, Lind set out to prove his hypothesis scientifically. During a voyage throughout the Bay of Biscay, he took 12 sailors with weak legs, putrid gums, and lassitude – all symptoms pathognomonic for scurvy – and divided them into six groups of two sailors each.[10] All 12 men subsisted on the same diet of water and gruel sweetened with sugar for breakfast, mutton-broth or pudding for dinner with occasional boiled biscuits with sugar, barley and rice, or wine. Lind then supplemented these epicurean meals with several potentially medicinal foods, each group receiving a different supplement: A) a daily quart of cider; B) 25 drops of sulfuric acid; C) six spoonfuls of vinegar; D) one-half pint of seawater; E) two oranges and a lemon; or F) barley water with a spice paste. Within six days, Lind had run out of oranges and lemons and had to cut the experiment short; however, he had already noticed that one of the men in Group E, partaking in the citrus fruits, was no longer experiencing his scurvy symptoms. The first group, supplied with cider, appeared to have improved physically as well. However, by the time they reached port at Plymouth roughly four weeks later, the man in the citrus group was so healthy that he was now serving as nurse for the other men. The other four groups were still stricken, unaffected by their compounds.

As the HMS Salisbury navigated around the Bay of Biscay, Lind's acidic theory of the cure for scurvy was disproved by what is now considered the first documented controlled clinical study. Simply viewing the associated benefit of citrus fruits for scurvy initially led to the incorrect assumption that acidic foods cured scurvy. Lind instead compared the different substances head-to-head, some simply with acid, others with more robust ingredients. Lind's trial would eventually prove that the ascorbic acid within the citrus fruits, known as vitamin C, was responsible for the treatment of scurvy (the term "scorbutic" means related to scurvy). What Lind did not realize at the time was that he had performed one of history's first clinical trials, a process that served as the basis for experimental research over the next several centuries.

The first randomized controlled trial would not take place until 1946. Doll's old boss and colleague Austin Bradford Hill tested the efficacy of streptomycin for tuberculosis treatment utilizing this novel method. While Lind served as the randomization technique in his earlier studies, Hill used a statistical determination based on random sampling to decide which subjects of the trial received the experimental treatment of the antibiotic streptomycin versus the prevailing standard of care – bedrest. Streptomycin was found to be significantly more effective at combating tuberculosis. This random selection technique to this day remains the gold standard in medicine and several other arms of scientific research.

In the early years after Hill's monumental randomized study, Doll's warning was still considered nothing more than an afterthought. As Doll cautioned, associations can suggest relationships between certain behaviors and cancer, but this suggestion forms nothing more than a hypothesis; further research is essential to confirm or dispute relationships before they become the "basis for preventative action." Finding coincidences within data is not uncommon, especially when the coincidences are related to an unseen factor and are no accident at all. Four decades later, however, Doll's final words may seem more germane: recent studies uncover conflicting relationships (i.e. coincidences) so often that they remain difficult to keep straight. Like any association, mechanistic evidence – in other words, human or animal studies that provide a physical or physiologic rational explanation for the association – must provide an explanation.

Be that as it may, animal studies back then were expensive, messy, time-consuming, and imperfect. These difficulties, combined with the propensity of certain countries and hospitals to evolve into more meticulous tracking of patient data, eventually ushered in an era where researchers were able to perform massive scientific studies while sitting at their office desks; Willett could analyze the data from thousands of his nurses without ever setting foot outside during the cold Boston winters. Furthermore, these studies sidestepped the ethical issues of purposefully altering individuals' habits by simply observing their behaviors and the eventual consequences of those behaviors. Despite the benefits, these studies were still plagued by limitations, even when compared to James Lind's rudimentary maritime clinical trial. These same limitations, in a sense, proved to be these studies' strength – at least in terms on production – as the ease of data acquisition would fuel a generation of countless scientific reports; and so was conceived the modern-day population study.

Many associations have been purported via the results of population studies, and many of us have fallen victim to overreliance on these associations to support our own personal biases and lifestyle habits. News and media sources constantly bombard us with study results, summed up through quick and catchy headlines. The latest and greatest population or epidemiologic study reveals that coffee "prevents" cancer, only to be replaced by a similar study days later claiming that coffee causes cancer. In reality, neither study soundly demonstrates that coffee causes nor prevents cancer, but rather that it may be associated with an increased or decreased risk, coincidentally or not. Often, these news releases are deployed as ammunition to support our lifestyle behaviors, and then ignored when they oppose them.

In medical school, I would track which substances were found to provide benefit or harm based on these studies, with the ultimate goal of creating a comprehensive online database accessible to the public. This database would provide some insights into which foods and lifestyle habits can lower the risk of cancer. The back-and-forth positioning from one study to the next, widespread dissemination of conflicting information, and the realization that most foods were found to both cause AND prevent cancer led me to abandon the undertaking. Instead of providing concrete answers, the results in these population studies, and especially those studies assessing risk of cancer, seemed to be consistently inconsistent. Each conflicting result further added to the mounting confusion among the general public eye. The recent expansion of internet accessibility to wider swaths of the general population coupled with the media's propensity to aggressively promote "latest and greatest" studies has further aggravated the misinformation problem. Although these population studies remain important for medical advancement reasons, their incessant back-and-forth results have fomented well-deserved skepticism among the public. According to a Gallup poll conducted in September 2016, only a third of nightly news viewers feel confident in the truthfulness of media news reports. For many, the nightly news is their primary first-pass source of health information, so between the heated politics and the health/safety scares, the flip-flopping nature of the results works to only further enhance public dismay. Furthermore, while population studies serve to identify connections among our activities and health outcomes, the majority reveal infinitesimally small associations. For instance, when Doll and Hill analyzed the risk of lung cancer and its association with smoking, they found an undeniable connection between the two. Those individuals who smoked 35 or more cigarettes per day were experiencing a death rate from lung cancer that was 40 times higher than nonsmokers.[10] The strong relationship between the two led to the view that "beyond a reasonable doubt" smoking was not only associated with lung cancer, it caused lung cancer. The study findings were immediately incorporated into public health measures. We were only midway through the twentieth century and one of the largest studies in the history of mankind had produced an undeniable relationship between a social habit and cancer. Doll and Hill were eventually knighted for their discovery, and their impact on public health would be immeasurable.[11]

The future was bright for the budding field of epidemiology; what other findings remain unearthed? Doll's next goal was to find out which if any foods were associated with cancer. However, the scientific field was unaware of just how high the bar was raised by Doll's initial work. This initial study had strongly implicated smoking as a cause of lung cancer, revealing a 40 times higher risk of contracting lung cancer in those who smoke (assuming lung cancer was uniformly fatal at the time). In actuality, these numbers reveal that the absolute risk of a lung cancer diagnosis is 16% – i.e. lung cancer occurs in 16 out of 100 smokers. This absolute risk certainly appears less daunting when compared to the relative risk of 40. However, context must be applied: the normal rate of lung cancer in the average nonsmoker is tiny. So, when this gets multiplied by the increased relative risk, that number still only rises to 16%. Yet, in the world of epidemiology, this increase is considered massive.

In fact, to this day, the link between smoking and lung cancer remains one of the strongest links ever observed in epidemiologic studies. Fast-forwarding several decades, the research field is now littered with population studies attempting to mimic these findings by observing other chemicals and foods in which humans are frequently exposed. For example, in 2012, researchers from the Division of Nutritional Epidemiology at the Karolinska Institutet in Stockholm, Sweden published a controversial study that quickly ignited a media firestorm when they linked processed meat with pancreatic cancer. In their study, the researchers found that the consumption of 50 grams of processed meat – just a few slices per day – was associated with a 19% increased risk of the often-deadly pancreatic cancer.[12] They did caution, like their patriarch Doll, that their findings may have been influenced by hidden coincidences known as confounders. Regardless of these concerns, The British Broadcasting Corporation reported that consuming just a couple of slices of bacon per day could increase pancreatic risk by 20%, while CBS news reported that only three sausages or six strips of bacon could increase pancreatic risk by 57%.[13]

Naturally, panic ensued as the public began questioning their physicians regarding this killer that could be found in the meat section of every grocery store. However, a closer examination of the Karolinska results shows just how far population studies have regressed since Doll's landmark study. The study revealed a 19% higher risk of pancreatic cancer, while Doll revealed that heavy smokers had a 40 times higher risk of dying from lung cancer. To put these numbers into perspective, we must account for the baseline risk of pancreatic cancer: 1 in 67 individuals are diagnosed with the disease. Therefore, the overall risk of pancreatic cancer is 1.5%, and factoring in the 19% increase based on this Swedish study, this risk would increase to 1.8%. If this risk was in fact more than a coincidence – which remains unresolved – comparing this 0.3% increase to Doll's 16% increase in lung cancer paints a vastly different picture of concern. Doll immediately stopped smoking upon exposing his lung cancer data, but whether this would have prompted him to go cold turkey on his breakfast sausage is doubtful. Regardless, it is highly doubtful whether this new risk number warrants media headlines questioning if processed meats are as bad as smoking (yes, this actually occurred!) – we may have reached a point where fear-mongering has overwhelmed actual science.

The current issue with using population studies to exaggerate small, coincidental, or flat-out incorrect associations has recently been brought into the spotlight. Even Doll's worldly food study from the 1970s yielded results that were incomparable to the association of lung cancer and smoking, likely prompting his concern with taking away any solid conclusions from the findings. A half-century later, current population studies rarely approach even a small fraction of this risk. We have seemingly reached the humbling realization that our exaggerated enthusiasm was more hopeful than it was reliable. The relationship that Doll and Hill had discovered was enormous compared to those of studies that would follow, and it began to set in that the gravity of the results of their epic study might be hard to reproduce, if not impossible. Per Willett's experience, not only were many associations small, several were starting to present in the opposite direction. After providing future researchers with an insurmountable precedence, what followed the initial study was a somewhat deflating understanding that correlation does not necessarily mean causation, and the clear majority of studies that followed Sir Richard Doll's work exposed a dwindling correlation. The sobering phrase "correlation does not equal causation" now serves to put those coffee drinkers in check when they gallivant around the office exclaiming to coworkers that their excessive coffee habit is defending them from cancer according to the latest and greatest study.

This lesson was thrust into the spotlight in 2013 when Jonathan Schoenfeld, a radiation oncologist and Assistant Professor at Harvard Medical School, and John Ioannidis, a professor of Medicine, Health Research, and Policy at Stanford University School of Medicine, joined forces to assess the impact of ingredients from random recipes in *The Boston Cooking-School Cook Book*. To add insight – not to mention a touch of humor – into the spiraling world of population studies, they published *Is everything we eat associated with cancer? A systematic cookbook review*, in the *American Journal of Clinical Nutrition*.[14] Taking the ingredients from the various recipes in the cookbook and available studies assessing them, they performed an array of statistical calculations, generating results providing associations with both an increase and decrease in cancer risk. Furthermore, as with the processed meat and pancreatic cancer study previously mentioned, the overall impact of these ingredients and foods was miniscule. Additionally, many of these findings became negligible when multiple studies were evaluated in what is known as a meta-analysis, again supporting the drastic deviation from the colossal impact Doll and Hill had found with lung cancer and tobacco. Ioannidis, also a Professor of Statistics at Stanford University, has since produced countless other studies exposing issues with many similar reports within the research world, particularly ones pertaining to health and nutrition. Many of these have helped fuel the massive controversy surrounding what the general population should be told to eat – if told anything at all – in order to adhere to a healthy lifestyle.

⁙

In 2008, investigative journalist Gary Taubes produced a controversial yet undeniably enlightening manifesto titled *Good Calories, Bad Calories*. His work exposed several provocative issues that had been implanted within our dietary guidelines and eventually disseminated throughout the medical community over the past several decades. Taubes argues that the chastising of dietary fat as the culprit responsible for weight gain and cardiovascular disease was the product of bias, a pandering to political and corporate special interest groups, shoddy research, and less than adequate population studies. While many of these population studies have introduced biases and preconceived notions into the cancer world, perhaps most illuminating was Taubes' systematic and scientific discussion of the major concerns with population studies, using the medical mistake of hormone replacement therapy as the benchmark of these issues. Taubes put the phrase "correlation does not equal causation" on the map.

This example is one of the few in science where the issues of population studies come full circle in almost less than a decade. In 1985, only two years before Willett's first major work examining the links between diet and breast cancer, his research group took part in another massive epidemiologic study in conjunction with the Harvard School of Public Health assessing the lifestyle habits of 122,000 women. They had uncovered evidence that the women within this group who were prescribed hormone replacement therapy (HRT) were experiencing significantly lower rates of coronary artery disease. Specifically, those women who were currently prescribed HRT experienced a 70% reduction in their risk, while former users experienced half the risk. [15] Ensuring this was not simply a coincidence, the researchers performed an array of statistics to limit those factors that Doll warned of, accounting for their interactions to limit false relationships or coincidences from factors like tobacco use, diabetes, hypertension, cholesterol levels, parental heart attacks, oral contraceptive use, and obesity. The findings held; simply taking HRT was significantly associated with a decreased risk of coronary artery disease in women.

The proposed benefits of HRT were welcomed with open arms by the medical field and embraced by women throughout the United States. As women enter menopause, normal levels of estrogen and progesterone begin to decline, ushering in a series of hot flashes, mood swings, fatigue, and several other nearly intolerable side effects. Hormone replacement therapy was frequently prescribed to reintroduce these hormones and mitigate the unwelcome side effects of this hormonal roller coaster. Rumors of a magical pill that would eradicate the debilitating symptoms that plagued menopausal women and enable them to feel decades younger ran rampant throughout the medical community. A pill that would make women feel younger while protecting their heart was a win-win for patients and doctors, and the more women wanted it the more physicians prescribed it.

Only after decades of this give-and-take relationship between doctors and their menopausal patients were these pills actually tested in a randomized study. In a similar vein as the study made famous by Hill decades prior, HRT was compared to a placebo in the controlled trial. To reiterate, randomized controlled trials – the gold standard of medicine – are the preferred method to test a hypothesis formed from a relationship seen in population studies; this study classification is more adept at accounting for differences between study participants to eliminate confounding factors, an all-too-common shortcoming of population studies. The massive study had taken place over seven years at 20 clinical centers across the United States.

As the lead researchers for this study sat down to analyze the results of the trial, their worst nightmare became a reality: not only were these magic pills ineffective at lowering the risk of coronary artery disease in women, but they raised it. And there was more to this nightmare, as it was discovered that hormone replacement therapy exacerbated the risk of several other adverse medical conditions in the study's participants. The subject group experienced a 30% increase in heart disease, a 26% increase in breast cancer, a 40% increase in risk of stroke, a 22% increase in risk of total cardiovascular disease, and a whopping 113% increase in risk of pulmonary embolism, which is a blood clot in the lungs that often proves fatal.[16]

Scientists were baffled; doctors and their patients were horrified. What could have possibly gone wrong? In the original wide-ranging analysis, statisticians accounted for every medical condition imaginable. However, all interested parties quickly realized that statisticians cannot account for all missing information, no matter how thorough their methods. When reviewing the initial HRT population studies, it was clear that the women who were prescribed postmenopausal hormones were generally healthier: they smoked less, exercised more, ate healthier foods, were generally wealthier, and were more educated. These factors were properly accounted for by the statisticians. However, combining all of these factors led to one glaring unaccountable characteristic: these women were more proactive when it came to their health. They were more proactive in eating well and following a healthy lifestyle, and their proactive dispositions led them to be more proactive in their desire to avoid the side effects of menopause... and ultimately led them to be more proactive in soliciting their physicians for prescriptions for hormone replacement therapy. The greatest statisticians the world over are always limited by the tools they are given to measure, and no tool was specific or powerful enough to account for this proactiveness. Unbeknownst to the scientists, the initial study had simply revealed the coincidence that healthier women used HRT more often, and HRT did not make women healthier. The data was tainted by a phenomenon known as healthy user bias; healthy users have a predisposition to follow their doctor's medical advice, exercise more, eat healthier, and generally live a healthier life. The study simply selected for these women, who happened to be on HRT, and applied their findings to all women, many of whom were not following their doctor's advice.

Correlation does not equal causation. One could say that the hormone replacement trial left us with a valuable lesson, but it merely confirmed the valuable lesson already given to us decades earlier by Sir Richard Doll. We can observe patterns, but until they are tested in randomized trials, it is anyone's guess as to whether they are causative – and even then, we still must remain cautious of findings and they may be disproven in later studies.[17] The world of epidemiology came full circle when Doll, now in his eighties, analyzed data revealing the risk of breast cancer after treatment with HRT as part of the Collaborative Group on Hormone Factors and Breast Cancer.[18] Their findings confirmed an increased risk in breast cancer during the usage of hormone replacement therapy (although to be fair, the study also revealed that risk decreased after discontinuation of the hormone treatment).

Epidemiologic and population-based studies are intriguing, and randomized controlled studies are expensive and often difficult, if not flat-out impossible, to perform in the real-world settings. Yet, these remain our strongest form of evidence despite their shortcomings. For instance, while scientifically it would be optimal to place several hundred individuals on closely watched diets within a hospital setting or metabolic ward, the accompanying astronomic price tag generally limits such attempts. Some studies have attempted to randomize women to different diet and lifestyle groups; however, these attempts have taken place in real-world settings, often relying more on subjects' ability to follow directions than their ability to test the actual intervention.

On the other hand, mice – the same creatures whose diets Rous, Tannenbaum, and Moreschi were experimenting with – can be kept in cages and eat the exact proportions of food served to them. While the ability to confine mice and control their feeding solves several major issues with human studies, it presents its own share of issues, including: 1) Mice are nocturnal, or in other words, they eat all night and sleep all day; 2) Mice forage and, while they generally eat most things, they rely on a primarily carbohydrate-based diet in nature; 3) Unlike humans, mice eat massive amounts of food in proportion to their weight. (Comparing an average-sized 45-year-old woman with a mouse, she would have to eat 26 pounds of food per day to equal in proportion the mouse's daily diet.)

Still, mice remain the best option for cancer prevention studies. We cannot guarantee the diet of a 45-year-old woman living and roaming in a free society, nor can we rearrange her genes so that she is prone to breast cancer, expose her to a toxic chemical that causes breast cancer, or (God forbid!) even purposefully give her breast cancer for purely scientific study purposes. However, we can do all of these things to a helpless mouse, in order to advance our medical knowledge of the human race and improve the lot of future generations. Scientists have known this well before Moreschi's experiment, the first of its kind, and the epic dawn of the recording and publishing of the epidemiologic study.

4

COUNTING DOWN TO CANCER

"Quantity has a quality of its own."

- Often attributed to Napoleon, likely incorrectly

"The basic scientific alphabet has been established. We should start learning how to put it into words."

- David Kritchevsky, Ph.D.

Takeaways:

Biosphere 2 was the largest enclosed self-contained simulated living study, where an 8-member crew spent just over two years isolated within an ecosystem that they would have to self-sustain. Unfortunately, after a series of mishaps, severe calorie restriction followed and resulted in physical and mental maladies.

The Minnesota Starvation Study evaluated 36 isolated individuals for a total of 14 months, arranged into 4 phases of varying dietary restriction and tracked for physical and psychologic distress.

David Kritchevsky, who was one of the most influential diet and cancer researchers in the latter half of the 20th century, was also one of the first to suggest and show that the impact of diet on cancer incidence and treatment was far beyond simple calorie restriction. His work set the stage for future research, illustrating that a variety of macronutrients and their influence on hormones within the body could largely affect cancer formation.

On September 26, 1991, eight individuals set foot into Biosphere 2, an enclosed self-contained simulated living environment built in rural Oracle, Arizona. Located not far from a gold mine owned by Buffalo Bill Cody, Biosphere 2 sits at the base of the Catalina Mountains, a short drive from Tucson. With a price tag of $200 million, the structure, eclipsing three football fields in size, completed construction in 1991 through funding from billionaire philanthropist Ed Bass. It remains the largest closed-living system ever constructed and is considered only the second fully livable biosphere (Planet Earth is the first). The project, which Discover Magazine described as "the most exciting scientific project to be undertaken in the U.S. since President John F. Kennedy launched us toward the moon,"[1] was created with the goal of studying the interactions between life systems within a closed system. These interactions and life systems included the eight participants and their interactions with each other, along with those between plants, animals, nature, farming, and technology. The underlying objective, many surmised, was to assess whether a similar enclosed living environment could one day be created on another planet to simulate earth's living conditions in otherwise inhospitable environments.

Roy Walford was the only physician of the eight study subjects in Biosphere 2, which early on was already being slammed by critical opponents of the experiment who felt that it lacked tangible scientific basis. Others applauded the impressive undertaking, hopeful of what new scientific lessons might be gleaned. A Professor of Pathology at the University of California Los Angeles School of Medicine who received his medical degree from the University of Chicago, Walford was considered by many to be a trailblazer within the world of calorie restriction and aging research. His work was integral in entwining scientific threads into a project that many felt to be more of a cultish fad idea than a scientific experiment – indeed, most of the other participants were part of a controversial group known as Synergia Ranch. The Ranch, a self-described ecovillage, was established by the original inventor and director of Biosphere 2. While it designated itself a private retreat and workshop center for small groups, Synergia Ranch had come under fire for its alternative cult-like nature and its influence on the creation and direction of Biosphere 2. This viewpoint of The Ranch as a radical organization influenced famous novelist Tom Clancy, who in his 1998 thriller *Rainbow Six* centered the plot around a team of elite soldiers battling a terrorist group aiming to exterminate the human race via bioterrorism while themselves surviving in a closed-off biosphere.

Like his predecessor Tannenbaum, Walford dedicated most of his career to studying the health effects of calorie restriction, but he focused sharply on its potential ability to enhance lifespan. He practiced what he preached, surviving on what is known as the CRON diet, which recommends a 20% calorie restriction or roughly 1,800 calories per day. Along with the seven other Biosphere 2 participants, he would be consuming a similar diet within the biosphere, one resembling the calorie-restricted diet that he often utilized in his research studies and touted in several of his books. This diet included beans, wheat, rice, bananas, and root vegetables like sweet potatoes and beets, all grown in an environment without toxic chemicals or pesticides (the use of these chemicals in a sealed environment would have disastrous consequences). The diet was also described as nutrient-dense, containing a proportionally significant number of vitamins and nutrients compared to calories. While overall their diet was considered low-fat, domesticated animals were also present for consumption in Biosphere 2, and goats provided milk as well.

However, as the Biosphere 2 experiment unfolded, unforeseen difficulties were encountered almost immediately, fueling the arguments of the many critics of the innovative project. Microbial life within the soil seemed to have been unaccounted for by the scientists, and also ignored was the thick layer of concrete curing beneath the biosphere dome. The soil microbes extracted valuable environmental oxygen from the crew and animals, slowly suffocating them, leaving them lethargic and functionally impaired. The concrete layer produced unexpected carbon dioxide, further hampering the breathing situation. Eventually, oxygen had to be pumped into the enclosed structure to ensure the crew and living organisms' survival.

However, the physical atmosphere might have been the least of the crew's problems: the social environment between the team members deteriorated faster than the available oxygen. In a scenario that mimicked *Lord of the Flies*, the crew began to argue incessantly, tensions rose, and they eventually separated into opposing groups. Walford's diet only served to worsen things, and issues with crop yields further lowered the eight members' available food, leaving them with an average 1780 calories each to consume daily. The calorically-restricted diet, combined with the daily work of farming and tending to the animals, left the participants in a constant state of hunger, further worsening their crumbling social order. As one crewmember, Jane Poynter, describes in her memoir *The Human Experiment: Two Years and Twenty Minutes Inside Biosphere 2*, tensions came to a head as the crew members began to experience the physical and mental states that often accompany hunger: fatigue, depression, mental fog, and an obsession with food.[2]

As relationships among the crew continued to dwindle, the population of insects continued to flourish; by the end of the study, the facility was overrun by ants and cockroaches. Undaunted, Walford persevered to compile his data on the health effects of calorie restriction. Other proposed and well-intentioned ecological studies on the plant, animal, and human interactions were all but abandoned by a crew desperate for survival. After the two years and twenty minutes of confinement, Roy Walford and the rest of the crew of the Biosphere 2 were ready to leave their temporary accommodations. The return to the normal world was bittersweet for the crew members; overall the project was considered a scientific success, but because tensions had reached such a boiling point, the media chose to have a field day with the mishaps. Superficial criticism of the project was easy – with so many moving parts within the massive undertaking, a few glitches were impossible to avoid. Attempting to get past the glitches was in and of itself part of the project.

While seven of the crew members ranged in age from 27 to 42 years, Walford was the outlier at 67. Yet during his time in the Biosphere and afterward, he paid no mind to his advanced age, spending countless hours dedicated to documenting his experience. He even produced scientific publications on the experience while captive in the dome. Although the overarching goals of the Biosphere 2 project remain murky to this day, the main ambition, or so it was reported, was to assess whether humans could survive in a completely enclosed and totally contained environment for several years. Roy Walford's goal was beyond survival; he wanted to quantify the physiologic effects of life inside the biosphere. As part of the study, the human lab rats agreed to have blood drawn prior to crawling into their cage, multiple times while inside the dome, and four times during the following 30 months when they were living freely outside of the bubble. The participants, it had been calculated, would consume approximately 2,500 calories per day as part of their typical diet. All food was to be produced within the Biosphere through farming and animal husbandry. The members engaged in physical activity through farming, facility repair, and raising livestock, which according to Walford totaled 3-4 hours per day, 6 days per week.[3] All food generated was, again according to Walford, apportioned equally between the members to simplify calculations.

Due to crop failures – perhaps the biggest punching bag target of the media's criticisms – participants found their diets dwindling to just over 1,700 calories in the first six months and were unable to increase their intake to 2,000 calories for much of the remaining time of the study. The ill-fated set of circumstances for the crew were clearly more fortuitous for Walford, who had already dedicated much of his life to researching calorie restriction. Of course, Walford's prior studies, much like those of his predecessors, were limited mostly to mice. With Biosphere 2, he had finally gotten the chance to perform his dream experiment on humans. After his time in the dome, Walford founded the Calorie Restriction Society and personally followed a calorically-restricted diet; needless to say, he was a believer in the potential benefits of calorie restriction. Such studies in humans were limited for many reasons, the most obvious one being that starving them either willingly or unwillingly was unethical. Furthermore, the inability to ensure that humans adhered to the diet without force brought about both ethical considerations and feasibility questions of whether such studies would be testing dietary changes or the participants' ability to follow the diet.

Prior to Biosphere 2, the largest documented human calorie restriction study in US history was performed by Ancel Keys during World War II. Keys, a physiologist with a keen interest in diet research, had created a formula for packaged meals for soldiers, branded as K-Rations. His war-based dietary studies would continue with the Minnesota Starvation Study, which was initiated three years after the US entered the war and ran from November 19, 1944 to December 20, 1945.[4] Thirty-six conscientious objectors were excused from battle in exchange for their cooperation in the study. Upon entering their temporary "biosphere" at the University of Minnesota, they were sworn to uphold perseverance in the project until completion. The participants resided in dormitories within the stadium at the university athletic building. All meals were consumed at a local hall, and they were free to use the library; study programs were provided as well. The investigation was broken into several phases: a three-month control period; the semi-starvation period lasting six months; three months for restricted rehabilitation; and the final eight weeks for the participants' unrestricted

61

rehabilitation period, where they could freely eat. A battery of physical and psychological tests during each phase of the study awaited the participants.

The diets were calculated to result in a 25% weight loss in the conscientious objectors, who were of normal weight at the start of the study. The participants initially subsisted on a 3,150-calorie diet containing 34% fat and 110 grams of protein. In order to simulate the starving conditions in famine-ravaged Europe during the war, participants entered a state of "semi-starvation" and watched their calories initially drop to 1,850 per day, and eventually to just over 1,700 calories, with fat reduced to 11% of calories and protein to 49 grams. Furthermore, participants engaged in physical activity, leading to further caloric expenditure. Their diet, which remarkably closely resembles the current United States Department of Agriculture's ChooseMyPlate, contained grains like oatmeal and whole wheat bread; vegetables including onions, garlic, celery, carrots, cabbage, lettuce, turnips; various legumes like beans and peas; and starches. However, to keep the subjects' diets consistent with those in famished war-torn areas, meat and dairy were limited and most protein came from vegetable sources and legumes. The diets did not, and could not, fully resemble the macabre diets in Europe, which contained 500-800 daily calories – an amount that would have resulted in significant health consequences and death, far beyond the ethical boundaries for a study that already bordered unethical conduct.

Nearly a century after Moreschi and his colleagues' groundbreaking studies, Keys found himself impersonating Tannenbaum as he calorically restricting his subjects – only for Keys, they were humans. The Minnesota Starvation Study diet was remarkably similar to the Walford diet, though it remains unknown if this was by design. In his publications afterward, Walford describes their low-calorie diet ranging from 1,750-2,100 calories per day, comprised of the exact same 11% from fat, small amounts of eggs, dairy, and meat, and large amounts of non-animal foods like fruits, vegetables, nuts, legumes, and grains. Walford does describe a diet containing significantly more fruit, both in number and variety. Additionally, the men in Biosphere lost 21% of their initial weight, quite similar to the 25% weight loss by subjects in Keys' study. While the Keys study subjects were engaging in physical activity, Walford describes intense physical labor for 3-4 hours per day, 6 days a week, totaling 18-24 hours. Furthermore, the issue of carbon dioxide accumulating within the Biosphere required the inhabitants to manage this issue via a carbon dioxide scrubber and collection of biomass from the savannah area of the sphere, requiring even more physical labor. Keys' subjects remained active via less intense methods including walking on treadmills and helping with housekeeping and laboratory operations; according to the report, these tasks initially occupied 25 hours per week. By the end of the semi-starvation period, the authors noted that all men were unable to continue this activity level as they succumbed to the weakness and fatigue that accompanies starvation; thus, activity levels at that point were unknown. Yet surprisingly, beyond this similarly painted picture, the reports describe drastically different outcomes between the Walford and Keys experiments.

During the Minnesota Starvation Study, most participants completed the study. Upon initiation of the semi-starvation diet, several had prolonged infections and persistent common colds, and another was removed for a severe urinary tract infection. An additional man was removed for "psychological reasons" and several others experienced "periods of emotional stress." However, according to the study team these individuals "responded well to simple psychiatric measures." By the second month of starvation, the physicians noted progressively visible swelling of the men's faces and lower legs. Some had an accumulation of fluid in their knees, others had decreased reflexes, and some even lost their reflexes. Joints creaked during normal activities. The gradual loss of protein was likely responsible for the fluid accumulation, known as edema from third-spacing.

By the end of the six months, the scientists and examining physicians noted that participants had appeared malnourished and emaciated. Furthermore, facial color was described as "sallow and pallid" with a patchy brownish pigmentation around the mouth and eyes, resembling the shape of glasses. Cyanosis, a purple and bluish discoloration, was seen around their nail beds and lips, indicating low oxygen saturation. Their eyes were eerily white without the hint of blood flow. The physicians even attempted to aggravate their eyes with soap to elicit the typical redness and irritation that follows but found none. The men's tongues had swelled, and an imprint of their teeth had formed around its edges. Their skin became thickened, a condition known as hyperkeratosis, with a tinge of brown throughout.

In the conclusion of their medical report, the physicians mentioned a general lifelessness seen in the men, further embellished by their lack of muscle. Men were described as progressively "silent, apathetic, and immobile." Their heart rates slowed significantly, and for some as slow as 30 beats per minute or below, a state known as bradycardia. Physiological changes showed a 40% decrease in basal metabolic rate – the men's bodies were shutting down both physically and psychologically. At the start of the study period, the men could push themselves to exhaustion on a treadmill for 245 seconds. By the end of the semi-starvation period, the average was 51.9 seconds, and the men were frequently collapsing; their hearts were unable to speed up and pump the required blood to the brain, and their muscles were equally unable to bear their weight when fatigued. The physicians described an additional strange phenomenon where the men would gradually lean farther and farther forward, as though expecting their feet to catch them from falling, but due to severe muscle loss and weakness, they would instead eventually tumble face-down.

In other words, the physicians were describing a horrifying report of individuals who were malnourished and losing their minds, conditions partially attributed to fat-soluble vitamin deficiency from the low amount of fat in their diet. Other vitamins and minerals accompany these foods as well, and the limitation furthered their deficiencies. Perhaps most dreadful to bear by the study physicians was the intense psychological impact that the diet had on the participants. They became obsessed with food, leading some to constantly talk of it and any topic related to food, like farming. Others became deeply resentful, further fueled by the incessant food conversations, and oftentimes these discussions would lead to violent outbursts. Eventually, the Minnesota Starvation Study participants stopped socializing with each other altogether, and like with the later Biosphere 2 experiment, the fabric of their social order unraveled.

Not surprisingly, excessive hunger was described by all men in the Keys' study, including "tiredness, fatigue…muscle soreness, apathy, general irritability, inability to concentrate, depression, dizziness, lack of ambition, moodiness, [and] sensitivity to noise." These complaints progressively increased; according to the observing doctors, by the last two months of the semi-starvation period, muscle cramps became endemic. The men also complained of the constant feeling of chills, even in the midst of a warm July; along these lines, the severe loss of muscle and body mass began to bother the men both emotionally and physically. For many it was painful to sit on unpadded chairs, and for others it was grueling to watch as their own bodies melted away and they began to resemble elderly men. The elderly depiction of the men was more than visual as most of them began to talk of feeling "old"; their listlessness, lack of libido, weakness, and depression simply made them feel decades older than they were. Depression gradually worsened, and eventually hysteria and hypochondriasis set in. Self-mutilation followed, and one participant, using an axe, severed three of his fingers, leading to amputation. When questioned later, he was unsure if the act was intentional or accidental. By the conclusion of the study, several of the men were hospitalized for further psychiatric care.

Months after the Biosphere 2 experiment ended, Walford published multiple reports describing the health changes he witnessed in himself and the other individuals that resided with him in the synthetic environment.[5] His scientific take on their own Minnesota Starvation Study paints a vividly different picture. Walford, who described the food mishap within the enclosed living space as a "serendipitous opportunity to study the responses of humans on such a diet and over a prolonged 2-year period under carefully monitored conditions,"[3] felt that his findings were fascinating.

As expected, all team members lost weight – holding onto fat, or even muscle, was nearly impossible on a 1,780 calorie per day diet, especially with the massive levels of daily activity that the crew was performing as they tended the land. Their blood pressures dropped well below the normal value of 120/80, dipping to 89/58. Their ratio of total cholesterol to high-density lipoprotein (HDL) remained the same, as both low-density lipoprotein and HDL decreased. HDL cholesterol almost halved, dropping from 62 to 38 mg/dl. Walford was also surprised to find that an unintended consequence of the rapid weight loss was release of chemicals from the breakdown of adipose tissue – significant amounts of toxins, including industrial chemicals and pesticides like DDT and PCBs, had accumulated within their fat after years of exposure and were being released as a byproduct into their blood as the fat was being metabolized for fuel.[6]

Other reports noted that "on a diet of beans, porridge, beets, carrots, and sweet potatoes, their weight plummeted, and their skin began to turn orange because of the excess beta-carotene within their diet." The diet – barring the large supply of fruit – and skin changes were unnervingly reminiscent of the Keys' reports. Observers from the outside peered in through the glass enclosure to encounter a scene that was eerily similar to the one described by the physicians in the Minnesota Starvation experiment decades before: faces were sunken, leaving the appearance of discolored and tent-like skin resting squarely on bone. Walford reported that all participants were given equal amounts of food, but other reports cite evidence that meals were initially served buffet style, only to be allotted equally after crew members began to go hungry, fueling already rising tensions. Walford was later quoted regarding the food situation: "I think if there had been any other nutritionist or physician, they would have freaked out and said, 'We're starving,' but I knew we were actually on a program of health enhancement."[7] This response was intended to rebut the outcry of the rest of the crew, who wanted additional food transported in once the situation worsened. Walford's multiple scientific papers make little mention of any psychological changes in his subjects, but the memoirs of other crew members seem to diverge drastically from his descriptions. Crew member Jane Poytner acutely described her own depression, excessive hunger, fatigue, and a preoccupation with food.[2] Her account paralleled that of the Minnesota Starvation Study physicians, and in a strange stroke of coincidence Poytner also amputated part of her finger while in the Biosphere, (though it was accidental during the cleaning of a rice-hulling machine). Always the optimist, Walford responded in a phone interview that the fingertip was reattached "within 15 to 20 minutes." She eventually had to leave Biosphere briefly for a surgical procedure to repair the finger.

Similar to the subjects in the Keys' report, the Biosphere participants began to obsess over food, and "their memoirs of the two-year project are filled with references to their recurring dreams of McDonald's hamburgers, lobster, sushi, Snickers-bar cheesecake, lox and bagels, croissants, and whiskey. They bartered most of their possessions, but food was too precious to trade. They became sluggish and irritable from lack of it and were driven by hunger to acts of sabotage. Bananas were stolen from the basement storeroom; the freezer had to be locked."[2] One member wrote a song, titled "Ode to Bananas," paying tribute to the sweetest fruit available within the Biosphere.

Time magazine judged Biosphere 2 as one of the 100 worst ideas of the twentieth century.[8] Walford published his medical findings throughout his two years and twenty days in Biosphere 2, but otherwise we are left with little other results from the undertaking except the foregone conclusion that it is difficult for humans to cooperate when in close isolation. The strangeness of the project was so comedic that it inspired the 1996 comedy film *Bio-Dome* starring Pauly Shore and Stephen Baldwin. (Much like the real Biosphere 2, *Bio-Dome* fell below expectations, losing $1.5 million at the box office.) While both the Keys and the Biosphere starvation experiments revealed the psychological issues with calorie restriction, they are two of our only scenarios where this dietary alteration – the same one that Tannenbaum and his colleagues found could decrease the emergence of cancer – was studied in humans. Does either study provide indications that the participants may have a lower risk of cancer? Did Walford's results, including laboratory and serum blood values, indicate that markers may have been altered in a way that would indicate a lower risk of cancer? Unfortunately, neither question can be answered from the studies.

Signaling the end of a strange series of experiments and in an unfortunate twist of fate, Walford passed away in 2004 at the age of 79, nearly a decade after exiting Biosphere 2. He would succumb to Lou Gehrig's disease, which he felt was precipitated by the elevated levels of carbon dioxide and nitrous oxide that he was exposed to during his time within Biosphere 2.[9] Adding a bizarre ending to a strange chapter in the history of calorie restriction research, his calorie-restricted diet may have hastened his demise, as mouse studies reveal that it can accelerate the progression of Lou Gehrig's disease.[10]

⁙

Some 6,000 miles away from the site of Biosphere 2 sits the Swiss Federal Institute of Technology, or ETH Zurich, a university specializing in STEM subjects (science, technology, engineering and mathematics). Since its establishment in 1855, ETH Zurich has been a beacon of education and research. The workplace of Albert Einstein in the early 1900s, it is now home to 21 Nobel Prize awardees and currently ranks 5th in the world in engineering and technology. Douglas Hanahan, an American cancer researcher, serves as the director of the Swiss Institute for Experimental Cancer Research, which is part of the ETH Zurich. Decades before accepting his esteemed position at ETF Zurich – and after receiving his Ph.D. from Harvard University – Hanahan developed a genetically modified mouse model used for pancreatic cancer experiments at Cold Spring Harbor Laboratory in New York. Hanahan's work described one of several initial transgenic mouse models created for cancer experimentation; these research tools can produce cancer for study simply by implanting specific genes within the experimental mouse's DNA genome. Simple in theory, his work was complex and novel, and his discovery was rewarded with a place in the renowned journal *Nature*, with Hanahan as the sole author.[11]

The pancreas, which is roughly translated from Latin into English as "sweetbread," is an endocrine organ that rests behind the stomach, tucked above the duodenum. The pancreas has quite the demanding role multitasking many physiologic processes within the human body; perhaps the most important of these is its full-time occupation supporting our blood glucose levels. This task, if not properly performed, may result in death from either low or high blood sugar levels. The pancreas produces an array of hormones during the regulation process, utilizing insulin and glucagon to lower and raise blood sugar levels respectively. These hormones are produced within the endocrine portions of the organ, while other areas of the pancreas produce enzymes that help with food digestion and to offset the acidic chemicals that coat food passed from the stomach. Furthermore, insulin is also considered the primary anabolic hormone in the body, increasing protein synthesis and signaling cells to build and repair organs and tissues, and potentially to grow (which is one of the reasons bodybuilders "carb load" after a workout in hopes that it will raise blood sugar, increase insulin, and signal muscle growth). The reduction of glucose within our blood occurs when insulin triggers our liver to stop producing glucose and our cells to draw it from the blood, utilizing it to support the synthesis of proteins and increase replication of our DNA.

Pancreatic cancer commonly arises within these "digestive" areas of the organ, and these tumors are known as pancreatic adenocarcinomas. These aggressive malignancies rapidly grow, releasing metastatic cancer cells that spread to nearby lymph nodes, the liver, and eventually distant organs. This spread causes painful symptoms and ultimately rapid death to its victims (the most prominent example being movie star Patrick Swayze who succumbed in less than 20 months). Pancreatic neuroendocrine tumors, or PNETs, on the other hand, form in the pockets of neuroendocrine tissue and slowly grow. These pockets are occupied by hormone-producing components like islet cells that help support blood sugar levels through their production of insulin and glucagon. PNETs are slowly progressive and behave entirely different than their more aggressive counterparts, illustrated by Steve Jobs' nearly decade-long battle with his pancreatic cancer.

Hanahan found that when oncogenes – the genes that signal to both our cells and cancer cells to grow – were implanted in his transgenic mice, they developed pancreatic tumors. He transferred manipulated insulin genes into the insulin-producing beta cells of the pancreas. The mice receiving this gene subsequently produced tumors, supporting the view that cancer was a genetic disease since the simple act of inserting a specific gene produced cancer.

Like Hanahan, Robert Weinberg, a Daniel K. Ludwig Professor of Cancer Research at the Massachusetts Institute of Technology, also serves as director of a renowned cancer center when not spending his time advancing the field of cancer research. Separated by almost 4,000 miles and the Atlantic Ocean, their work overlaps in scope and is equally innovative. Weinberg spends his free time teaching introductory biology at MIT; his course is affectionately known as 7.012. (Students at MIT refer to all classes and courses by number, and Course 7 signifies a class in the biology department.) Hanahan, before graduating with a bachelor's degree from MIT in 1976, took a similar introductory biology class. In keeping with Hanahan's research on the genetic influences on cancer, Weinberg discovered *ras*. *Ras* are a group of cellular proteins that signal to activate other cellular proteins and processes. Insulin, the hormone that is released from the pancreas that Hanahan studied intensely during his experiments, signals to *ras* and activates them during the process of cellular progression. This signaling triggers genes to promote cellular growth and survival – two necessary processes in healthy cells, but also requirements for the growth of cancerous cells. Genes that have the potential to endorse cancerous processes are called proto-oncogenes, and *ras* are one of the most famous of these cancer-promoters. *Ras* presents the double-edged sword of cellular progression: a mutation can occur in the proto-oncogene, switching on the proverbial light switch of cancer growth and turning it into an all-out oncogene (onco meaning tumor).

Weinberg's work illustrated how a simple mutation can permanently activate a cancer-promoting oncogene, triggering a cascade of cancer initiation and growth. In theory, the inactivation of an opposing tumor suppressor gene could result in the same cancerous endpoint of unchecked cellular growth. Retinoblastoma, or *rb*, is one of the most famous tumor suppressor genes. Several years before Hanahan would be awarded his Ph.D. from Harvard, Weinberg – from a laboratory just one subway stop away in Central Square in Cambridge, Massachusetts – discovered that cancer-producing genes could be directly implanted into normal cells to flip their cellular switch from Jekyll to Hyde and turn them cancerous. Prior to this, research was generally conducted by using viruses to implant and activate cancer genes, research no doubt inspired by Rous' Nobel Prize-winning work. Following this discovery, Weinberg would isolate *ras* and publish his groundbreaking findings, only to isolate the tumor suppressor gene *rb* shortly after, revolutionizing cancer knowledge on both ends of the spectrum.

The *rb* gene creates a protein that works to inhibit excessive cell replication and cancer by blocking our cells from progressing through the cell division cycle – a natural process painstakingly memorized by most of us in high school biology only to forget it moments after the final exam. The cell cycle contains several checkpoints through which a cell must proceed like a travel-weary passenger at the airport to ensure it is functioning normally and not a threat. Furthermore, these checkpoints ensure that the cells are only allowed to replicate when necessary. Inactivating *rb* can allow damaged or unsafe cells to bypass one of these checkpoints and possibly enter into unrestricted replication, eventually forming a malignant tumor. Just as oncogenes act as the gas pedal for cancer growth and reproduction, *rb* and tumor suppressor genes act as the brakes, halting potential cancer emergence and growth. For instance, human papillomaviruses, or HPV, can inactivate *rb* in cervical cells, allowing them to replicate without control and eventually culminate in cervical cancer. HPV can be picked up on pap smears and treated before it enters the cell, binds to *rb*, and inactivates it.

It was only a matter of time before Hanahan and Weinberg, both powerhouses within the burgeoning field of cancer research, would cross paths. As fate would have it, the two joined forces in January of 2000 to produce the scientific article *The Hallmarks of Cancer*, which, as titled, is a discourse on the potential causes of cancer based on the current available research.[12] Published in the journal *Cell*, the article has been cited or referenced nearly 20,000 times by other research articles, and predictably most cancer researchers have referred to it at one time or another in their careers. Between Hanahan's genetic mouse model and Weinberg's discovery that cancer can be initiated through simple insertions of "gas pedal" genes and deletions of "brake pedal" genes, the sentiment of the article strongly suggests that cancer was almost entirely a genetic process. A simple misstep in our programming code, the first in a row of dominoes, could fail, which would catapult into a series of downstream changes, rapidly increasing the risk of cancer as more dominoes continued to fall. Perhaps paralleling this metaphor, the initial sentence of the Hanahan and Weinberg manuscript greets the reader with a strong feeling of the strictly genetic basis of cancer at the time: "After a quarter century of rapid advances, cancer research has generated a rich and complex body of knowledge, revealing cancer to be a disease involving dynamic changes in the genome."

Overall, the article plays out like a well-constructed prosecution, scientifically building a case against those criminals guilty of accessory to cancer. These dynamic changes in the genome that they refer to include the activation of Hanahan and Weinberg's oncogenes and the inactivation of Weinberg's tumor suppressor, *rb*. Both were a straightforward method of producing cancer, and both directly implicated our genes as a hallmark of cancer – they may not have committed the original crime, but they are certainly guilty of aiding and abetting. The scientific trial expanded far beyond these two simple changes, providing six requirements for a normal cell to turn vagabond, go rogue, bypass normal cellular checkpoints like *rb*, and become a full-fledged cancer. These included:

1. Proliferative signaling – the cell is signaled to rapidly reproduce (from proteins like *ras*)

2. Evading growth suppressors – the cell can ignore stop signals (like *rb*)

3. Resisting cell death – the cell resists normal programmed death

4. Enabling replicative immortality – the cell can replicate unhinged

5. Inducing angiogenesis – the newly cancerous cells sprout vessels, much like plant roots, and begin to hoard blood, oxygen, and nutrients

6. Activating invasion and metastasis – the rogue cells invade neighboring cells and virally spread to distant cells

These six aspects of cancer initiation can be translated as scientific verbiage that describes the ability of normal cells to morph into precancerous cells and eventually bypass those safety checkpoints to overcome the body's regulatory and stop mechanisms, leading to full-blown cancerous cells that no longer obey the cellular laws embedded within our biology. Jekyll becomes Hyde after an array of missteps lead to this final offense, and these missteps can be hastened by the number of insults that our cells and genetic material experience on a daily basis. Cancerous chemicals, background and ultraviolet radiation, inflammation, and other toxins continually bombard our cells like a lightning storm. The damage can be minor and easily fixable, simply harming the surface of the cells. However, irreparable damage can also occur to the core of the cell, harming the DNA and genetic code within its mainframe. Several cellular components can sense this irreparable damage and activate a series of processes that command the cell to sacrifice its own life by programmed cell death. These processes, known as apoptosis, program the cell to fall on its sword – a cellular *seppuku* so to speak. A similar process known as autophagy triggers the cell to find any damaged parts and recycle them.

If the dangerous cell somehow circumvents this selfless act for the greater good of the organism, it can instead experience another of Weinberg and Hallahan's hallmarks of cancer. One misstep, one wrong gene turned on or off, and a normal functioning cell suddenly becomes a Manchurian candidate, plotting our cellular demise from within as it increases in size and number, begins to steal nutrients from our healthy cells through angiogenesis, and eventually infects surrounding cells before it infiltrates the whole body in a viral-like spread known as metastases. At this point, the cell has acquired all the hallmarks of cancer.

⁂

Shortly after Moreschi reported on his groundbreaking study linking diet with the growth of sarcomas, Jacob and Leah Kritchevsky gave birth to their son, David, in Kharkov, Russia. David emigrated to the United States with his parents only three years later in 1923. A bright and ambitious scholar, David earned a master's degree in chemistry and then a Ph.D. in organic chemistry during the 1940s. Both were awarded in Chicago, not far from the labs where Tannenbaum had performed his dietary studies at the Michael Reese Hospital.

Blessed with sharp wit and abundant intelligence, Kritchevsky eventually worked his way up to become Associate Director and Professor at the Wistar Institute in Philadelphia, Pennsylvania. He was also awarded full professorship at the University of Pennsylvania. He began his career as a student of the pioneering diet researchers, only to find himself joining their ranks during the latter half of the 20th century. Studies had markedly advanced beyond the trailblazing efforts by Moreschi, Rous, and Tannenbaum, and some of the earlier experiments had revealed that heating fats before feeding them to different mouse strains could enhance their cancerous potential. Kritchevsky's initial study assessed the physical and structural changes within these heated fats and oils that may have accounted for this change.[13]

As Kritchevsky began to accumulate his share of vital data from experiments testing the impact of different foods on preventing and triggering cancer, his preconceived notions left him surprised at the results. One of his earliest studies found that restricting calories by 40% in mice on a diet high in coconut oil completely blocked the ability of a carcinogen to cause breast cancer.[14] Shortly thereafter, Kritchevsky was experimenting with a compound formed while frying beef known as conjugated linoleic acid, or CLA. While these experiments were initially constructed to study the cancerous chemicals formed during the process of charring meat, known as heterocyclic amines, the fortuitous discovery of CLA unearthed a natural compound in our food that seemed to provide anti-inflammatory and anti-cancer benefits. The fatty acid CLA had proven itself able to inhibit both atherosclerosis and the initiation of cancer in animal studies.[15] Kritchevsky also began to notice innate cancer-reducing properties from placing his mice on a limited diet, regardless of whether it was achieved through dietary restriction or over-exercising them to create a calorie deficit. He, like others in the field, also realized that the rotund control mice used in these experiments were anything but normal. Perhaps his most important contribution to the field of diet research was his work proving that in many of these mouse studies, a high calorie diet was a prerequisite to *increase* cancer rates, regardless of whether it was a high-fat or high-carbohydrate diet.[14,16] In other words, Kritchevsky's predecessors had been comparing apples to oranges when they calorie-restricted the overly indulgent mice; they may have been merely correcting the cancer-promoting properties of food overconsumption in a group of mice that were already fattened for the kill.

Advancing the work of his predecessors, Kritchevsky attempted to understand why calorie restriction was interfering with cancer development and decreasing the cancerous capability of carcinogens, pushing for an understanding of the impact of the quality of foods not just quantity. He worked with carcinogens, like those in chemicals from burnt food, hypothesizing that several mechanisms were accounting for the decrease in cancer risk attained through calorie restriction, even in the presence of these harmful cancerous chemicals. Studies had suggested that decreasing overall food intake led to a corresponding decline in hormone production within the body. Less food triggered less compensatory release of hormones to deal with the excess food. For instance, less sugar within the diet would require less insulin produced by the pancreas to lower that sugar once it entered the bloodstream. Countering this, it was surmised that excessive amounts of food would drive the body to generate more of these hormones. For instance, dietary protein seemed to drive the body to produce more of a certain growth factor known as insulin-like growth factor 1 (IGF-1). Many of these hormones, especially growth hormones like IGF-1, stimulate the growth of our cells, and much like Weinberg's example with *ras,* excessive stimulation of this growth can by definition result in cancer.

It only stood to reason that if excess food led to excess hormones which in turn led to excess growth of cells, then limiting food would limit cancer. However, as Kritchevsky heated his oils, he was imparting on them a significant amount of oxidative damage from free radicals. When he then overfed the mice the damaged oils, he was hormonally and physiologically priming them to get cancer and, adding insult to injury, bombarding their cells and DNA with free radicals that promoted further molecular damage. Through these experiments, however, Kritchevsky realized that underfeeding the animals provided their cells and DNA the ability to better withstand and repair the bombardment of free radicals and damage from carcinogens like heterocyclic amines. Finally, he introduced discussion on the role that insulin, a specific hormone that was increased by a specific macronutrient, was playing in tumor development and growth.

Kritchevsky was asked to give the Quartercentenary Lecture for the Nutrition Society in 1993. During his address which he titled *Undernutrition*

74

and Chronic Disease: Cancer, he began to surmise about the reasons why calorie restriction was working in these mice.[17] With strong undertones of disappointment, he voiced to the crowd that the "mechanisms by which energy restriction affects carcinogenesis are moot." He later regarded that this may have been due to a lack of interest within the medical and scientific fields, resulting in an inability to take the effects of dietary studies seriously. Unlike most scientists at the time, Kritchevsky was intrigued by the relationship between diet and health and dedicated his life to furthering our understanding of it. It has been said that quantity has a quality of its own, but the inability to describe the exact mechanisms behind the vague process of calorie restriction left Kritchevsky discontented at the lack of quality of dietary research attempting to solve this enigma.

During his mission to unravel the mystery of calorie restriction, Kritchevsky also surmised that simple dietary changes might enable these mice to successfully battle the cancerous free radicals that were being hurled at them from the heated vegetable oils in their diet, noting that several studies revealed an increase in cellular antioxidant pathways such as superoxide dismutase and glutathione peroxidase in mice consuming a restricted diet. Antioxidants are produced by our cells as they attempt to offset the potentially cancerous and lethal damage from free radical bombardment. Furthermore, several studies, Kritchevsky noted, reported a decrease in the number of free radicals present within the livers of these diet-constrained mice. Was the reduction in their food causing a compensatory stimulation in their defense against free radical damage, a major cause of cancer, he wondered? He also saw an improvement in the ability of these animals to repair damage to their DNA from both free radicals and cancer-promoting chemicals, thus effectively thwarting the potential activation of one of the hallmarks of cancer. Bringing his work full circle to collide with that of Hanahan and Weinberg, Kritchevsky found that dietary restriction also decreased the expression of oncogenes. Starving mice also appeared to starve the genes that could promote cancer. A target was in sight, but support at this point was still shrouded by speculation, and the research world was unable to pull the trigger on what would soon be a foregone conclusion.

As Kritchevsky closed out his lengthy lecture, he briefly mentioned several studies published within the last two decades about the role the hormone insulin might play in cancer promotion. While insulin serves many vital physiologic roles, in excess, it can interfere with optimal cellular function, thus promoting high blood pressure, obesity, and a plethora of medical issues. Insulin was not even discovered until a decade after Moreschi's groundbreaking study that implicated diet's ability to promote cancer growth. This discovery provided a lifesaving treatment for Type I diabetics, as it eventually led to the production of an external source of insulin to account for their pancreas' inability to produce it, ultimately extending their otherwise shortened lives. It would take another 40 years before human insulin was chemically synthesized in Germany, and fully synthesized human insulin was not produced until 1975.[18] Recombinant DNA insulin, or true "human" insulin, was not even tested until 1980. In other words, insulin was never even on the radar of the early researchers.

Insulin was a relatively new addition to the medical world, and its recent introduction into the science world was a slow one. Kritchevsky briefly described that one study in the 1970s and a second additional study in the 1980s revealed that animals deprived of insulin experienced an inhibition of cancer growth. Furthermore, when scientists triggered tumors in mice by exposing them to DMBA, a potent carcinogen with some similarities to heterocyclic amines in burnt food, 90% of these tumors were dependent on insulin, a result that foreshadowed a handful of subsequent studies. When insulin was removed, many of the tumors rapidly regressed in size.[19] Restricting the body's insulin supply paralleled the earliest studies on dietary restriction, and by 1989 studies began to connect the dots by illustrating that the often initially overfed and then calorie-restricted mice experienced an immediate and severe drop in their insulin levels.[16] However, these studies were unable to pinpoint an exact mechanism to implicate insulin, and studies incriminating certain foods and their ability to raise insulin – and potentially cancer risk – would not surface until years later. The other similar hormone known as insulin-like growth factor I would also decrease with dietary calorie restriction, but Kritchevsky and his colleagues found that, unlike insulin, IGF-1 would gradually rise back up to normal levels.[20]

By the 1980s, studies had indicated that both insulin and IGF-I would bind to cancer cells, feeding their thirst for growth and allowing them to embody several hallmarks of cancer; this was reinforced in several prominent breast cancer studies in both petri dish and animal experiments.[21] Kritchevsky concluded his lecture with a final comment: "How these events affect tumour growth is unclear." But as the science began to delve deeper into the mechanisms of the interaction between energy restriction and cancer incidence, fueled by novel studies within the field, something was amiss. The amount of insulin secretion from the pancreas, along with IGF-1 production, was not equally proportional to the consumption of the three macronutrients of fat, protein, and carbohydrate, with a wider disproportion in favor of the latter two. Such findings suggested that there was more to the equation than simply considering calories, as the type of calorie consumed could promote markedly different hormonal responses. The chemical interactions resulting from mixing the three macronutrients of fat, carbohydrates, and protein – which is usually the case in the real world – further complicated an already complex and contentious area of study.

Kritchevsky passed away in 2006 at the age of 86 and continues to be regarded as one of the most influential diet researchers in the latter half of the twentieth century. His final article *Diet and Cancer: What's Next?* was published three years before he passed.[22] His ultimate message cautioned against vilifying one dietary component in isolation. He warned us of "our tendency toward reductionist thinking, dating to the days when one drug killed one bug. We could learn something by trying to reconcile the differences." His article went on to expound on the importance of nutrients, suggesting that it would be interesting to combine energy restriction with nutritional treatment. Kritchevsky did not have the mechanistic answers as to why calorie restriction reduced cancer in the famous mouse studies, but he knew that others within the field who were vilifying certain nutrients lacked answers as well. Furthermore, due to an earlier lack of understanding of biochemistry, the late development of insulin, and the knowledge of its ability to stimulate cancer growth – not to mention the fact that nearly all experiments were performed on obese and unhealthy "control mice" – it is possible that we may have been led down the wrong path for the better part of a century.

While the first half of the twentieth century marked the initial dietary study linking food and cancer, the latter part would be exemplified by the exhaustive search for the unknown mechanisms to describe this link. Kritchevsky, among others, played a vocal part in rousing enthusiasm within the field to support further research to establish this link. He promoted additional research to assess the mechanisms, incorporate them into practice, and supply the general population with tangible, evidence-based dietary recommendations. The clear path forward for future researchers was summed up best by Kritchevsky: "Dietary approaches to inhibition of carcinogenesis have focused on one compound or class of compounds at a time, which belies the complexity of the problem. The basic scientific alphabet has been established. We should start learning how to put it into words."[22]

5

STEEL, RUST, AND CANCER

"I have legs of iron, but to tell you the truth, they're starting to rust and buckle a bit."

- Jeanne Calment,

Born: February 21, 1875, in Arles, France

Died: August 4, 1997, in Arles, France

"There is absolutely no impact of a low-fat diet on weight loss at one year, as confirmed by many studies...The overall evidence suggests more that low-fat diets are less successful in maintaining weight loss."

- Walter Willett, M.D., Dr.P.H.

Takeaways:

Bridges rust from oxidative damage when not properly sealed or preserved, providing a metaphor for how our cells and bodies corrode from similar damaging processed when not properly maintained.

Carbohydrate intake and insulin are looked at in relation to cancer growth, utilizing studies from the controversial weight loss world.

I spent the first 18 years of my life driving over bridges, listening to discussions about the issues with the steel industry and its decline, and watching the Steelers on television most Sundays during the football season. My childhood was by no means unique: several other million individuals who grew up in Pittsburgh in the 1980s will likely describe a similar childhood and adolescence. In the city birthed by US Steel, strewn with steel bridges and steel mills, and home to the NFL's Steelers, Pittsburgh's locals are no strangers to steel. And, as anyone acquainted with steel knows, familiarity with steel must necessarily be accompanied by awareness of rust. Driving across the Roberto Clemente Bridge to the North Side and Heinz Field or traversing the David McCullough Bridge to the Strip District, one cannot avoid catching a glimpse of burnt-orange rust breaking through the yellow paint-coated steel beams.

Pittsburgh's Roberto Clemente Bridge was named after the famous Pittsburgh Pirate and the first Latin American inducted into the National Baseball Hall of Fame, who died in a plane crash at age 38 while transporting aid to earthquake victims in Nicaragua. His namesake bridge replaced the original bridge, a massive, innovative work created by Brooklyn Bridge designer John Roebling. Roebling and his family emigrated from Prussia due to a lack of job opportunities in the aftermath of the Napoleonic wars; they settled just outside of Pittsburgh in a German colony called Saxonburg. In a strange intertwining of fate, Saxonburg is only a stone's throw away from the Allegheny-Ludlum Steel Corporation where John Allen, the inventor and director of Biosphere 2, originally got his career started in the 1960's developing alloys. Almost three decades later, Allegheny-Ludlum would supply the steel for the Biosphere 2 project.

Allen currently runs a company that produces sustainable ecological projects; so, he would likely blanch at the fact that his old partner Allegheny-Ludlum Steel Corporation holds the record for the second-highest fine in United States history for violating the Clean Water Act. They were ordered to pay $8,244,670 for dumping toxic chemicals from their mills located along the Kiskimenetas and Allegheny Rivers, the latter of which is spanned by the Clemente Bridge. Two decades later, they were charged with further violations for dumping chromium, zinc, nickel, other harmful metals and oils into nearby rivers. I spent my childhood crossing the toxic three rivers of Pittsburgh via the city's myriad bridges and it is not lost on me that, at the time of writing this, cross the Allegheny every morning to administer toxic treatments to cancer patients from this same area.

Like many Pittsburghers of his time, Roebling spent most of his career fighting rust. Steel was favored as a primary metal used in bridge design for its strength, permanence, and malleability; these physical features allowed it to be manipulated to meet the demands of large-scale projects. Furthermore, with a fresh coat of paint applied every few years, a steel bridge can appear brand new. When Roebling made his first bridge, he needed to account for gravity, wagon and train weight, wear and tear, and of course the corrosive rust that would inevitably form on the surfaces of the steel girders. He combined ingenuity and intellect with his unmatched knack for design for the former three, but combating the latter was nearly impossible.

The beams and wires supporting Roebling's bridge were made from steel, a supple metal mixture created by blasting pig iron with carbon. This process, known as smelting, is a cost-effective one that results in a metal alloy that is strong yet flexible, thus making steel a natural pick for structural design. However, there is also a downside: the iron in the steel eventually forms rust from its constant exposure to oxygen. This flaky reddish/brown material, known also by its chemical term iron oxide, forms when iron interacts with oxygen and water or moisture in a process aptly termed oxidation. The presence of large steel structures residing in or near water is the exact recipe for the unavoidable onset of rust. During oxidation, acidic compounds form and begin to degrade the iron, and over a long enough exposure time the entire steel structure can corrode and turn to rust.

Due to rust damage, Roebling's third and final bridge in Pittsburgh was eventually replaced in 1892 by a temporary structure, and then finally by the Roberto Clemente Bridge which still stands today. The replacement bridge was floated down the Ohio River and ultimately used in the construction of the Coraopolis Bridge, which 100 years later allowed me and countless other Pittsburghers easy access to Neville Island (and its memorable Roller Rink where I had my grade school roller skating parties). During all those trips across the bridge, I would always notice the moldlike rust creeping along the edges of the structure, but never once did I contemplate that the same process was occurring within my body. Just as Roebling's steel bridges were constantly being bombarded with water and oxygen to produce rust through the process of oxidation, so too were my cells. When iron is exposed to oxygen, the oxygen molecules eventually tear away electrons, which are the negatively charged particles rotating around atoms. The loss of electrons produces hydroxide, a reactive chemical that causes corrosion, rust, and ultimately, destruction of the steel.

Interestingly, human cells rely on a process quite similar to rusting, except with the goal of creating energy instead of corrosion and destruction.

The cellular process is known as oxidative phosphorylation and occurs in the cell's mitochondria, which when exposed to oxygen, breaks down nutrients to produce energy. A highly efficient method of energy derivation, this metabolic operation is not entirely free of glitches. It takes place within the microscopic cells of our body – which are composed of 60% water – in the presence of oxygen. Additionally, because electrons are passed around during this process, things can sometimes get off kilter and gummed up much like the spread of rust affecting Roebling's bridges.

The microscopic details of oxidative phosphorylation are not critically important to understand; however, it is imperative to note that oxidation arises from the process and that there is not much that can be done to stop it from occurring. Atoms dislike the gain or loss of electrons as doing so makes them unstable and releases radicals, or highly reactive molecules with one or more unpaired electrons in their outer orbit. (In the oncology world, we use this to our advantage when we bombard cancer cells with free radicals, tearing away pieces of their DNA in the hopes that damage inflicted on the wayward cells is fatal.) In this scenario, the pulling of electrons and subsequent reaction with oxygen produces free radicals and byproducts like superoxide, hydrogen peroxide, and hydroxyl. Similar to the rust that damages the mighty steel bridges throughout Pittsburgh, these reactive substances inflict corrosion and damage to the DNA of our cells and tissues, leading to aging and cancer. As there is an inescapable need for steel's strength and flexibility in bridge design that invites rust buildup, so too is there an absolute requirement of oxygen and oxidative phosphorylation by our cells to produce vital energy that necessarily exposes us to a double-edged sword whereupon free radicals age our cells and eventually lead to our demise.

While not technically a free radical, hydrogen peroxide is formed alongside free radicals within our cells during the production of energy. Though harmless in isolation, in the presence of an oxygen radical and an iron compound, hydrogen peroxide forms a reactive hydroxyl radical. If this process sounds familiar, it should – our cells, upon exposure to this compound, are beginning to rust. Perhaps most concerning is the ability of these free radicals to bind and damage polyunsaturated fatty acids located on the surface of our cells. Much like in Kritchevsky's heated oils, the free radicals bind to the fats, then steal electrons, damage their structure, and initiate a process called lipid peroxidation whereby the free radical parks itself within the fat. For instance, a pan left with vegetable oil cooking for too long eventually begins to smoke, and – like a steel bridge exposed to the elements – oxidizes and turns brown. Free radicals are teeming within and these same free radicals act like grenades, blowing holes in the protective fatty membranes of our cells.

Although free radical damage, also known as oxidative damage, from our own cellular processes is an unfortunate form of self-destruction, these free radicals are also utilized as messengers and are important components of cellular signaling. Over millions of years, our cells have evolved to be able to channel these potential dangers for benefit, often weaponizing them to kill infectious agents. However, external sources of free radicals appear to affect our cells differently, as they can cause similar oxidative damage by attacking our proteins and fatty cellular components. For instance, free radicals attack cholesterol along the walls of our arteries, leading to atherosclerosis.[1] By far the worst type of free radical injury is oxidative damage to our DNA. Damage occurs to the pairs of nucleotides within DNA, and in the worst-case scenario, breaks between the DNA strands form errors when that DNA is transcribed for protein construction.[2] Free radical damage can also inactivate certain parts of DNA while promoting others. Similar to the observations from Weinberg and Hanahan's research, deactivating a gene that signals for cells to stop replicating – i.e. a tumor suppressor gene – or activating an oncogene could lead to unchecked cellular reproduction that is a hallmark of cancer.

Newer steel production techniques have adapted to combat rusting. Painting the steel to limit the exposure of water and oxygen or coating it with chromium to produce stainless steel can minimize oxidation and rust. An older and cheaper technique known as galvanization electroplates the surface with zinc. (However, the vision of brown water pouring out of a faucet may jog your memory as to one of the several performance issues of galvanizing steel pipes.) Additionally, rubbing oil or other chemicals on steel can provide a small measure of protection, as can running an electric current through it or using rust inhibitors (which are generally ineffective). Not surprisingly, our cells have also adapted to the barrage of free radicals produced during energy derivation over the past several thousand years of our existence. They have developed the antioxidant defense system, which senses elevated free radical levels and then activates certain enzymes like catalase, superoxide dismutase, and peroxidases to neutralize these damaging radicals. The process is so vital for life that inactivating it in mice leads to a swift death. Some evidence suggests that based on the type and amount of free radicals, our cells may produce a larger than necessary amount of antioxidants to detoxify these harmful substances and halt oxidative damage.[3,4] Additionally, like the protective layer of yellow paint covering the bridges of Pittsburgh, fat-soluble antioxidants like vitamin E are placed along the fatty surfaces surrounding our cells to provide protection directly where free radicals attack.

Similar to the inevitable rusting of steel, free radical damage is guaranteed to plague us for as long as we are breathing and inhaling oxygen. Furthermore, as with the failed attempts to stop rusting via galvanization, oil coatings, and rust inhibitors, supplementing our diets with antioxidants has failed to aid in this battle and, like the brown liquid pouring out of a galvanized faucet, may lead to damaging side effects for these supplement users.[5,6] Paralleling the need to continually repaint the golden bridges – 446 bridges in total! – jutting across the three rivers of Pittsburgh, a little maintenance can go a long way to stop the rusting of steel and the accumulation of free radicals in our cells. Several lifestyle activities and dietary strategies provide the body with the building blocks to create antioxidants, but also stimulate the body to produce those antioxidants ahead of time.

⁙

By the time they published *Hallmarks of Cancer: The Next Generation* ten years later, Hanahan and Weinberg's initial work had been cited over 15,000 times. While the initial *Hallmarks of Cancer* was an attempt to simplify a massively complicated process, since then newer studies had emerged, exposing additional mechanisms that largely influenced the emergence of cancer compared to the initial six hallmarks. Segueing from prior discussions emphasizing the genetic basis of cancer, newer studies suggested that the emergence of cancer was prompted through several mechanisms that expanded far beyond that simple genetic view, including:

1. Deregulated metabolism – i.e. the breakdown of substances within cells to derive energy

2. Immune system evasion – i.e. the ability of cells to avoid assassination from our cellular security system

3. Genome instability – i.e. a plethora of cancer-causing mutations within our genes have been discovered

4. Inflammation – i.e. the necessary cellular and chemical response to cellular irritation, infections, foreign objects, and trauma; inflammation is often present near tumors and may increase the risk of cancer

The progression from discussions of the hardwired computer-like code within our cells destining us to cancer to the impact of the atmosphere surrounding this genetic code suggests that cancer expands far beyond simple genetics. Perhaps our genes dictate whether we are one of the unlucky future victims of cancer, but the impact and interaction of the milieu surrounding these genes may be the impetus to push them in one direction or another. Or as the authors described, the "biology of tumors can no longer be understood simply by enumerating the traits of the cancer cells but instead must encompass the contributions of the 'tumor microenvironment' to tumorigenesis."[7]

The illustration of a genetic mishap that presses on the cellular growth pedal or releases the brakes fails in its greatest attribute: its simplicity. What triggers this push on the gas? Why was the genetic alteration not repaired before it led to a release of the cellular brake pedal? This discourse was absent from the original hallmarks discussion, but the cancer world was scurrying to answer these questions. Clearly, the microenvironment serving as a home for our cells and genetic material has an immense impact on the optimal function of our cells, their ability to repair damage, and the constant avoidance of cancer. The microenvironment is the soil in which normal cells are nurtured. Feed them too much, and the vines turn weed-like, growing incessantly and reaching abnormal lengths without producing healthy fruit. Feed them too little, and the cells grow slower, struggling for life.

The newer hallmarks indicate that beyond our genetics, we have a cellular security force that patrols our cells from above, much like the security team in an airport. If any individuals appear to be a threat, a healthy security system tags them as so, eventually carrying them off into the back room for questioning. A healthy metabolism and cellular environment ensure that our security force is at its best to find these threats. These rogue cells are then broken down and recycled via the process of autophagy, where they are programmed to fall on their sword via apoptosis. Two situations, however, could be extremely detrimental in the fight against cancer; 1) Cells able to elude our innate security system can become a cancerous threat, and 2) Our security system is not functioning optimally to recognize these threats. Similar systems serve as rehabilitation for these would be criminals, as they exist to repair DNA damage before it signals to the cell to go rogue and become cancerous.

The scientific description of the new hallmarks of cancer elegantly, albeit indirectly, wove in the work of Kritchevsky and the studies tracking back to the turn of the twentieth century. For instance, Moreschi was exploiting these hallmarks when he placed his sarcoma cells in overfed mice, an ideal "soil" environment encouraging the cancer cells to proliferate like over-nourished weeds. This overabundance of nutrients, which satisfied the first of Hanahan and Weinberg's next-generation cancer hallmarks, fueled the deregulated metabolism that frequently occurs in cancer cells, supporting their rapid replication and feeding their massive growth.[8] This massive growth, scientifically referred to as biomass production, often results in palpable tumors, similar to those growing along the muscles of Moreschi's mice. Furthermore, the mechanisms that Kritchevsky so strongly coveted were finally being discussed within the scientific world, signaling that his efforts to garner enthusiasm were perhaps successful, and the scientific alphabet was finally being put into words.

The impact of Rous, Tannenbaum, and their colleagues and the accompanying century of research on energy restriction came full circle in Hanahan and Weinberg's second analysis. Autophagy, the process of programmed cell death, is activated during times of cellular stress. The "most obvious" cellular stress, they noted, is nutrient deficiency which results in the breakdown and recycling of malfunctioning and unnecessary cellular components. The recycled material can then be reused for energy or cellular building blocks. Could simply decreasing available food neutralize a hallmark of cancer?

In the original *Hallmarks of Cancer*, the beneficial effects of nutrient restriction were never mentioned, as the tone remained sharply focused on the genetic aspects of cancer induction and growth. However, in the decade leading up to the publication of *The Next Generation*, something changed. The growth-fostering environment throughout the body, the cancerous fuel-like effect of inflammation, and the importance of a healthy immune system to rid the body of potentially cancerous cells took a front seat in cancer prevention. Furthermore, newer data have revealed that epigenetic changes – or the turning on and off of genes – can be accomplished through different foods, nutrients, and vitamins, along with activities like sleep, relaxation, meditation, and exercise.[9]

The shift in focus became clear in the decade between the two publications: while the initial *Hallmarks of Cancer* favored the circumstance where a genetic switch is turned on, allowing continued and unchecked cellular growth, the *Next Generation* of hallmarks favored the metabolic environment that fosters the development of cancer cells. Researchers now sought to answer what turns on that switch in the first place. While the initial hallmarks may be viewed as the mechanisms by which the cancerous seed sprouts and grows, the next generation represents the soils and fertilizers that foster that germination. The first of the revisited hallmarks, the reprogramming of energy metabolism, further reiterates this view. Cancer cells alter normal cellular metabolism to rely on specific macronutrients, and to burn through them on overdrive to support cancer growth and biomass production.

This phenomenon was originally conceived over a half-century ago by Otto Heinrich Warburg. Warburg had recently completed Nobel Prize-worthy work on mitochondria, the powerhouses of our cells, and their ability to burn nutrients for energy in the presence of oxygen, known as cellular respiration. Warburg and other researchers, like Herbert Grace Crabtree, found that cancer cells were particularly greedy when it came to metabolizing sugar as fuel for energy. Furthermore, they tended to utilize it as the brick and mortar for cancer cell construction during the process of biomass production. In this respect, cancer cells differed drastically from our normal cells. They instead behaved more like a breed of anaerobic cellular organisms present on Earth billions of years ago when oxygen was not yet at high enough concentrations for organisms to utilize during energy production. Cancer cells, like yeast feasting on grapes in a barrel of aging wine, chose to ferment glucose for energy derivation.

Traditionally our cells break down glucose into an energy source called acetyl CoA. Acetyl CoA is then shuttled into the mitochondria for the efficient process of oxidative phosphorylation, which produces adenosine triphosphate (ATP), the energy currency of our cells. When our quadriceps muscle rhythmically contracts while sprinting or our biceps contract repeatedly during a set of dumbbell curls, minimal amounts of oxygen are present. As a result, the local cells are forced to break down glucose to pyruvate for energy production in the absence of oxygen via a process called anaerobic glycolysis (literally, the breakdown of glucose without oxygen). This process is inefficient and produces lactic acid, which has traditionally (and incorrectly) taken the blame for the burn we feel within our muscles during an intense workout. The process, however inefficient, rapidly provides the muscles with energy via ATP. The successful survival of our human species across our long stretch as part of the planetary food chain owes itself to this mechanism, which has allowed us to outrun and outlast bigger and stronger potential predators.

When oxygen is present, on the other hand, our cells engage in aerobic respiration. Glucose is completely broken down into acetyl CoA, which is then shuttled into the mitochondria for the significantly more efficient process of aerobic respiration.

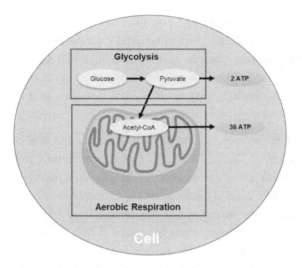

Figure 5: *Glucose is broken down into pyruvate in the cytoplasm of the cell. No oxygen is required. However, the breakdown of pyruvate to acetyl-CoA within the Krebs Cycle requires oxygen.*

As first discovered by Warburg, regardless of the presence of oxygen, cancer cells for unknown reasons prefer the less efficient process of glycolysis and largely ignore the powerful mitochondria with their ability to generate significantly more energy.[10] The cells appear to forget about the efficient process of oxidative phosphorylation and instead return to their less efficient billion-year old primordial methods of energy derivation. Some believe this irrational tendency of cancer cells to rely on less efficient glycolysis is due to defective mitochondria in cancer cells, but this hypothesis remains a contested one. Crabtree found the similar process occurring in yeasts produced alcohol (as opposed to lactate as in our cells). Coined the Crabtree Effect, this process occurs in *saccharomyces cerevisiae* yeast present during the process of winemaking and is partly responsible for that higher amount of alcohol in your nightly glass of red.

In a true affirmation of the importance of his work, Warburg was awarded the Nobel Prize in Physiology for his research on cellular respiration in 1931. Warburg, a friend of Albert Einstein, was serving as director of the Kaiser Wilhelm Institute for Cell Physiology when World War II erupted. Remarkably, Warburg, of Jewish ancestry, was able to remain in Berlin performing experiments during all but three weeks of Adolf Hitler's reign. In total, Warburg published 105 scientific articles during the control of the Third Reich. Many believe that one of the few things that superseded Hitler's disdain for Jews was his fear of cancer (oncophobia), so he allowed Warburg to continue his research that showed promise to find a cure for, or at least successful prevention of, cancer.[11]

Similar to the segue witnessed from Hanahan and Weinberg's first to second edition of *The Hallmarks of Cancer*, the genetic-centric view of cancer pushed Warburg's work aside for decades, only for it to be resurrected upon full consideration of the energetic requirements of cancer cells. A series of researchers have helped propel this reemergence over the past several decades. One of these researchers is Michael Ristow, who, like Hanahan, is a professor at the ETH Zurich. Ristow specializes in energy metabolism studies, and his work has indicated that providing cancer cells with a special protein called frataxin to awaken those same dysfunctional mitochondria inactivates one of the initial hallmarks of cancer, as these cells begin self-imploding through the process of apoptosis.[3] The simple change in mitochondrial function triggers this process of programmed suicide, thereby withdrawing the potentially harmful cells their ability to resist cell death – freedom from enslavement by the third hallmark of cancer. Cancer cells may have deregulated metabolism according to the next generation of hallmarks, but some thought it possible to correct their deregulated metabolism and turn them back to normal cells, or even prevent them from becoming cancerous in the first place.

While this hypothesis remains the subject of debate, the metabolic propensity of tumor cells has led some to question genetics as the root cause of cancer. Later research building upon Ristow's work points to the antitumor activity of mitochondria, partially from their collaborative efforts with tumor suppressor genes like *p53*.[12] Scientists such as Thomas Seyfried and Adrienne Scheck have shown in animal studies that drastically restricting dietary carbohydrates via a high fat ketogenic diet can offset many of the original and next generation hallmarks by cutting off a cancer cell's blood supply (angiogenesis), thereby activating the immune system to battle these cells and thus amplifying the effects of current cancer treatments like radiation therapy in a coordinated strike on cancer cells.[13,14] Other critics cite studies suggesting that the genetics of a cancer cell dictate which diet will fuel them or starve them, and not the other way around. For instance, mutation and activation of a gene family known as PI3K within cancer cells leaves them insensitive to the effects of dietary restriction.[15] Solving the issue of rust on steel has surely proven difficult for decades, but it pales in comparison to understanding and solving the metabolic aspects of cancer.

⁜

The consequences of being overweight – more specifically, having excess adipose tissue – and its connection to higher cancer risk are by now well publicized. Obesity also renders cancer cells more difficult to treat: as adipose tissue accumulates throughout the body, it acts like an endocrine organ, secreting excessive and potentially harmful sex hormones and inflammation that lead to blood glucose and insulin imbalance, hormonal imbalance, deregulated metabolism, and genomic instability.[16] To put it simply, excessive adipose tissue ushers in several of the hallmarks of cancer, leaving our cells not only less adept at fighting cancer but also more prone to support cancer's growth and development.

While the link between obesity and cancer was recently established through a plethora of formal scientific studies, knowledge of a connection is anything but new. Being overweight increases the risk of cancer, and in those who already have cancer, it increases the chances that it will come back after treatment.[17] In fact, it is estimated that for every 10 pounds increase in body mass index, men with prostate cancer have about a 20% increased risk of recurrence and dying from their prostate cancer.[18] The excess fat in obese men is also associated with an increased risk of their disease spreading via the process of metastases.[19] So, what is it about excess fat that increases the risk of cancer, fuels its growth, and prompts it to spread throughout the body?

Peering into the inner workings of the human body, we observe an intricate interplay of chemicals and hormones secreted from our organs and cells, orchestrating other organs and cells to function properly and react to external signals. Any signal that throws this elaborate interchange out of whack could create a butterfly effect with dire consequences. The body is not accustomed to excessive fat tissue, as its purpose (as a warmth and energy source) would dictate the necessity of only a limited supply. Some adipose tissue is necessary to help the body function optimally, but too much will harm the joints and our innate physiology. For instance, obesity is characteristic of metabolic syndrome.[20] This syndrome, also known as insulin insensitivity syndrome, is characterized by central obesity – the famous belly bulge – along with two of the following five risk factors: elevated blood sugar, insulin resistance (requiring more insulin than normal to lower blood sugar), elevated triglycerides, high blood pressure, and low HDL cholesterol.[21] This metabolic state has been shown to provide cancer cells with hormones, chemicals, and signals that ultimately offer them an environment rich in fertilizer that is more conducive to their growth and development. Obesity leads to a disorganized and unorchestrated metabolic state of varying levels of testosterone, estrogen, insulin, insulin-like growth factor 1 (IGF-1), and leptin.[22] All of these alterations are associated with an increased risk of cancer. During Kritchevsky's time, data emerged from studies that implicated the reduction of insulin as a factor more powerful in its links to cancer than calorie restriction. For instance, mice that no longer produce substantial insulin experience regression of their tumors and inhibition of new tumor manifestation.[23] Furthermore, excessive secretion of leptin, a hormone that inhibits hunger, by adipose tissue can cause the body to eventually become desensitized to its effects, leading instead to ravenous hunger. Beyond simply having excess fatty tissue, normal signaling becomes broken in many ways from metabolic syndrome.

Perhaps the most damaging attribute of excess adipose tissue is the inflammatory hormones it releases that irritate and inflame otherwise healthy cells and organs. These hormones interfere with insulin's ability to function properly, creating a vicious circle that leads to insulin resistance, elevated blood sugar, and even more inflammation as a consequence.[24] Adipokines, like leptin, are other necessary hormones secreted by our adipose tissue that can quickly become damaging when present in excess. These hormones promote the unchecked growth of our normal cells, the stimulation of aberrant blood vessel formation (angiogenesis), and the remodeling of the normal tissue surrounding our cells known as the extracellular matrix, which facilitates cancer progression.[25] These inflammatory hormones are plentiful, with the most well-known being tumor necrosis factor alpha (TNF-α) and interleukin 6 (IL-6), which not only promote the formation of cancer,[26] but worsen survival in cancer patients by promoting its growth and spread throughout the body.[27] A third common inflammatory factor released by adipose tissue is C-reactive protein, or CRP; CRP can be overproduced due to obesity, and in particular from the central bulge. Excess levels of CRP correlate with poorer outcomes after treatment for men with prostate cancer[28] and women with breast cancer.[16]

Perhaps most damaging from a cancer point of view, excessive adipose tissue fosters a state of insulin resistance within the body. In other words, the normal amount of insulin no longer works to lower blood sugar after the ingestion of carbohydrates, and increased amounts of insulin are secreted by the pancreas to counter this insufficiency. Central obesity – the trademark "tire" around our midsections – appears to be much more effective than general obesity at triggering insulin resistance. Over time, individuals with this physical condition eventually experience elevated levels of insulin, blood sugar, and IGF-1, forming the perfect cancer cocktail.

While adipose tissue can directly act to create a hospitable environment for cancer cells, its indirect effects are also damaging: it wears down insulin sensitivity over time, eventually allowing blood sugar levels to gradually creep upward, rendering our normal defense mechanisms less alert and less able to pick the cancerous cells out of the crowd of normal cells. Fatty tissue even releases a hormone known as resistin, named as such since it literally causes the resistance to insulin.[29] Over time, fat accumulates between our organs and muscles, and fatty acids begin to collect within our blood. The vicious feedback eventually leads to an inability of our cells to extract glucose from the blood; the cells then send out signals that they are starving, and the liver responds by producing even more glucose, exacerbating the overall situation.[30] Finally, fatty tissue has an innate ability to decrease the amount of proteins available to bind and inactivate these hormones, like sex hormone-binding globulin, or SHBG.[31] While the body may not always be able to lower its hormone levels, it uses SHBG as a fail-safe mechanism to incapacitate excessive hormones. Shutting off this fail-safe can have dire consequences.

In summary, an excess of fat leads to an abundance of health issues. This excess of fat has generally been felt to be best avoided and treated by simply cutting calories. Scientifically, this strategy makes sense – eat less or as much as you burn, and you will not add weight. This simple strategy obeys the laws of thermodynamics as energy must be conserved. In other words, energy in equals energy out; this holds for all life on earth, including humans, our activities, and our diets. If we eat too much, we gain weight, and to lose weight we must burn weight. For weight loss, we must obey Newton's law by simply eating less and exercising more. This traditional view of weight loss remains a central tenet of the dietary world. However, what these truths tell us about maintaining an optimal weight and body type is less clear. Why do some people eat as much as they please yet never gain weight, while others seem to be constantly dieting yet constantly overweight?

Eat less and exercise more. This advice is so ubiquitous to the medical and diet field that few would doubt its effectiveness. Simply resist temptation, eat less, and exercise, and the trials and tribulations of weight gain will be avoided. But is it that simple? What if certain foods gradually made us fatter, and this increase in adipose tissue and fat cells, along with the cancer-supporting metabolic and unfettered hormonal changes, commanded these fat cells to consume us from within? What if the fat cells – like aggressive cancer cells in their propensity to grow and expand – began to steal our food, making us feel hungrier and causing us to eat more food and gain more weight until ultimately, we find ourselves obese?

I sat in a lecture hall and watched as Dr. David Ludwig asked the audience these same questions. Ludwig, author of the New York Times' Bestseller *Always Hungry*, argued that certain factors have signaled our fat cells to take in glucose and nutrients, causing them to swell and slowly grow out of control. Ludwig, physician and nutrition researcher at Boston Children's Hospital and Harvard Medical School, explained that many factors increase the risk of obesity, including sleep, stress, exercise, the genes our parents passed to us, and of course, the food we eat. One hormone, however, appears to play a large and previously underappreciated role in obesity: insulin. The same hormone that the pancreas secretes to lower blood glucose and support several vital physiologic processes when present in excess leads to the accumulation of nutrients within our fat cells. Furthermore, foods that potently stimulate insulin seem to play the largest role in the recent obesity epidemic. If true, this theory would place the crosshairs squarely on those simple carbohydrates and sugary sweets that have the largest impact on the release of insulin, or "the Miracle-Gro for your fat cells" as Ludwig referred to it.[32] Less refined carbohydrates allow a slower and less drastic release of insulin. Proteins cause the release of even less insulin, and dietary fat seems to result in very little change in insulin levels. Perhaps most worrisome, since the late 1970's and the US's adoption of the Food Pyramid, we have largely replaced dietary fat with the most insulinogenic food: simple and refined carbohydrates.

Like most physicians, Ludwig has witnessed numerous diabetics injecting excess insulin and gaining weight over the past several decades, while those that are deficient in insulin lose weight. Marking insulin as the main culprit responsible for obesity is not a new phenomenon but has certainly gained increasing support in the last decade or so. The Carbohydrate-Insulin Model of Obesity, or CIM, is the more recent explanation for this phenomenon – the excessive consumption of foods that increase our blood sugar leads to excessive insulin secretion from the pancreas, triggering our fat cells to pull in excess calories and grow disproportionately. Ultimately, the fat cells continue to consume more nutrients, become fatter and then starve other cells of nutrients which, contrary to logic, leaves the body feeling hungrier and more prone to overeat. The problem is likely more than simple willpower and the avoidance of calories and overconsuming food; certain foods drive us to overeat, gain weight, and become severely obese, and the population has been advised to eat those exact foods over the past several decades. The current rates of overweight and obese individuals speak volumes in making the case of proponents of the Carbohydrate-Insulin Model of Obesity.

History is littered with examples of individuals who popularized a diet that capitalized on the CIM, or at least the simple view that carbohydrates – either indirectly or through the stimulation of overeating – are inherently fattening. One of the first references came from a quite unexpected source. William Banting, an undertaker on St. James Street in London, England during the 1800's, struggled with obesity for years. He had helped conduct funerals for two King Georges (III and IV), along with many other royal figures including Prince Albert in 1861. Yet, he was so massive that he had to walk up his stairs backwards – too large to bend over, he also had to use a specialized hook to aid him in placing his shoes on his feet. Two years after Prince Albert's service, Banting completed his most famous embalming when he released his *Letter on Corpulence, Addressed to the Public*, a first major effort in establishing the view on the benefits of carbohydrate restriction for weight loss.[33] Banting struggled after years of failed doctor's advice and treatments, including failed diets, fasts, and eccentric treatments like sea air, gallons of physic (a cathartic medicine of the era), and liquor potassae. He was repeatedly told to exercise more and eat less. He ended up exercising more, but this was followed with increases in his appetite from the activity, and so he ended up eating more and gaining even more weight. He even tried extreme calorie restriction, which did little to help his weight problem but did cause boils to form on his skin in very uncomfortable places.

The rather simple advice of one physician was finally successful for Banting. He crossed paths with an ear surgeon named William Harvey, who had recently attended a lecture by French physician and researcher Claude Bernard. Monsieur Bernard was a proponent of blind experiments and, like James Lind, was one of the first to suggest implementing this revolutionary type of clinical study. He first discovered glycogen, the storage form of carbohydrates within the liver.[34] From his research with sugar, he eventually narrowed his focus onto the study of diabetes, the pathologic state that results in elevated sugar within the blood, eventually spilling over into the urine. The strategic aspects of dealing with the body's inability to manage dietary sugar by eliminating starches and sugars within the diet was where Bernard's studies flourished. He eventually lectured on these possibilities to a room full of spectators in Paris, leaving a strong impression on William Harvey who would later see Banting in his practice.

Banting met Harvey while his other physician was on vacation for the holiday. Harvey, an ear specialist, commented that Banting's ear canals were obstructed by excessive fat which muffled sounds as they attempted to enter the inner ear, leading to Banting's hearing loss. An immediate change to his diet was required and, following Bernard's hypothesis, Banting's diet was changed to several servings a day of green vegetables, fruit, meat, and dry wine. Banting also avoided pork and butter as he thought they contained starch. The changes resulted in gradual weight loss, so long as Banting avoided sugar, starch, and similar foods. His weight dropped from 202 pounds to a remarkable 167 pounds, averaging about a pound lost per week. Banting published his manifesto, not as a means for profiting – his family business was quite successful at that – but rather in "earnest hope it may lead to the same comfort and happiness I now feel under the extraordinary change," and as thanks that "Almighty Providence" directed him "into the right and proper channel."[33] He eventually sold around 63,000 copies in Britain, donating all profits to charity. Neither he nor Harvey ever attempted to patent or copyright their successful diet.

Banting died at age 81; he is immortalized as one of few people whose name is an official verb in the English Dictionary. Another figure who popularized "banting" was cardiologist Robert Atkins, who created his own commercialized version of the diet in 1972 and steadfastly adhered to it until his death in 2002. The Atkins diet plan was initially much stricter but followed the same premise; Atkins allowed for less carbohydrates than Banting (and did not include Banting's frequent six or so glasses of claret, wine, sherry, or Madeira – sweet wines like port and champagne were forbidden).

Much like the mystery behind the mechanisms of Tannenbaum, Rous, Moreschi, and other "calorie" restriction studies, exactly how these diets were resulting in miraculous weight loss remained unknown, especially since followers ate demonized high-fat foods and ignored calorie counting. Attempting to further the science on low-carbohydrate diets, researchers in the twentieth century generally attempted high protein and low carbohydrate diets, which misconstrued some of the potential mechanisms. However, several years before Atkins' death, physician-author duo Michael and Mary Eades furthered the discussion of the science and mechanisms that supported why this lifestyle was so successful in their 1997 book, *Protein Power*. While the title is deceiving, further illustrating the anti-fat attitude during the 1990's, the book focused on the role that carbohydrates play in the diet, the effect they have on insulin, and their mechanism to signal to the cells to accumulate excessive adipose tissue. When Gary Taubes published his New York Times' Best Seller *Good Calories, Bad Calories*, the theory was brought into the popular spotlight, along with an exposé by Taubes on the social and political reasons why the theory – with its potential benefits of significantly increasing dietary fat consumption – was met with so much opposition.

Apart from the battles that continue to be waged in both scientific communities and popular online forums over the competing dietary theories, studies supporting the CIM continue to accumulate. Ludwig became a thorn in the side of the CIM opposition when in 2004 he published a study illustrating that feeding two groups of mice the same number of calories while increasing the amount of dietary starch in one of the groups resulted in almost double the accumulation of fat in the starch-fed mice. By the end of the study both groups weighed the same; in one sense this was a victory of the proponents of the simple caloric model of obesity. However, the result that diets of the same caloric content could result in one group of fattened mice and another group with a significantly higher amount of lean body mass – a major marker of health – was a huge initial step in chipping away at the simple caloric model of obesity.[35] It was also one of many studies signaling that perhaps we should focus on body composition instead of merely considering weight.

In an extension of the same study, Ludwig and his group removed part of the pancreas for some of the mice, producing a study subgroup unable to fully secrete the necessary insulin required to lower blood sugar after a meal. This physiologic state represents insulin insensitivity, which is currently threatening a large portion of the population as a condition known as prediabetes. With continued worsening of pancreatic function and decreased insulin sensitivity, type II diabetes develops as the insulin is no longer able to pull sugar effectively from their blood and into their cells. Following the pancreas surgery, these mice were placed on similar diets as those in his initial experiment. The higher starch diet, though containing similar calories, led to significant increases in both body fat percentage and weight in the rats. In fact, to maintain a similar weight between the groups it became necessary to restrict the calories of the high-starch rats, as they began to gain more weight than the low-starch group. Furthermore, the diet higher in starch led to significantly larger upswings in blood sugar and insulin in these mice, revealing that similar caloric diets may result in dissimilar physiologic responses by the body when insulin sensitivity is suboptimal.

As with the cancer dietary research pioneers of the early twentieth century, we need to remind ourselves that these later experiments were performed in mice and rats, and furthermore, some were surgically altered. A randomized study in humans would be necessary to fully answer the question, but such a study would require the placement of participants in a metabolic ward for months with a price tag in the millions. Instead, Ludwig and his group of researchers turned to an epidemiological method known as mendelian randomization. Instead of taking a discovery and working backwards to remove associations and potential confounding factors that are often impossible to account for in the search for causation – think of proactive women asking for hormone replacement therapy – the mendelian method accomplishes similar results via genetics. Genotypes, our genetic snippets passed to us by our parents, are given to us in a randomized fashion from either parent as we develop within the womb. One can then look at a gene to see if it portends a certain outcome, such as obesity, to assess if the gene is associated. While this method has its limitations, those shortcomings pale in comparison to those of the initially overly simplistic cause-and-effect population studies.

In a special edition of the journal *Clinical Chemistry* in January 2018, Ludwig and his group published their study utilizing this technique to further support the CIM. The group used genetic predeterminations for insulin release 30 minutes after a carbohydrate meal that predicted for body mass index. In other words, those individuals that are predestined to secrete a larger amount of insulin after consuming carbohydrates generally weigh more than individuals who secrete less insulin – 10 pounds more on average to be exact. They checked for the reverse as well – a finding that would support the traditional view on weight gain – and genetic predisposition to a high body mass index did not foresee increased insulin secretion. In other words, being overweight does not mean one necessarily over-secretes insulin after eating carbohydrates, but being an "over-secretor" of insulin does place one at a significantly increased risk of being overweight. While the traditional theory on obesity can be simplified as "excessive calories promotes excessive body fat which promotes excessive insulin secretion," Ludwig's multiple studies support a view that excessive consumption of carbohydrates leads to excessive insulin secretion which leads to excessive body fat, and then corresponding excessive eating is the final scene in this cascading metabolic tragedy.

Regardless of which theory is right – and, judging by the strong opinions on both sides, we will likely be without an answer for decades to come – the current traditional theory provides few tangible solutions to the obesity crisis. Current obesity statistics would lend credence to the view that dietary dogma is failing miserably, as the rate of obesity continues to climb. As Ludwig pointed out in an editorial for the *New York Times*, only one in six overweight or obese Americans has reported losing ten percent of their weight and maintaining it for a year. Simply restricting calories has been an epic failure for weight loss, and the numbers do not lie. We now have several plausible reasons for this failure, including a 1995 study from the Laboratory of Human Behavior and Metabolism at Rockefeller University in New York.[36] Study subjects that lost ten percent of their body weight experienced a ravenous increase in hunger and an associated drop in metabolism; when the body loses weight, it flicks on a switch to counter the weight loss via a process called homeostasis. Studies from the 1960's revealed the opposite effect, as overeating participants experienced an increase in their metabolism.[37] In other words, feeling "fatigue, depression, mental fog, and an obsession with food," like the participants in Biosphere 2, or feeling "silent, apathetic, and immobile," like the men in the Minnesota Starvation Study, would stop the strongest-willed individuals from continuing on a significant calorie-restricted diet. This inability to follow strict calorie restriction and "simply" eat less and exercise more is playing out in our society, and we desperately need a solution.

The CIM theory remains contentious, with many followers and equally as many critics. And like the traditional theory, it also remains unproven. Dozens of randomized studies have compared a calorie-restricted, low-fat diet – a diet like most weight-loss recommendations based on the traditional view – to a carbohydrate-restricted, calorically *unrestricted* high-fat diet that was effective for Banting. While the latter restricts carbohydrates, the fact that participants can eat until they are satisfied is an attractive component. In an analysis of the randomized studies at the time of this publication, the high-fat diet has been victorious over the low-fat diet 29 times, and 28 times the results have been even. The low-fat diet on the other hand has never been victorious. Furthermore, participants on the high-fat diet appear to spontaneously decrease their caloric intake as their appetite drops, even as they lose weight. If we truly wanted individuals to simply reduce their calories, this last point should be strongly considered.

At the time of this writing, a recent randomized trial found that at one year, participants on a low-carbohydrate, high-fat, and calorically unrestricted diet lost significantly more weight than those on a calorie-restricted and low-fat diet that followed traditional weight loss recommendations.[38] Furthermore, as predicted by Ludwig and others' research, dieters that restricted carbohydrates watched as their typical blood sugar levels dropped, and they required less diabetic medications as their insulin sensitivity rose. While these studies reveal some of the many reasons for the inefficacy of low-fat and calorie-restricted diets and provide some clues as to why current dietary recommendations have failed on such massive proportions, they by no means prove the CIM. Whether it will, like Banting's diet, allow "Almighty Providence" to direct us into the "right and proper channel" remains unknown.

Individuals who have found that a high-fat diet leaves them satiated and able to maintain a healthy weight can at least rest assured that the bulk of data supports this approach, while individuals plagued by the feeling of disappointment over their inability to follow a low-fat, calorically-restricted diet can feel assured that they are not weak-willed and gluttonous failures; rather, they are battling ingrained physiologic mechanisms and genetics with inadequate weapons. Within the cancer world, however, diet remains an intriguing subject to examine due to its potential ability to modify several metabolic pathways that are important for cancer initiation and growth, including lowering insulin. Not only does this anabolic hormone appear to stimulate fat growth, but a multitude of studies support its ability to stimulate cancer growth as well. Ludwig's "Miracle-Gro" for fat cells seems to have similar extraordinary abilities to do the same with respect to cancer cells. If the general public has been instructed to eat a diet that increases the release of a hormone that can potentially fuel cancer cells, there are major ramifications for the cancer landscape in individuals following those same dietary orders.

6

OIL, SPOIL, AND TOIL

"Food is all those substances which, submitted to the action of the stomach, can be assimilated or changed into life by digestion, and can thus repair the losses which the human body suffers through the act of living."

- Jean Anthelme Brillat-Savarin, Author of *Physiologie du goût* (*The Physiology of Taste*)

Takeaways:

Not all fats are created equal; here, we explore unsaturated and saturated fats, cooking oils, the potential health-related effects of heating them, and the free radical damage that can ensue, promoting oxidative damage like the rust on a bridge and the potential activation of cancer-prone pathways.

One of the largest studies to date testing vegetable oil and its effect on our health is discussed. Is cancer simply luck? This question is thoroughly addressed.

A frigid breeze swirled across the horizon, pulling with it tufts of snow, blending with fumes from the steel mills in the distance. It was a cold Pittsburgh day; snow, smoke, and soot permeated the air, coalescing into a muddy concoction that settled onto the fabric of white shirts, turning them grey and eventually black. The color of Leonardo's thick coat matched the hue of the sky, with its heavy fabric dutifully keeping the frigid cold out. After accumulating so much dust from the steel mill exhaust, the coat now seemed to double as an air filter. Leonardo was on his way home in one of his most difficult trips of the winter – the wind ripped across his face like a razor blade, eliciting extreme pain with each gust. The McKees Rocks and West End Bridges had yet to be built; the new Sixth Street Bridge, which replaced Roebling's old Sixth Street Bridge after it was demolished in 1892, would make Leonardo's journey far too long and the razorblades far too unbearable. Leonardo may have been a poor Calabrese shop owner, but even he knew that the closest distance between two points is a straight line. In what seemed like a geometrically ingenious plan, Leonardo pulled his horse-drawn buggy onto the thick ice of the Ohio River and began to cross.

He had just filled his wagon with provisions from the 20 blocks of food stores and markets, wholesalers, and auction houses that made up the Strip District. Tucked between downtown Pittsburgh, the Allegheny River, and a multitude of industrial buildings, foundries, and iron and glass factories, the district served as the central marketplace of the city. Store owners like Leonardo were able to supply their local ethnic neighborhoods with many of the same foods they consumed in their homelands. The Strip District was the heart of commerce in metro Pittsburgh, and eventually Westinghouse, Heinz, ALCOA, and US Steel would be located there.

Upon approaching the small town on the south bank of the Ohio River, Leonardo once again felt the earth beneath his wheels as he pulled his horse and buggy onto the terra firma known as McKees Rocks. The "Rocks," as it was known to locals, was at one point considered to be the future site for Fort Pitt, but it was later decided it would be easier and cheaper to build it on the destroyed French Fort Duquesne. Instead, Alexander McKee was deeded the land, and so the plot bounded by the rocky shoreline along the Ohio River was berthed the name McKees Rocks in 1792. It was incorporated as a borough in 1892; in the decade following, Italian immigrants flocked into the area for work. Most of them ended up at its biggest employer, the Pressed Steel Car Company. Part of McKees Rocks, known as Presston, was even owned by the company and housed many of the workers in serfdom-like conditions. Functioning as a banana republic – or in this instance a "steel republic" – several similar bogus cities were formed around Pittsburgh, where workers were treated more like indentured servants than paid employees. Work at Presston was so tough and dangerous that the plant eventually earned the unflattering nickname "The Slaughterhouse." By 1909, the Slaughterhouse was averaging nearly one causality per day. While Andrew Carnegie was the business titan who took the most local heat for his poor work conditions, nearly all steel mills in the Pittsburgh area treated workers as expendable commodities. Tensions would gradually rise at Presston Steel until they culminated in the infamous McKees Rocks Strike of 1909.

As a former farmer and cheese monger from southern Italy, Leonardo, who was always afraid to slaughter his own sheep, decided that working in the Presston slaughterhouse was also not for him. Now a shepherd in search of a new flock to feed in the urban town of McKees Rocks, Leonardo returned to what he knew best and began operating an Italian grocery store at night. Instead of producing milk and dairy products from the sheep he raised, he opened a store that specialized in sourcing traditional Italian food products and the same foods that he grew up producing from his sheep's milk in Calabria. Not long after writer Upton Sinclair conducted his clandestine visits to the slaughterhouses to write *The Jungle*, his famous tome denouncing the American system of meat production, Leonardo had left his own slaughterhouse in his rearview mirror to begin selling produce, meat, and groceries to his fellow Pittsburgh neighbors. He still produced his own cheese, sausage, eggs, and even wine (though according to his family, the latter may have been less than appetizing). He would frequently take trips to the Strip District to replenish his supplies of Italian goods, leaving the slaughterhouse butchering and quartering of meats to others with stronger stomachs for it.

On this day, however, the weather was not cooperating, forcing Leonardo to take his shortcut over the Ohio River. He eventually made it to the grocery store and parked his wagon to go inside and unload his provisions. His sacks contained cheese, prosciutto, soppressata, olive oil, and lard. Lard was the major cooking source for Leonardo and his fellow Italians in McKees Rocks. Olive oil was used for garnishing, but lard – produced from pork fat – was cheaper and easier to make, could be heated for cooking on the stove, and rarely smoked or became rancid due to its sound chemical structure. Leonardo knew that lard was a stable fat, and that property made it ideal for cooking.

At that time, production of vegetable oils was experiencing a sharp increase. In 1911 Proctor and Gamble began marketing cottonseed oil, a product created through the intense chemical processing of unused cottonseeds, turning their former waste into a new cash cow. (P&G even doubled down on the investment when they began using the industrial waste from the vegetable oil process as animal feed.) They eventually attempted to replace the customary usage of lard with Crisco. Crisco, a trans-fat vegetable shortening, was cheaper than lard and seemed like the perfect solution to the media frenzy over the proposed view that saturated fats were clogging arteries. Shortly after, researchers like Tannenbaum and Rous were using corn oil and other similar vegetable oils like cottonseed oil as carcinogenic compounds in their experiments. They could assess how dietary changes would impact mice consuming large amounts of corn oil, which like DMBA and other carcinogens would cause high rates of cancer. It was known that these vegetable oils would become inundated with free radicals during their time on the shelf, and these free radicals would damage and degrade the oils, leaving oxidative products like lipid peroxides. Applying a tiny bit of heat to these oils created an ideal environment for a Kritchevsky-approved cancer study.

Like my great-grandfather Leonardo, these researchers were aware that polyunsaturated fats and vegetable oils, unlike heavier and more stable partially saturated fats like lard, were susceptible to structural damage from heat. For Leonardo, no scientific explanation was necessary – cooking with these unsaturated fats would cause them to turn brown, smoke, and ruin the foods to which they were exposed. Leonardo's wife Philomena was a tough-as-nails Italian woman and an incredible cook with high culinary standards; imparting any taste of burnt oil onto her food left Leonardo in the dog house. In fact, he and other poor Calabrians often relied on lard, and not the more expensive olive oil.

Researchers at the time were well aware that polyunsaturated fatty acids, or PUFAs, became laced with free radicals during the browning and smoking process known as oxidation. In this process the PUFAs undergo a change that is quite similar to rusting both visually and structurally. Furthermore, as these oils turn rancid, they begin to decompose, releasing potentially harmful and volatile chemicals. Heating fats and oils, even for a short amount of time, appeared to change their chemical structure.[1] Lavik and Bauman, who performed one of the original studies illustrating the cancer-promoting effects of fat, ran several experiments at the University of Wisconsin exposing a doubling of the cancerous effect when vegetable oil was first heated at 572°F for 1 hour.[2] Kritchevsky also compared regular and heated corn oil with Leonardo's favorite olive oil, and he found that heated corn oil produced significant atherosclerosis along the arteries in mice; free radicals accumulated within their arterial walls, attacking normal cells, causing oxidation, arterial rusting, and eventual blockages.[3] Kritchevsky even began to refer to these oils as "vehicles" since they were responsible for driving free radical damage into the body.

While Leonardo needed no scientific explanation for why his lard was a better alternative for cooking than newfangled oils, a simple explanation does exist, albeit one involving a basic understanding of a complex subject: organic chemistry. The different structural properties of saturated and unsaturated fats largely lead to their chemical differences, which gives context to both Kritchevsky's "vehicle" nomenclature for driving up oxidation and Tannenbaum's references to a "direct property of fat" to produce cancer. It also explains why certain fats along the skin of mice would accelerate tumor production in the presence of carcinogenic chemicals.

Fatty sources such as pork fat (lard), butter, and coconut oil contain higher amounts of saturated fats and thus remain solids at room temperature due to their more stable and more saturated molecular structure. This simple observation has been made for thousands of years and explains one of the major reasons why such sources were used for cooking in many cultures across the globe. All fats have a chain of carbons that are connected as their backbone, similar to thee vertebral bones that make up our spines. These carbons then connect to other atoms, and the degree of saturation is based on how many of these carbons are free or saturated with hydrogens. Saturated fat is completely saturated with hydrogens, as shown in the picture below.

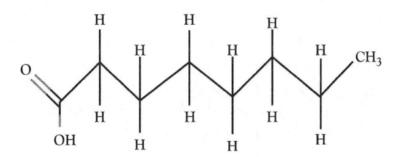

Figure 6: The carbon backbones of saturated fats are fully saturated with attached hydrogens.

This stabilization keeps saturated fats solid at room temperature and requires a significantly higher temperature for them to melt (i.e. become a liquid fat or oil). Unsaturated fats, on the other hand, have one or many unbound parts of their carbon backbone, thus making them less stable. Nearly half of lard is comprised of monounsaturated fat, while olive oil is about 75%. Unlike PUFAs, monounsaturated fats only contain one unsaturated link, as illustrated in the diagram below:

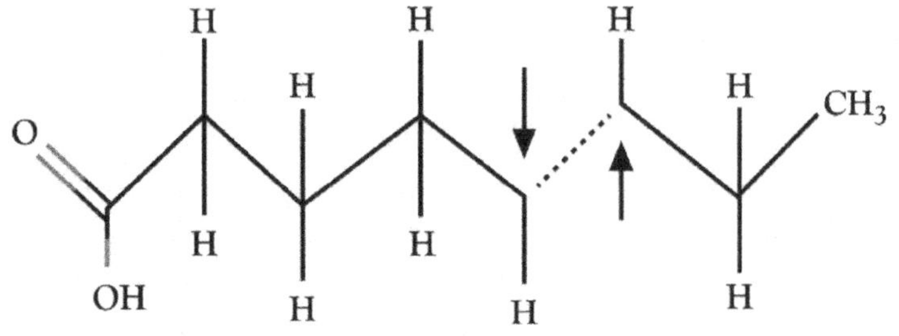

Figure 7: This monounsaturated fat has one unsaturated link along the arrows.

Finally, polyunsaturated fats have several unbound carbons along their backbone, as shown below:

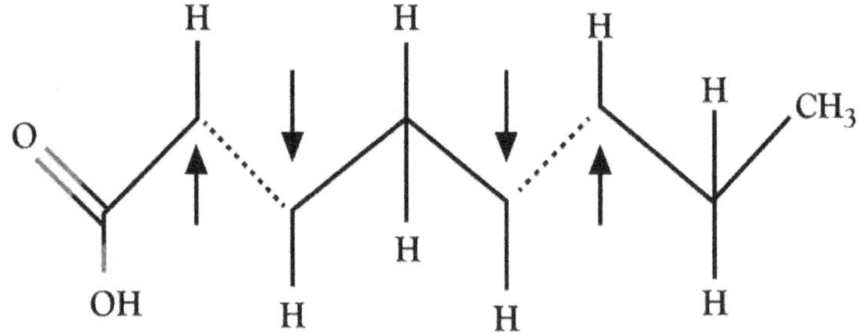

Figure 8: This polyunsaturated fat has four unbound carbons along its backbone.

The dotted line connection between the two arrows represents a double bond, which accounts for the lack of hydrogens bound to its ends. The polyunsaturated fat structure above has four unbound areas, one at each end of these double bonds, but the number can be much larger. The unbound nature of these areas leaves them vulnerable to attack by free radicals, like the exposed steel in the bridges that Leonardo could have crossed during that cold winter day in Pittsburgh. Instead of an attached hydrogen molecule as in a saturated fat, the polyunsaturated fat leaves room for an attached free radical in its place. When the radical attaches, the oil is then considered oxidized. As unpainted areas of steel are more susceptible to moisture and oxygen damage, the more unbound and vulnerable areas of a fat or oil, the more susceptible it is to becoming oxidized.

Like the corn oil used in many studies during the first half of the 20th century, this oxidized dietary source becomes a vehicle for free radicals to enter the body. While our cells create mechanisms to offset free radical damage, the process appears to differ when free radicals are produced by our own machinery such as our mitochondria, as opposed to being introduced from an outside source. Adding further fuel to this fire, the process by which these polyunsaturated fats are created – there are trivial amounts of fat in corn to make corn oil – involves processing them at high heats and exposing them to a handful of chemicals which can further bombard them with free radical damage. This is another characteristic that distinguishes healthy monounsaturated olive oil from potentially carcinogenic and atherogenic corn oil.[4] The compounding damaging effect of incorporating oils with free radicals reflects why the early scientists were finding that heating oils increased their ability to promote cancer, and in many instances increasing dietary fat led to an increase in cancer in mice.

If you are wondering how these same oils could have been (and still are) promoted as healthy, consider the health recommendations of hydrogenated oils. The formation of hydrogenated oils – known as trans-fats, the most familiar of which are Crisco and vegetable shortening – has been an adulteration of an attempt to derive the benefits that Leonardo saw in lard through the utilization of leftover waste components from industry production. Both the Wesson Corporation and Proctor and Gamble found that they could create Wesson Oil and Crisco by processing leftover cottonseeds. The remains from this process were then used as animal feed to provide these corporations with financial benefits at the previously unmonetized final step of their production chain. The detriments of these products on our health did not seem to stand in the way of their profiteering approach. During hydrogenation, an unprotected vegetable oil is bombarded with hydrogens to artificially saturate its many unsaturated carbon backbones and produce a trans-fat. The result is a grotesquely monstrous Frankenstein fat – "frankenfat" as we in the industry like to say – that visibly resembles Leonardo's lard, but structurally resembles a PUFA with hydrogens fixed into place. These fixed hydrogens later cause havoc as our body attempts to digest and process them. Further illustrating the spectacularly disastrous collision of controversy, corporate profits, and health was the involvement of the 1980s mainstream media in the chastising of animal and saturated fats like lard with claims that they damaged the arteries, ushering in a prolonged period of promotion and praise for trans fats. During that decade, they largely replaced the usage of saturated fats in many popular dining settings, the most notable of which was to cook McDonald's famous golden fries. Studies now confirm that trans-fats bombard the body with inflammation, damaging our cells, organs and, most ironically, our arteries.

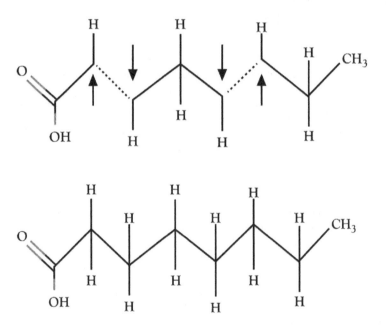

Figure 9: A polyunsaturated fat is bombarded with hydrogen at each arrow to produce an artificially saturated fat.

Free radicals naturally occur within our body and, considering their potential for damage, are surprisingly utilized as part of many normal physiologic and cellular processes. They are, however, a double-edged sword due to their extremely reactive nature and potential for damage. For instance, the caustic nature of free radicals is used by our cells as a defense against infectious agents. On the other hand, free radicals are produced within our mitochondria during energy derivation, and as mentioned before, these free radicals damage our cells like rust to iron via oxidation. Knowing the potential harm of these reactive substances, our body has evolved to channel this effect and has also created several mechanisms to combat this potential cellular self-mutilation.

Exposure of our cells to some degree of free radicals is beneficial, as the compensatory production of disarming antioxidants helps to fight the daily free radical and oxidative damage to our cells. However, as opposed to bombarding our cells with external sources of free radicals, the production of free radicals by our internal cellular processes triggers several inborn mechanisms to reduce potential damage from these reactive substances. For instance, when scientists push mitochondrial activity to overdrive in mice, diseases caused by free radical and oxidative damage like cancer and heart disease actually *decrease*.[5] Free radicals also serve as their own chemical switches, turning naturally occurring physiologic processes on and off. For example, platelets release free radicals after injury which message for help, attracting other platelets and immune cells to the damaged site to aid in repair. Free radicals may serve other purposes as well, many of which are yet to be discovered.

On the other hand, free radicals are chemically charged compounds that are extremely reactive with anything they encounter, and their potential danger is to be appreciated. When present in large quantities, they can bind to our cellular membranes, proteins, and, perhaps most importantly, our DNA. This damage can inhibit the normal function of our cells, and damage to the DNA can lead to cancer. The damage can be so intense that cancer treatment techniques often channel the damaging effects of free radicals: ionizing radiation works by lobbing free radicals at cancer cells like grenades to tear apart their DNA, often leading to irreparable injury and cellular death.

Free radicals are arguably one of the largest threats to cellular well-being, and throughout our evolution, our cells have adapted several processes to protect against this threat. The antioxidant defense system creates chemicals like glutathione that serve as free radical neutralizers by absorbing the brunt of their potential damaging effects to disarm them, similar to how buffers are poured onto surfaces to neutralize a toxic chemical spill. The introduction of excess free radicals from sources external to the body can overwhelm this defense system – much like in Tannenbaum's mouse studies, where he bombarded the mice with oxidized substances – leading to cellular damage and cancer. In many of the older studies, described by Kritchevsky decades later, these free-radical laden fats were acting as a Trojan Horse, transporting the threats within. Once released, these radicals could attack and bind to the fatty acids that comprise the membranes surrounding our cells. Many of these past studies mentioned that fat per se was likely not the cancer-promoting element of food, but more so the vehicle carrying carcinogens. These passengers – oxidative, cancer-causing free-radicals – were the real perpetrators. Like the mythical character Keyser Söze played by actor Kevin Spacey in the Oscar-winning 1996 screenplay The *Usual Suspects* (one of my favorite movie villains of all time!) the focus by Tannenbaum and his colleagues was erroneously cast upon the elusive and at times ambiguous character of fat, yet the real culprit was lurking right under their nose.

By the time Leonardo pulled up to his shop on that frigid day to empty his precious cargo – absent of vegetable oil and processed food, mind you – his prototypical Roaring 20's moustache was frozen onto the inside of his coat. He was unable to even lift his head, leaving him in the conundrum of whether he should leave his goods unguarded outside while he went in to thaw out, or wait for help to arrive. This story has been retold in my family for decades, but the crazy thing is that nobody in the older generations of my family seems to know or remember how it ended. It is a legendary larger-than-life yet verifiable tale that my grandfather crossed the frozen Ohio River one day with his wagon full of produce, and the minute details (such as his frozen moustache) likely came from Leonardo himself or his close friends and family who had heard him recount the story hundreds of times. The story has been handed down to me from my grandmother Rose; as I hear it now (and every past winter season when I was home for the holidays), the thing that always sticks out to me is how Leonardo was oblivious to the fact that he was supplying the kind of unadulterated, natural, real food to his McKees Rocks neighbors that would one day in the distant future be heavily chastised by the society-at-large in which his grandchildren and great-grandchildren have been raised.

⁙

Nearly 1.7 million people will find themselves contemplating treatment options for their newly diagnosed cancer next year in the United States alone.[6] Worldwide, another 11 million individuals will be victims of cancer, and it will take the lives of over half of them. Throughout our entire lives, we can expect around a 40% chance of experiencing it ourselves, and due to several overarching factors – like longer lives and higher rates of chronic diseases like obesity and diabetes – this risk of cancer is poised to increase.[7] For some of the population, the frequent diagnoses seen in friends and relatives have led them to expect a diagnosis at some point in their lives. These staggering numbers speak for themselves: cancer is a modern-day Goliath, and while modern medicine is relentlessly, cleverly, and valiantly fighting like the young David did, it has yet to slay the beast.

As my patients begin their journey and arm themselves to wage war, a common question often surfaces: "What aspects of our lifestyle influence our risk of cancer?" A recent study helps provide some insight into the answer, although the answer is a frustrating one to cancer prevention researchers. This study may question whether the winner between David and Goliath is even dictated by skill and strategy, or rather a simple matter of luck. The massive rates of cancer experienced throughout the US and the world beg the question as to whether lifestyle is causal to cancer contraction or if these 12.7 million individuals simply drew the short end of the stick. Even Rous wrote in his research findings that some unlucky mice grew tumors regardless of his most extreme dietary regimens and seemed predestined to get cancer irrespective of how much he starved them.

In 2015, two researchers from Johns Hopkins University fanned the flames of the theory that cancer contraction is mostly due to bad luck of the draw. Drs. Burt Vogelstein and Christian Tomasetti attempted to provide some clarity to this question through intense mathematical modeling and an in-depth analysis of cancer incidence based on different cell types. Not surprisingly given the hot-button topical relevance and widespread global interest in this common question, their results were published in the eminent

113

journal *Science.*[8] They found that, according to their calculations, over two thirds of all cancers appear to be the result of sheer bad luck, and the bad luck was proportional to the number of times a cell replicated. As they described, "the more often stem cells within an organ proliferate throughout our lifetime, the greater chance of that organ acquiring cancer." With each replication, the cell and its genetic material is exposed to an opportunity for an error to occur. If this error goes unfixed or involves a gene that could enable a hallmark of cancer, its owner may experience an unlucky case of cancer. More replications expose more chances for errors and increase the chances of bad luck. Following this logic, since cell division is generally predetermined – some cells replicate more often than others – Vogelstein and Tomasetti concluded that cancer risk is largely out of our hands: the mathematical models showed that 65% of the time there was nothing a patient could do to avoid getting cancer.

As the latest addition onto the conveyor belt of hastily reported health studies sure to ignite a media frenzy, the Vogelstein and Tomasetti report was to the surprise of no one, immediately, widely, and inaccurately circulated by mass media sources. The confusing results of the scientific report led to subsequent second-hand media reports that were even more puzzling to audiences. The news spread rapidly like wildfire, and soon the public was under the impression that all cancer was formed from bad luck and we were all left helpless – David was slain before the battle began. Vogelstein had even tried to give cautionary pause before jumping to these rash conclusions; when questioned about the study, he responded: "All cancers are caused by a combination of bad luck, the environment, and heredity, and we've created a model that may help quantify how much of these three factors contribute to cancer development. This study shows that you can add to your risk of getting cancers by smoking or other poor lifestyle factors."[9]

Tomasetti's feelings were mutual; he provided an insightful context by reversing the perspective. As he put it: "If two-thirds of cancer incidence across tissues is explained by random DNA mutations that occur when stem cells divide, then changing our lifestyle and habits will be a huge help in preventing certain cancers, but this may not be as effective for a variety of others." Yet even if some of us are predestined to get cancer, other questions remained unanswered: 1) If cellular and DNA errors happen more frequently in cells that replicate more often, how can this be directly affected by improving our body's ability to correct these errors? 2) Can we limit the sources of this damage? 3) Daily DNA damage and replication errors are expected, but is it a prudent strategy to reduce the exposure to carcinogens like tobacco, environmental hazards, and excessive inflammation to maximize our luck?

Interestingly, their analysis did not include breast and prostate cancer. Breast cancer occurs in one of eight women and is the second most common cancer in women (second only to skin cancer) with nearly 233,000 cases in 2014.[10] It kills more women than every other cancer except lung cancer. Prostate cancer affects one in three men and is slightly more common than breast cancer according to the National Cancer Institute. Furthermore, both cancers have been intimately linked to lifestyle habits, including diet and exercise.[11,12]

And so, it was that Vogelstein and Tomasetti attempted to answer some of the criticisms of their first report during the spring of 2017, when the updated version of their work was published again in *Science*.[13] Their findings held, and they still considered nearly two-thirds of cancers to arise from bad luck. In the two years since 2015, other data was published confirming their findings, with the caveat that external damage to cells could activate stem cells to replicate more, creating a "perfect storm" for cancer initiation. In other words, it is likely that Vogelstein and Tomasetti's luck-versus-behavior risks were related, and external factors could damage and convert cells into those unlucky ones that often turn to cancer.[14] Other data have paralleled this view, as has the controversial scientific field known as epigenetics, which is the mechanism that changes how genes are expressed without actually altering our DNA sequence.[15] Epigenetics allows our lifestyle activities to leave a lasting impression on our genes, albeit in an indirect manner. One epigenetic process, known as DNA methylation, leads to the silencing of a gene by the addition of a methyl group to one of the base pairs of its DNA. Another of these processes is histone acetylation, whereby chemicals known as histones that package and organize our DNA can be regulated by the addition or subtraction of an acetyl group. Histones protect our DNA from damage and stand guard like a bouncer at a nightclub refusing or allowing access. Foods, substances, and activities that inhibit histone deacetylase (HDAC) unlock the cell's DNA, allowing expression of the genes within. The exact mechanisms are quite nuanced, and the field of epigenetics remains novel and exciting, yet also controversial like Vogelstein and Tomasetti's work.

For instance, an animal study suggests that even a short spurt of high blood sugar after a meal can lead to epigenetic changes, including the transcription of an inflammatory protein that persists for days after blood sugar drops back to normal.[16] Butyrate, the anti-inflammatory fatty acid in butter that colon cells preferentially utilize for energy, works as an HDAC inhibitor.[17] Similarly, consuming a cup of broccoli sprouts inhibits HDAC for three hours afterwards.[18] Furthermore, butyrate is oxidized for energy in normal colon cells but due to the Warburg effect in cancer cells – the reliance on glucose for energy production – is inefficiently used as an energy source by cancer cells. It instead, accumulates in their nucleus, the computer hard drive of the cell, interfering with normal gene function.[19] Other dietary sources of HDAC inhibitors include garlic, onions, selenium-rich foods like Brazil nuts, resveratrol in grape skins, red wine, green tea, and the spice turmeric.[20]

So, it seems that when it comes to cancer, the "luck" of our genes may be directly affected by a variety of foods and lifestyle habits. The influence of epigenetics may again place more emphasis on lifestyle and environment, though this relationship is anything but straightforward. Vogelstein and Tomasetti's updated work did little to soften the critics, who felt that the paper was a "reductionist approach to a complex problem."[21] *Science* magazine later covered the debate, coming full circle as they traversed the dietary controversy within the cancer world when they turned to Walter Willett, who, according to the article, "speculates that something as simple as weight loss or stopping hormone replacement therapy in menopause might inhibit random mutations from ultimately causing a life-threatening tumor." Once again, random mutations may result from bad luck, but still we may be able to decide how many times we get to roll the dice. Conclusions remain unresolved, but new studies that expose the link between our food and lifestyle choices and their influence on cellular functions continue to accumulate. However, a split is ever present between those within the medical field who believe in luck and those like Kritchevsky and the generations of subsequent researchers like Willett who consider our diet and lifestyle intimately related to our risk of cancer.

⁘

By the middle of the 20th century, the rapid changes in the landscape of Leonardo's small Italian-American community in southwest Pennsylvania paralleled the rapid changes within the scientific and medical community. Eventually, Leonardo would have to close down his grocery store due to slowing business. His shop was somehow able to survive the Great Depression, feeding many of the local starving families who were out of work free of charge. However, store owners like Leonardo faced many obstacles between the Great Depression and the second World War. In 1930, McKees Rocks would reach its largest population of 18,116 but soon thereafter began its rapid decline. Pittsburgh experienced a catastrophic flood on St. Patrick's Day in 1936 that caused an estimated $3 billion of damage and left over 60,000 steelworkers without jobs. World War II led to a sharp decrease in population numbers, food shortages, and subsequent rationing across the country.

By the 1950s, the U.S. steel industry began to crumble due to poor planning, overexpansion, and outdated methods of manufacturing that were exposed by foreign competitors. As many of the steel mills closed their doors, so too did Leonardo shutter his shop. A simple farmer sheltered from the world of social sciences, Leonardo did not anticipate how the global economics and politics would put his modest store under financial attack, prompting its closure. Nor could he gasp how his traditional foods were now coming under attack by the scientific community. Both the lipid hypothesis and diet-heart hypothesis were giving dietary fat a bad name, chastising his beloved lard and olive oil and criticizing his cherished cheeses and meats.

The continuing fallout led to a series of studies attempting to connect heart disease with lipids in our blood and fat within our diet. The results of these studies were mixed and continue to be one of the most contentious areas in modern medicine. The wide range of data collection methods of the reports have led some scientists to suggest that they have succeeded in connecting the three, while others believe that the available data disproves the connection. While there is a possible connection between saturated fat and heart disease, however subtle, how did these findings impact the relationship between diet and cancer? Willett's data, albeit not randomized, had suggested that fat is unrelated to cancer, and perhaps even protective against breast cancer.

Shortly after Leonardo closed his shop doors in the 1950s, scientists Morton Lee Pearce and Seymour Dayton began accruing individual subjects to participate in a groundbreaking one-of-a-kind study at the Veterans Hospital in Los Angeles. In total, 846 men would enroll and agree to be randomized to a control or intervention arm. The control arm allowed these men to eat their typical diet, which at the time was thought to represent Leonardo-endorsed quantities of lard and saturated fat. Overall, 40% of their diet came from fat, and most of this was animal fat. The intervention arm of the study continued to eat about 40% of their calories as fat. However, these animal fats were replaced with polyunsaturated vegetable oils like corn, soybean, safflower, and cottonseed oil, which were at the time thought to lower cardiovascular risk. The diet of the intervention arm also contained significantly higher quantities of vitamin E and omega-3 and -6 fatty acids.

By 1971, Pearce and Dayton reported their results on the first randomized controlled clinical trial studying the impact of a diet high in polyunsaturated fat.[22] The primary endpoint of the study was to assess the impact of the diets on coronary events – defined as sudden death or definite myocardial infarction, known more simply as a heart attack. While they were able to lower blood cholesterol values in the experimental group, the trial was initially deemed unsuccessful; mortality rates were similar between the two groups of men, as were overall rates of cardiovascular events. However, when pooling several unplanned endpoints together, they did find a slight decrease in atherosclerotic events in the intervention arm. Yet because this unplanned follow-up analysis was executed after they observed their initial negative primary endpoint, it was met with criticism and initially discounted.

Criticism aside, the intervention group in the study was experiencing less cardiac events. However, men in each group were living just as long as each other, a shocking revelation to Pearce and Dayton. Furthermore, when Pearce and Dayton examined the differences between the groups, the control arm was comprised of double the number of moderate and heavy smokers – a statistically significant difference that according to Doll and Hill's data would have predicted for a higher rate of lung cancer and fatal diseases before any intervention even took place. If anything, this group should have been dying significantly more often than the intervention group, but for unknown reasons it was not playing out as predicted.[23]

Upon further analysis, they found that – much like Tannenbaum and Kritchevsky's mice – men partaking in the high vegetable oil diet were dying of cancer almost twice as often as the control group, with a large portion of these deaths from lung cancer. The overall differences were small and borderline statistically significant, but by the end of the study cancer rates began to rise rapidly in the group consuming vegetable oil.[24] Consistent with this study, a study from the same year revealed that a dietary switch from saturated to unsaturated fats in mice led to a significant increase in cancer rates,[25] and several similar randomized studies revealed increases in deaths and reduction in survival within groups consuming higher amounts of vegetable oil.[26,27] Dayton was so concerned with his findings that he immediately published on the potential dangers of polyunsaturated fats. Furthermore, with the rapid increase of cancer rates, Dayton was concerned that these rates would continue to rise exponentially but would no longer be tracked due to the completion of the study. Echoing the concerns from Willett's initial report on fat and cancer, Dayton and Pearce cautioned that future trials should be planned for well over eight years as opposed to the traditional five years, as cancer takes longer to transpire.

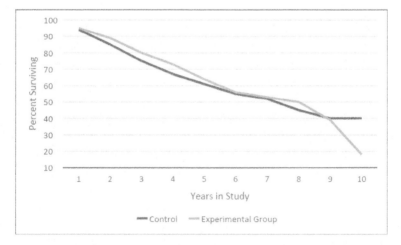

Figure 10: Survival within the experimental group took an unexpected drop by the end of the study.

Consistent with Kritchevsky's scientific discovery, the likely culprit responsible for the late increase in mortality in the individuals consuming the vegetable oil-laden diet pointed to oxidation. Chris Masterjohn, who holds a Ph.D. in nutritional science, has pointed out while writing for the Weston A. Price Foundation that men in the intervention arm were supplied with more than polyunsaturated fats; the vegetable oils contained significantly larger amounts of vitamin E, along with omega-3 fatty acids, both of which act as anti-inflammatory mediators and antioxidants.[28] The fat-soluble antioxidant and fatty acids were likely to have been incorporated within the fatty membranes of the study participants' cells, buffering and disarming the free radical damage from the vegetable oils. However, once these membrane antioxidants are exhausted from the consistent bombardment by the oxidizing free radicals over the course of several years of the study, the oxidized polyunsaturated fats eventually overwhelm these mechanisms and become incorporated into our own fatty tissue. A similar phenomenon was described in Baumann and Lavik's initial study on fat and cancer. Over time, a vitamin E deficit arises once supplies are exhausted, oxidation and free radical damage increases, and eventually cancer ensues. The process can take years to develop, explaining the delays in time between cancer diagnosis and death in these men.[29]

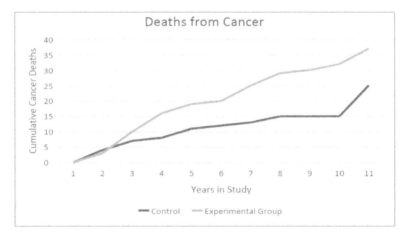

Figure 11: The deaths from cancer were unexpectedly higher in the group consuming the vegetable oil.

Furthermore, polyunsaturated fats, and specifically vegetable oils, are laden with an omega-6 fatty acid known as linoleic acid. Beside containing multiple areas for free radicals to attack, these fatty acids when present in excess can promote inflammation within the body. While omega-6 fatty acids are physiologically required by our cells to function optimally, when present in above-normal concentrations they can promote the overproduction of eicosanoids, like prostaglandin, and COX-2 (the same pathway that is blocked by many anti-inflammatory and pain medications). Similar to omega-3 fatty acids and vitamin E, omega-6 fatty acids are incorporated into the fatty membranes surrounding our cells and accumulate within our fatty adipose tissue over a period of several years. Omega-3s, on the other hand, support several beneficial physiologic processes, including reducing inflammation by lowering the body's production of proinflammatory cytokines, lowering potentially harmful serum triglycerides, and reducing the risk of blood clots.[30,31] Furthermore, they support the function of organs like the brain and heart.[32]

The balance of omega-6 and omega-3 fatty acids provides further insight into the issues with vegetable oils and our health. An elevated ratio of omega-6 to omega-3 fatty acids tilts our cells towards a proinflammatory state and, unsurprisingly, has been associated with an increased risk of multiple cancers.[33] Additionally, omega-3 fatty acids compete with omega-6s to reduce the overexpression of inflammatory eicosanoids, like prostaglandin, and COX-2, to reduce the risk of cancer. Several animal studies even reveal that omega-3 fatty acids may provide a lethal blow to microscopic cancer cells,[34] further illustrating the potential anti-cancer benefits of increasing consumption of foods rich in omega-3 fatty acids.

At the end of Dayton and Pearce's study, it was unclear if this accumulation of omega-6 to omega-3 fatty acids in the observed subjects was complete, or if the ratio of omega-6 to omega-3 fatty acids would continue to increase even after the trial observation period ended. This accumulation of linoleic acid draws in vitamin E to offset some of the oxidative damage; however this does bring about two major problems: 1) This potentially necessitates an increase in vitamin E to offset this damage which, if inadequate, may pull the rug out from under our cells, eventually bombarding them with oxidative damage and an accompanying risk of cancer, and 2) The omega-6 fatty linoleic acid also competes with omega-3, thus decreasing availability of this anti-inflammatory fatty acid. Over time, this recipe supplies all the inflammatory ingredients for a health disaster, which played out quite consistently in Dayton's study, along with several others.

The strategy that might have proven more effective for Dayton and Pearce would be to maximize dietary sources of omega-3 fatty acids as opposed to overloading the cells with omega-6 linoleic acid. Furthermore, as has previously been pointed out, the control arm was given a diet quite deficient in vitamin E that potentially impacted cardiovascular risk, which was already elevated in smokers within the control group (defensive compounds are needed to offset the constant bombardment of damage from smoking).[35] Had they been supplied a fat with a dense source of vitamin E – for example, butter made from the milk of grass-fed cows – the group may have likely experienced even lower rates of cancer, even though they smoked significantly more than the members of the experimental vegetable oil group.

Epidemiologic studies from multiple countries have suggested that those cultures consuming considerable amounts of omega-3 rich sources like fish, and thus lower amounts of omega-6 fatty acids, experience lower rates of cardiovascular disease and cancer.[36] While supplementing diets with fish oils and other sources of omega-3s has produced mixed results, higher dietary intake of naturally occurring omega-3 food sources is associated with lower rates of several diseases, including cancer,[30,37] a finding that is backed by significant mechanistic support. Eggs, dairy fat from grass-fed ruminants, and fish and marine animal oils contain significant amounts of two important omega-3 fatty acids, docosahexaenoic acid (DHA) and eicosapentaenoic acid (EPA). Fish produce these vital fatty acids from alpha linoleic acid (ALA) found in marine plant life. While ALA is present in leafy green vegetables, humans are much less able to synthesize DHA and EPA from these sources, further illustrating the importance of animal sources of these fatty acids within our diet, particularly fish. Finally, studies reveal that DHA, more so than other omega-3 fatty acids, is vital in supporting both brain function and resilience, enabling cells to offset harmful damage.[38]

Dayton and Pearce's trial did little to slow the changes being rapidly promulgated by the forces at-large within the dietary world, and so Leonardo could only stand by and watch helplessly as the world around him began to crumble. Years earlier, he had removed the last remaining cocoon-like slab of cheese hanging from his shop's ceiling and tossed it into the back of his wagon, packed up the remaining inventory and furniture from Pesce's, and locked up the storefront doors one last time. During his final solemn ride home, he reflected on how far his life had taken him: from a young shepherd in the rural mountains overlooking Southern Italy, to a hardy steelworker in the big city, to an Italian grocery store owner serving the quiet suburban communities along the banks of the Three Rivers. Waxing nostalgic, Leonardo felt a twinge of sadness creeping into his heart, but relief and excitement for his future soon washed over him. He would continue venturing down into the Strip District regularly, but now as an artisanal craftsman instead of a shopkeeper. These frequent market trips were instead for dairy staples and grapes for his most beloved of hobbies: producing homemade soppressata, cheese, and his favorite, red wine, several of the villainous food products on the hit list of dietary experts at the time.

÷

By the late 2000's, Mark Mattson must have abruptly come to the realization that nearly all of his experimental mice were obese. As he described in a 2009 article in the *Proceedings of the National Academy of Science of the United States of America*, these animals under "standard laboratory conditions are relatively overweight, insulin resistant, hypertensive, and are likely to experience premature death."[39] Mattson had also noted, like Tannenbaum and others, that restricting food intake in these mice by 20-40% would improve their overall health and reduce their risk of cancer, type 2 diabetes, and multiple other diseases, thereby increasing their lifespan. The health issues of these chubby mice provided an angle of examination that was rarely considered throughout the past century: was calorie restriction allowing these experimental subjects to live longer with lower rates of cancer simply by undoing the massive amount of harm inflicted from being overfed and kept in crowded cages while they awaited their fates as laboratory rats? An abundance of studies have since confirmed the health issues in obese and overweight individuals with an excess of fatty adipose tissue and all the issues that accompany this.[40] This fat secretes many inflammatory chemicals and other hormones that can stimulate and fuel cancer growth, and any method to decrease it may help avoid cancer and other diseases. Furthermore, when mice are kept in what is referred to as an "enriched environment" – meaning they are provided exercise wheels, ample light, and adequate space to run around – this simple change leads to greater health and the promotion of several anti-cancer genes within the mitochondria.[41] Yet, as humans continue to crowd into smaller and smaller living and working quarters, obesity continues to rise and activity levels continue to fall, these mouse models may indeed be segueing to a more applicable research model, albeit for the wrong reasons.

However, Mattson, unlike Tannenbaum, did not focus the bulk of his efforts on cancer prevention, or even on weight loss in his fattened mice. Rather, he found utility in dietary methods to foster healthy aging of our brain. Furthermore, his research touched on methods to offset the brain damage that occurs after traumatic events like strokes, or slowly progressive yet devastating conditions like Parkinson's and Alzheimer's Disease. For Mattson, his research was more than an occupation: his father was a victim of Alzheimer's, and Mattson lived through the experience of supporting him as his memory faded. The Chief of the Laboratory of Neurosciences at the National Institute on Aging in Maryland, Mattson holds a Ph.D. from the University of Iowa, is a Professor at Johns Hopkins University School of Medicine in the Department of Neuroscience, and is also a master gardener. His research interests span across a handful of seemingly unrelated genres, but his focus on lifestyle choices intertwines them all, with significant attention dedicated to dietary strategies for offsetting disease.

Mattson's innovative work has revealed that metabolic pressures on our cells – such as intermittent fasting, exercise, and occasional stresses – train and enable them to offset future damage more effectively, ultimately encouraging them to function optimally without disease. Stressing brain cells through intense exercise and fasting upregulates free radical defense mechanisms, and much like normal cells inhibiting the formation of cancer, brain cells can avoid damage and mutations that may lead to neurologic disorders like Alzheimer's Disease. Fasting and other dietary strategies can initiate the eventual breakdown of fat to an energy source known as ketones, which may further enhance this process. On the other hand, Mattson's work has also revealed that excess blood sugar, elevated insulin, and diabetes work in opposition, damaging the special cells within our brain known as neurons. Mattson's work has complimented the dietary research pioneers, as it has revealed that these activities jump-start the pruning process of autophagy within our neurons and other cells, allowing them to salvage unhealthy cells and parts.[42] This salvage process prevents the accumulation of cellular junk within the brain, which can hinder cognition and promote aging. Furthermore, it enhances mitochondrial health and sharpens the cells' DNA repair mechanisms, restoring damaged DNA caused by occupational exposures, cancerous chemical encounters, and/or unlucky mutations that can occur in frequently replicating cells.

Vogelstein and Tomasetti may have led some to believe that lifestyle had little to do with cancer, but even they emphasized that almost 40% of cancers were potentially preventable, and more recent studies may raise that estimated number even further.[14] However, a major underlying point of emphasis in their work was that we still have a long and perilous journey ahead of us in our quest to slay the Goliath known as cancer. As Tomasetti admitted, "It's the best that can be done today." Mattson's research may beg to differ when it comes to brain health, and if still alive, Kritchevsky and Tannenbaum would likely question the luck assertion as well – there was a clear difference in cancer incidence between the underfed mice that were exposed to their carcinogens. While studies in humans are difficult and most often are limited to population studies (i.e. Willett's initial studies), researchers are still capable of providing mice a dose of "bad luck" by exposing them to carcinogenic chemicals.

That being said, Mattson's research may also simply be pondering whether excess body fat, blood sugar, and insulin – all risk factors for cancer – that we inflict upon our research mice is just a lot of bad luck. While Moreschi and his contemporaries realized a clear connection between diet and cancer that seemed hardly due to luck, it is unclear how the numbers that Vogelstein and Tomasetti calculated would have affected their studies. These questions are unanswerable, but the early researchers clearly noticed that cancer rates in their mice climbed proportionally with this "unlucky" carcinogen exposure, with some of these included in the list of chemicals that modern humans encounter on a daily basis. Furthermore, the researchers noted that distinct eating behaviors significantly impacted cancer rates.

Yet, while predicting cancer in humans is limited to controversial population studies, experimenting with mice also has its fair share of shortcomings. In 2007, it was estimated that 90% of clinical trials testing a novel drug failed as a result of the mouse model testing it; scientists were unable to predict the medication's effect in humans.[43] Additionally, some observers have questioned whether these results were in large part due to the metabolic dysfunction of the obese, diabetic mice. This dynamic plagues the mice with inflammation and many other hallmarks of cancer, perhaps exaggerating any preventative measures in mouse studies when translated to humans. Even the way mice are handled can influence study results: lifting them by their tail produces anxiety, triggering release of the stress hormone cortisol, which subsequently raises blood sugar. Studies have revealed that male scientists appear to cause more mouse anxiety than females, and even the smell of men can trigger the release of cortisol in research mice.[44] Unexpected toxicities remain a concern as well; the diabetes drug Troglitazone was pulled from shelves after humans were experiencing liver toxicity that was unseen in initial animal studies.[45]

Beyond the superficial differences, mice and humans share nearly an identical set of genes. Currently some 4,000 genes and counting have been identified and studied, and less than 10 are exclusive solely to mouse or man. Over 90% of our DNA is considered junk DNA with code that appears to fill space with no practical purpose and remains unused for gene transcription and protein production, complicating calculations. Furthermore, the portion of human and mouse genes coded are around 85% identical, but this number can range from 60-99%. All things considered, humans and mice are extraordinarily similar based on our genetic codes, which is why they are so often used as experimental test subjects in pursuit of advancing human health.

Of course, the lifestyles of these two creatures are not so comparable. While humans spend our nights asleep and days at work, mice are nocturnal animals that roam and forage for food at night. They have an aversion to bright light and so they spend 12-13 hours per day asleep, as opposed to our 7-8 hours per night. While most mice primarily feed on plant sources of food, they will also consume animal products. They will even eat their own feces to gather nutrients and butyrate, the source of fat found in butter and also produced by bowel bacteria when fermenting fibrous food sources. (Aside: there are whispers that Milton Hershey used butyrate as his secret ingredient in his chocolate.) A mouse has a significantly higher metabolism than a human, with heart rates up to ten times that of humans (up to 600 beats per minute). In total, mice eat 15-20 times per day and consume around 10-15% of their body weight per day. To put this into perspective, a 200-pound human with this metabolism would have to eat around 20-30 pounds of food per day just to provide adequate calories.

These differences of mice and men are only compounded by the problems highlighted in Mattson's work. Obese laboratory mice are produced *en masse* using assembly-line techniques similar to that of the feedlots that fatten cattle with unnatural corn and grains. The "metabolically morbid" mice as Mattson has referred to them are anything but normal.[39] When comparing wild mice with the laboratory specimens, nature's version appears to eat less and live significantly longer.[46] Perhaps calorie restriction was simply pushing the reset button for these mice and more closely mimicked their natural environment? Mattson and other researchers, acknowledging the issues with calorie restriction such as the difficulty in maintaining it and concerns over whether it is even effective in healthy individuals, were motivated to explore alternative approaches. Intermittent fasting has been one of these approaches; contrary to popular belief, it is not a harbinger of constant misery but rather a technique of discipline that confines one's hunger to several periods throughout the week. These fasting periods are also accompanied by distinct metabolic and physiologic changes, including a profound lowering of insulin and the production of alternate energy sources known as ketones. Further research suggests that we may be even able to derive the same benefits from simply keeping carbohydrates relatively low, fasting intermittently, or periodically engaging in a ketogenic diet.[47,48]

While mice – genetically engineered or not – are imperfect as experimental models, they remain the best option within the cancer world, as exposing humans to carcinogens in research experiments would violate the boundaries of ethics. In other words, when it comes to forming scientific hypotheses mice remain an ideal starting point, but the end point must be the humans themselves. Even in some of the earliest studies, researchers found that while large quantities of vegetable oil were effective at triggering cancer in mice, they were much less effective when they transitioned to rat experiments.[2] Scientists began to wonder how such data can be taken seriously as we climb the species ladder: how do we translate these findings to humans if they cannot even be translated between mice and rats? Comparing the diet of mice and humans is nearly impossible due to the metabolic differences described previously. Instead, scientists can assess metabolic and laboratory changes in humans to compare mice and men, in conjunction with Mattson's work.

In 2016, Mattson formed a team conducting a clinical trial comparing general calorie restriction with alternate daily fasting in humans.[49] The scientific world had recently become enthusiastic about the prospects of health benefits from different forms of intermittent fasting, as the approach avoided the dreadful experiences of significant calorie restriction seen in the men in Minnesota or the Biospherians. Furthermore, this technique can provide a periodic depression of blood sugar and insulin while metabolizing fat and producing ketones, those energy sources produced by our liver by breaking down fat when blood sugar levels drop, during periods of low amounts of food, or when the diet is low in carbohydrates. As an added bonus, early studies have suggested that ketones provide protection to the brain from damage and aging. Furthermore, fasting is a state that was commonly experienced by humans throughout our ancient history, so it is plausible that we possess ingrained cellular mechanisms to cope with extended periods without food. While fasting for an entire day would be difficult for most people, intermittent fasting – defined as not eating for an extended period of eight or more hours – is felt to be a more natural and easier method of eliciting the metabolic changes that accompany reducing calories in mice. Furthermore, if the fast includes time asleep, the hours without food can quickly add up. Perhaps most important, multiple beneficial physiologic changes are achieved via the intermittent fast. These changes appear to mimic another physiologic state that many humans experience in colder climates or during the winter months – significant and even extreme carbohydrate restriction. In Mattson's study, the researchers were assessing the diet for weight loss, and as the fasting individuals lost an average of 17 pounds in eight weeks, it was successful. Unfortunately, the metabolism of the study participants decreased significantly as well, which was an expected byproduct of the weight loss.

While intermittent fasting has proven successful for the goal of weight loss, the metabolic benefits expand far beyond simply helping to prevent obesity. After measuring the metabolic changes during extended fasts, scientists have found that they lead to a significant drop in insulin levels. During a prolonged period without food, less insulin is necessary to manage nutrient processing, thus less is produced and secreted by the pancreas, and the body becomes more adept at utilizing these smaller amounts, resulting in increased insulin sensitivity. With less dietary sources of glucose, blood sugar gradually drops until the study participants' livers began to produce significantly more ketones, relying on these water-soluble products of fat metabolism to fuel the brain when blood sugar drops. A similar effect can be elicited by eating a very low carbohydrate and moderately low protein diet, known as a ketogenic diet. These ketones are rapidly extracted by our cells and shuttled to their mitochondria for energy derivation. Mattson's array of studies revealed that this increase in mitochondrial metabolism was partially responsible for the benefit of intense exercise on brain function. Furthermore, fatty acids within the blood of the participants rose as glucose dropped, and their cells began to utilize the breakdown of fat for energy. Finally, as the study progressed, the fasting participants gradually began to burn fat rather than carbohydrates for energy. In other words, their mitochondria – the energy-producing intracellular factories studied by Warburg – began to take over for the majority of energy production, which in turn promoted several cellular changes. As mentioned, these cellular mechanisms aid in the pruning of faulty cells and correcting damaged DNA, potentially helping to prevent cancer. In a further attempt to make these dietary habits feasible, the researchers even recommended a small mid-day meal several times per week to break up the hunger that accompanied all-day fasts yet still glean the positive effects of the technique.

The reduction in carbohydrates, followed by the reduction in protein, is most responsible for the stimulation of ketogenesis and lowering of insulin. This change does not require a calorie deficit, nor is it present with general calorie restriction, providing some insight as to where the metabolic consequences of each may diverge. Both fasting and calorie restriction may result in weight loss; however, fasting in conjunction with both carbohydrate restriction and a high-fat/low-carbohydrate ketogenic diet appears to result in distinct metabolic and cellular changes that are not connected solely to calories. While data are limited and at times mixed, these changes have led many contemporary oncologists to question whether such dietary strategies can enhance cancer treatment or improve the chances of preventing cancer in the first place.[47,50,51]

In our rearview mirror is a century of population studies rife with dubious findings, millions of sick, overweight, and diabetic mice that get leaner and less cancer when starved, and two large-scale experiments revealing the utter misery of attempting calorie restriction in humans. We are pulled over on the side of the road, and we check our fuel gauge and scratch our heads while glancing at our roadmap and recalibrating our compass.

Where do we go from here?

PART II

THE TANGIBLE

7

A DIRECTIONLESS PATH

"It is important not to have a calorie level [less than] 1200 without an evaluation by a dietician or physician."[1]

- Handbook of Clinical Nutrition and Aging, Humana Press, 2009

"The Marine Corps does not want robots. The Marine Corps wants killers. The Marine Corps wants to build indestructible men, men without fear."

- Private Joker, Full Metal Jacket (1987)

Takeaways:

A historical view is provided, exploring many great philosophers' views on diet and sustenance. Plato is deeply reviewed due to his impactful message largely influenced by his interest in foods and eating patterns. However, his often-contradictory statements and considerations regarding what composed a nutritious diet may be partly responsible for this continued confusion today. He mentally quarreled with the merits of filling the mind with knowledge versus the stomach with food, instead of considering both to coexist peacefully. By reviewing these historical views, we come to understand that diet has always been linked to health, religion, and philosophy, but for better or worse, these factors have left the debate on a healthy diet as tenuous.

The role of insulin, insulin-like growth factor-1 (IGF-1) and its receptor (IGF-1R) are discussed. While IGF-1 is necessary for healthy growth and development during adolescence and repair and regeneration later in life, excess IGF-1R activation can trigger cells to forgo their natural pruning process potentially leading to cancerous conversion and growth.

Government guidelines recommend that 25% of the diet includes fruits and vegetables. However, a deeper look at the science behind how our body reacts to different plant foods reveals the potential benefits of distinct vegetables; in particular, cruciferous, green leafy vegetables may yield the greatest anti-cancer benefits. Their mechanism further links our diet and cancer.

Just months after his Biosphere crew penned their "Ode to Bananas," Walford wasted no time compiling his data upon mission completion, publishing the results in an array of medical journals. His reports proselytized the healthful changes in his cohabiters: they lost weight, blood pressure bottomed out, and cholesterol plummeted. Yet throughout all his manuscripts, Walford failed to make mention of his colleagues' obsession over food (culminating in a song dedicated to fruit), the bartering of prized possessions for basic nourishment, or the locks that had to be placed on the freezers to prevent desperate hoarding. Instead, Walford's descriptions seem to more closely resemble the utopian society described in depth throughout Plato's *Republic*. Walford, however, is not alone in his selective disclosure when discussing the more miserable aspects that accompanied his cherished diet or the psychological toll that ensued.

If the participants in Biosphere 2 were so miserable on the forced restrictive diet, how could Walford have concluded that the real-world inhabitants outside of the steel-and-glass jail containing his hardy crew could have possibly followed this diet? Additionally, why did Walford fail to describe any of these issues in his work? Several decades separated the studies by Keys and Walford, and while Keys was studying the miseries of starvation, Walford seemed to be happily engaging in it. The dissimilar views between Walford's reports and the individual accounts of the rest of the crew in Biosphere 2, in addition to the accounts from the previous Minnesota Starvation Study, illustrate a hidden force that seems to permeate throughout the nutrition and dietary world. Why did the results of the Minnesota Starvation Study remain undisclosed for half a century? Why do nearly all dietician and nutrition textbooks continue to recommend extreme calorie restriction for weight control? Dietary textbooks continue to promote severe calorie restriction for weight loss close to the methods tested in both studies. The *Handbook of Clinical Nutrition and Aging* only cautions to alert a physician when lowering calories to 1,200 per day. They also advise a diet of 1,600 calories per day as a normal daily caloric amount for elderly individuals, an amount far less than both the Minnesota Starvation Study and Biosphere 2, and less than the amount that weakened men to the point where they were falling down face-first. How can these sources and the field of nutrition and dietetics recommend a strategy that provoked severe psychological distress – including driving a man to amputate his own finger! – and uniform misery described by all?

The answer may have nothing to do with scientific studies, dietary strategies, or sound medical advice. This underhanded influence is difficult to quantify, but seems to occur repeatedly across many decades, numerous medical studies, and within the hallways of most modern medical institutions. A bias continues to linger within the indoctrinated world of calorie restriction; an invisible hand seems to propel this bias to propagate throughout the research and scientific world. Just how far back this invisible hand has influenced the medical world remains unknown, but evidence suggests it tracks back thousands of years to around the time of the Roman Empire.

Marcus Porcius Cato, more widely known as Cato the Elder, was born in 234 BC in Tusculum. Part of the region of Latium, Tusculum was an ancient city whose remains were a fragment of the largest enduring Roman Empire ruins in central Italy. Tusculum, resting 300 miles north of present-day Calabria in central Italy, was founded by Latins several hundred years before the Trojan War. Shortly after 400 BC, Tusculum was annexed by the Roman Empire and unlike Leonardo Pesce's impoverished birthplace eventually became a favorite retreat city for wealthy Romans. The famous politician and philosopher Cicero spent significant time in Tusculum, pensively staring out at its landscape through the windows of his villa as he wrote several of his classics. Cicero would eventually leave to promote a return to a traditional republican government after Caesar's death, but ultimately, he would join Caesar in the afterlife when he was decapitated under the order of Mark Antony. Tusculum would eventually be ravaged by war, covered by time, and overgrown by trees. Lucien Bonaparte, the younger brother of Napoleon and an amateur archeologist, would unearth the remaining ruins of the city over a millennium later during his excavations in the early 1800s.

Cato, like Cicero, was a famous Roman politician and statesman, compiling many significant works across wide-ranging disciplines from philosophy to politics. In 160 BC, Cato created what is considered the oldest surviving Latin document to this day. The essay-turned-book *De Agri Cultura* is also by default one of the first cookbooks. Perhaps more a manual on animal husbandry and a guide for city dwellers who wished to rough it in the farmland, Cato's *De Agri Cultura* provides an exploration of farming and agriculture in ancient Rome. However, the claim of the oldest and perhaps first cookbook in existence goes to a Greek named Archestratus. The Greek Sicilian created his work *Hedypatheia* in 350 BC, centuries before Cato was born. Translated as "Pleasant Living," Archestratus' cookbook provides recipes accompanied with instructions on where to acquire certain foods throughout the Mediterranean. He also recommends that meals provide strong flavors known as *opsa* to "provide extra proteins and herbs or cheese and onions," and comments on the influence of personal traits on eating, further noting that "greedy people might eat too much carbohydrate, luxurious people too many *opsa*, particularly highly-prized fish."

While Mesopotamian tablets containing recipes date back as far as 1700 BC, the Greek and Roman cooks, statesmen, and philosophers provide some valuable insights into the view of food during their contemporary times. Only several thousand years before Cato and Archestratus – a small blink in the history of humans – the mere thought of a cookbook was nonexistent. Beyond a manual for preparing food, the thought of dealing with an abundance of food was also unfathomable during both the early days of civilization and the hunter-gatherer days of humanity.

Further south and across the Ionian Sea, the eminent philosopher Plato founded the Academy of Athens in Greece. Around the same time, increases in trade and wealth throughout the Mediterranean ushered in an era of open distribution of spices, wine, and foods that were previously unknown to locals. While Plato preached his philosophy, food progressed from a simple instrument for survival to a commodity that could be altered to satisfy the greatest of epicurean wants and desires. Furthermore, abundant fertile land and agriculture aided in producing larger yields of foods, supporting the transition from a society that once hunted and gathered for all nourishment to one that was freely able to overconsume due to the abundance of easily accessible foods. It also led to the mass migration of once-unknown foodstuffs like spices, peppers, and herbs to places like Calabria, where thousands of years later Leonardo would use them to make his soppressata in his cave-like basement. Such globalization also led to the creation of new literary genres and works like Archestratus' *Hedypatheia*, which only centuries before would have been an impossible concept to fathom.

With the introduction of these new foods, another novel concept was born: the necessity to control oneself and one's gluttonous tendencies by defeating temptations from pleasurable foods. Gluttony, a once unknown phenomenon, had now taken center stage to be analyzed by some of the world's most famous philosophers and religions. Plato, like several other philosophers, held the view that while cooking was not a medical art, promoting a healthy diet was one of the most important roles of a physician. Furthermore, Plato believed that food was more than nourishment: it served as a form of medicine. The medicinal view of food was further emphasized by physicians and philosophers from Hippocrates, the Greek "father of medicine," to Galen, the centuries-later physician of the Roman philosopher-emperor Marcus Aurelius. The lack of other successful medical treatments during this time further emphasized the rule of food as medicine. While definitions vary based on time and text, Galen would refer to *opsa* as medicinal foods that provided flavor and superfluous nutrients. He would later categorize foods like pepper, cumin, and coriander as drugs, emphasizing their medicinal properties. Even over a thousand years later, the famous Jewish philosopher and physician Maimonides uttered the often-quoted adage "no disease that can be treated by diet should be treated with any other means."

With the newfound easy access to gluttony – one of the seven deadly sins! – and the contemporary worldview of food as medicine, both philosophers and physicians saw an opportunity to push upon the public their services and expert opinions. Plato felt that the Greeks were obsessed with food and supposedly referred to Greece as "a gluttonous place where men eat two banquets a day and never sleep alone at night,"[2] further conflating eating behavior with other immoral vices and sins like lust and fornication. Plato felt that while "knowledge is the food of the soul," the food of man could often get him into trouble both spiritually and physically. Such perceived connections from an esteemed scholar further fueled public contempt for overeating and indulgent foods.

Plato was not the only philosopher who thought that food and philosophy were inseparable. Cato, a strict follower of stoic philosophy, interlaced his philosophical views throughout his writings, and his cookbook was not free of these influences. Gluttony and the seven deadly sins were popularized by Dante when he wrote of them as layers of hell in the *Divine Comedy*. Cato's *De Agri Cultura* provides in-depth detail on the subjects of grazing livestock and farming, including cultivating vineyards, and also delves into the transition to larger farms occurring at the time in Campania, the area of southern Italy that draws nearer to the mountains where Leonardo tended his flock of sheep. Cato's work advised herders like Leonardo on the best practices of the area. The only recipe present in Cato's *De Agri Cultura* pays homage to Leonardo's success as an Italian meat and cheese shopkeeper, and is incredibly close to the recipe that has been passed down through generations in Italian families including my own. In the first known recipe for curing meat, Cato advises:

"You should salt hams in the following manner, in a jar or large pot: When you have bought the hams cut off the hocks. Allow a half-modius of ground Roman salt to each ham. Spread salt on the bottom of the jar or pot; then lay a ham, with the skin facing downwards, and cover the whole with salt. Place another ham over it and cover in the same way, taking care that meat does not touch meat. Continue in the same way until all are covered. When you have arranged them all, spread salt above so that the meat shall not show, and level the whole. When they have remained five days in the salt remove them all with their own salt. Place at the bottom those which had been on top before, covering and arranging them as before. Twelve days later take them out finally, brush off all the salt, and hang them for two days in a draught. On the third day clean them thoroughly with a sponge and rub with oil. Hang them in smoke for two days, and the third day take them down, rub with a mixture of oil and vinegar, and hang in the meat-house. No moths or worms will touch them."[3]

At the same time that Archestratus produced his novel cookbook, Plato, the famous pupil of Socrates and teacher of Aristotle, began promoting his now-famous philosophical views throughout Athens. Arguably one of the most significant philosophical figures within the history of the western world, Plato's metaphysical reach expanded from medicine to the natural sciences. Yet somewhat surprisingly, his strong views on food and dietary predilections often go unnoticed within the philosophical world. Some could argue that Plato saw food as above all else in importance. For instance, in the written account where Plato, speaking through the character of Socrates, describes the ideal philosophical city, *The Republic*, he states that the "first and chief of our needs is the provision of food for existence and life." Without survival, philosophical musings were worthless; according to Plato, our priority should consistently fall upon food to nourish the mind, and sound philosophical reflections only present themselves after hunger pangs have been satiated. Plato's consistent utilization of food as a metaphor to explain his philosophies serves to further emphasize its importance to him.[4] Plato's approach was followed by a similar strategy utilized by the famous philosopher known as Jesus of Nazareth, who made water out of wine and fed several thousand from a few loaves of bread and fish according to the accounts in the *New Testament*.

Plato's later works continued to produce strong views on food, eclipsing his metaphorical vehicles and instead entwining the issues of the soul and gluttony – to him, it was as if gluttony encircled the soul, strangling it constantly like a serpent. As the soul was always challenged by pleasures, food and drink naturally became both friend and enemy of the body and soul, with gluttony always lurking only steps away. That being said, Plato acknowledged the importance of certain foods, and especially animal foods, which were some of the most nutrient and vitamin-dense foods available. These foods were perfect according to Plato for "existence and life." Nutrients and the building blocks of our body were viewed as additive in nature to Plato: "flesh is added to his flesh and bones to his bones," and "in the same way the appropriate thing is added to each of his other parts."[5] Plato recognized that to fuel our muscle and bones, we needed an adequate source of vitamins, minerals, and nutrients, and this was most easily accomplished via dense dietary sources like animal flesh. Plato's assessments were remarkably correct anatomically: for instance, CoEnzyme Q10 helps the heart to function optimally. Confirming Plato's logic, the largest source of dietary CoQ10 can be found within animal heart – flesh is added to flesh.

The anatomic aspects of food are where this author might agree with the great Greek philosopher's viewpoints, had this been the actual source of Plato's disdain with nutrient-dense foods. Countless times after slicing through formaldehyde-soaked flesh during my anatomy training in medical school, I vowed to never eat meat again. There was a reason Leonardo would run for the hills when it was time to slaughter his sheep. The visceral response to open flesh, the kind that Michael Pollan describes in *The Omnivore's Dilemma*, could understandably push the strongest willed away from consuming meat. Yet each time, I found myself clawing back to it after abstinence left me feeling undernourished and underperforming in both athletics and coursework. My body requires the dense vitamins and fuel within animal sources of foods. Plato described the benefits of such foods, only to later abandon them.

Plato's views on the benefits of many of these foods would seemingly stop here. Like many philosophers of his era, he cautioned against the indulgent nature of the "denser" foods, even recommending the limitation of fatty foods like olive oil and advising their replacement with lighter foods like grains and cereals including wheat, barley, and corn. Plato was less concerned with the visceral and moral response to the slaying of animals for food and more preoccupied with the indulgent nature of these foods. According to Associate Professor of Humanities and Plato scholar Daniel Silvermintz, three major themes arise in Plato's works on the soul, pleasurable aspects of food, and gluttony: "(1) Plato considers gluttony or intemperance to be such a pervasive condition that it typifies most men's souls, (2) the over-weaning desire for pleasure prevents individuals from apprehending the rational world of ideas, and (3) there is a complementary passion for knowledge that is accessible to an individual that is able to master his or her appetites for bodily pleasure."[6] Plato feels that we as humans are rational creatures constantly tempted by the pleasures of food, but gluttons on the other hand are "chained prisoners."

In the eyes of Plato, gluttony obstructed the soul's path to enlightenment. Perhaps Plato was on to something: as of 2016, the prevalence of obesity has reached alarming levels among adults in the United States.[7] If Plato was correct, many souls are on a path to be damned. However, by the final chapters of Plato's masterpiece, *The Republic*, a Walfordian twist emerges. Plato begins to strongly advise the avoidance of denser foods and replacement of these with vegetables and grains, in turn unearthing inconsistencies between his earlier-presented views on the "first and chief of our foods" and the consumption of nutrient-dense foods like "muscle and bones" to fuel our muscle and bones. Furthermore, several accounts of Plato's work reveal his view of reincarnation, which may have been responsible for his philosophical tendencies to promote the avoidance of animals within the diet – it is not morally or philosophically correct to eat your friends after they are reincarnated. Plato even later endorses that milk and cheese comprise a considerable portion of the diet, further consistent with a common vegetarian strategy to provide several nutrients densely found in animal fat without consuming meat. Plato's work continues to advise his readers that "first and chief of our needs is the provision of food for existence and life," and yet seems to advance inconsistent views, in a similar manner to the inconsistent recommendations that prestigious cancer institutions have been providing to cancer patients during and after their treatment.

The pleasure that accompanies food leads to overeating, and gluttony ensues. In the Platonic view, our minds should be filled with the densest knowledge possible to satisfy our wants and desires. Filling our minds may require emptying our bellies, particularly of dense and satisfying foods. Plato ultimately describes gluttony as the result of ignorance, and with the help of physicians and experts the common person can be instructed as to which foods are healthy and nutritious and which merely serve to feed gluttony. Plato even recommends objectively measuring the benefits of pleasurable foods versus the potential issues, one of history's first mentions of the intake of food as a mathematical problem detached from its nutritive benefits. At the hand of Plato, calorie counting is born… and so is born a classic centuries-old conflict.

⁜

The tug-of-war between nutritionist and glutton is a pervasive theme across Plato's writings. Plato may have birthed the double-edged view of food regarding health on one side and gluttony on the other, but the current state of modern food science continues to perpetuate this interpretation thousands of years later.

Plato advises us that dense foods nourish us and support our bodily structures but also fill our bellies, the latter of which should be left hollow so that we can better focus on filling our minds with knowledge. To Plato, it is as though both minds and bellies cannot be filled at the same time – either the body or the soul can be nourished, but we must choose one. Cato, among other philosophers, wrote recipe books for handling dense foods like cured meat and soppressata, and Archestratus – who was more a gastronomic poet and less a philosopher – warns us that "greedy people might eat too much carbohydrate." Many modern views on health, especially ones dealing with diet and nutrition, have transformed over time based more on folklore and philosophy than scientific evidence. Much like Plato's opinions on philosophy and their propensity to override those on food and health, a similar propensity often trickles down to the current medical field, where philosophical and historical interpretations can permeate throughout society at-large and override science. Perhaps best illustrating this schism within the medical research field is a mundane hormone that signals to our cells, muscles, and bones to repair and grow. This hormone is insulin-like growth factor 1 (IGF-1), a subject of heated debate that may be the modern-day reincarnation of Plato's opposing views on both beneficial and risky aspects of nourishing foods.

In the 1990s, some 70 years after the discovery of insulin, several researchers, including Dr. Renato Baserga, noted a particular receptor embedded within the protective cellular membrane that encapsulates cancer cells. Cellular receptors are periodically scattered along the surface of cells; they encounter multiple passing hormones within the blood, some of which can bind to them like a key settling into a matching lock. Once bound, the hormone-receptor combination turns on an array of processes that signal the cell to perform a specific action. Human growth hormone, for instance, signals cells to grow, promoting the large muscles of bodybuilders and jutting jawlines seen in many of our Major League Baseball home run champions at the turn of the century. In both instances, muscle and bone growth was signaled by this hormone after binding to its respective receptor. From his laboratory in Philadelphia, Pennsylvania, the Italian-born Baserga realized that this particular receptor was strangely similar to the same landing point along the surface of cells where the hormone insulin would bind, signaling growth.

Insulin has many invaluable roles within the human body, but its most important may be its ability to signal cells to extract glucose from the circulating blood supply. This task, in effect, prevents its accumulation within the blood which, if too high, can leave us in a near-fatal state known as hyperglycemia. Upon binding to cells, insulin also signals to them to grow, which allows them to make use of the recent influx of glucose. This also makes insulin a member of a group of growth factors known as anabolic hormones, though not quite as potent as the more famous performance-enhancing anabolic steroids. Cancer cells, whose prime objective is unchecked growth, are well aware of this anabolic potential, and most display their own insulin receptors on their surface. Upon embracing the hormone, the insulin receptor triggers a cascade of glucose influx for utilization by the cancer cell as a fuel supply, along with a potent anabolic signal beckoning it to grow and spread.

The receptor that Baserga dedicated most of his career to studying, known as the IGF-1 receptor (IGF-1R), was remarkably similar – about 70% similar in properties and chemical makeup – to the insulin receptor. Not surprisingly, insulin and IGF-1 are also structurally similar – in fact, so similar that many earlier scientists felt IGF-1R was simply a redundant version of the insulin receptor. However, progressive studies revealed that both insulin and IGF-1 could bind to this receptor signaling growth, with a comparative advantage to IGF-1. Eventually, the landing pad for IGF-1 was named the insulin-like growth factor 1 binding hormone receptor, or IGF-1R. Besides the many similarities with the insulin receptor, some key differences were noted; while both were found on cancer cells, the IGF-1R seemed much more important for signaling the uncontrolled growth of normal cells, their conversion to cancer, and their protection from the body's natural process of pruning damaged and suspicious cells through the mechanism known as apoptosis.[8] In essence, when IGF-1 bound to the IGF-1R, these cells were provided the ability to bypass the checks on Hanahan and Weinberg's Hallmarks of Cancer. It was as if IGF-1R activation provided them a hall pass to evade the multiple checkpoints along the way to full-blown cancer. Baserga and others found that IGF-1R was so vital for cancer induction and growth that cells without the receptor were practically resistant to transformation to cancer.

Similarly, blocking the IGF-1R in cells that had already become cancerous was a potent method of hindering their growth and ability to dodge apoptosis. It appeared that simply blocking the IGF-1R and stripping their hall pass would also prevent the cells' ability to disengage the hallmarks of cancer. Initial enthusiasm for targeting IGF-1R as a cancer treatment was immense, and the potential of this treatment to target cancer cells while sparing our normal cells further ignited that enthusiasm. The connections between the IGF-1R and the insulin receptor only helped strengthen the view that blocking these targets – or at least decreasing the amount of substances that signal their activation – could tame the metabolic dysregulation described by Hanahan and Weinberg to decrease cancer growth, or perhaps prevent it in the first place.

The basics of IGF-1 help to illustrate the current double-edged viewpoint that prevails regarding its importance to a properly functioning body, and also its implication in cancer. IGF-1 was first isolated and characterized in the 1950s, when two scientists discovered a mysterious factor within the blood that incorporated sulfur into cartilage, thereby supporting its growth.[9] This mysterious factor was driven by growth hormone, the anabolic protein that prompts cellular sprouting and regeneration and also, like insulin, has a remarkable ability to pull glucose from the blood and into cells. Not surprisingly, the structure of IGFs would later be found to closely resemble insulin. Furthermore, insulin stimulates our cells to extract the glucose after a similar lock-and-key binding to cellular receptors. During this binding, it engages an "open" switch on the protective fortress wall that is the cellular membrane, opening the drawbridge to allow sugar to come pouring in. IGF works similarly, and there are several different IGF ligands (which bind to substances) and receptors (which substances bind to). The most common of each of these is IGF-1 and the IGR-1R (R for receptor), respectively. While there are more elements to IGF than these two, the pair takes the lion's share of responsibility and will be highlighted within this discussion.

A nuanced discussion of IGF-1 is not essential, but a brief description provides insight into its links to cancer. Release of growth hormone from the pituitary gland, the endocrine organ resting at the base of our brain, signals to the liver to secrete IGF-1, which then commands the growth of nearly every cell within our body. The signal affects our bones, cartilage, muscles, nerves, blood cells, and organs. Other cell types can produce IGF-1, but the liver handles the majority of production; promoting growth is the main action of IGF-1.

IGF-1 also signals back to the pituitary to stop releasing growth hormone. This naturally occurring method of self-regulation to prevent excessive hormone levels is known as negative feedback. IGF-1 levels are highly dependent on growth hormones and their levels can be abnormally low due to growth hormone deficiency and malnutrition.[10] Other normal activities like sleep increase IGF-1 levels.[11]

Typical teenagers illustrate the "growth" in insulin-like growth hormone as they consume massive amounts of food to satisfy their large appetites, increasing circulating IGF-1, which thus commands the bones to grow larger and longer. IGF-1 levels are high during these years, reach a plateau around age 30, and begin to drop off quickly at age 60 until our final resting days. This drop in IGF-1 may be partially responsible for our ultimate fate, as low rates of IGF-1 in the elderly are associated with an array of the signs of aging: weak bones and fractures,[12] a higher risk of dying,[13] increased body fat, thinning of the skin, and decreased muscle mass.[14] These associations are largely responsible for the numerous internet popup ads featuring incredibly muscular old men with younger bikini-clad women in one hand and a bottle of IGF-1 in the other.

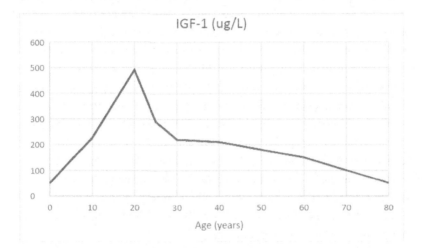

Figure 12: Levels of IGF-1 sharply increase early in life, then drop off as we age.

This ability to stimulate bone and muscle growth is vital for adequate growth during childhood, and IGF-1 levels are proportional to height in children.[15] Through its ability to signal neuron growth, IGF-1 also supports brain development and function, and to no surprise, children with higher levels of IGF-1 are taller with generally higher IQs.[16] After childhood, IGF-1 continues to support the brain by repairing and aiding neuron function and survival.[17] IGF-1 also helps to degrease the brain of amyloid, the tiny plaques that can accumulate within folds to hinder proper brain function, leading to Alzheimer's Disease and dementia.[18]

Finally, IGF-1 supports our heart and blood vessels and dilates arteries to protect them from damage;[19] further reports suggest that IGF-1 also decreases arterial plaques. Other studies indicate that it decreases inflammation by reducing the inflammatory factors known as IL-6 and tumor necrosis factor (TNF).[20] While IGF-1 supports development during youth, it may also support the metabolic function of aging individuals by aiding in the breakdown of sugar and fat by our cells for energy derivation.

With all these potential benefits, the advertisements with muscular geriatrics touting the benefits of IGF-1 are less surprising, along with the claims – incorrect or not – that it works as an anti-aging supplement. Yet beyond the benefits of IGF-1, the body understands that cancer can be a very unwanted consequence of excessive cellular growth, and as such has created several mechanisms to keep this potential menace in check. It creates IGF-binding proteins (IGFBP), which work as handcuffs restraining and incapacitating IGF-1, in effect disabling its growth-signaling potential. Furthermore, cancer cells are left no longer able to use it as a hall pass to avoid the normal cellular growth checkpoints. IGFBP-3 is the most common of these inhibitors and binds to around 75-90% of the IGF-1 in our blood. When the pituitary gland secretes growth hormone, which nudges the liver to release IGF-1, the body also produces IGFBP-3 as an insurance policy. Excessive amounts of insulin, however, jeopardize the entire operation by raising levels of IGF-1, decreasing binding proteins, and leaving excessive bioactive IGF-1 hanging around.[21] In other words, insulin, a growth hormone, can further increase IGF-1, another growth hormone.

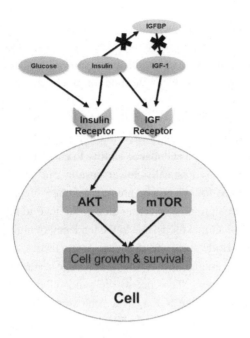

Figure 13: Glucose, insulin, and IGF-1 can stimulate cell growth and survival, while IGFBPs bind and inactivate IGF-1. Consistent with its similarities with IGF-1, insulin can bind and stimulate both the insulin and IGF-1 receptor.

These combined issues have led many nutrition and cancer researchers to consider the combination of insulin, IGF-1, and the ratio of IGF-1 to its IGFBP-3 to be the most important predictor of cancer risk.[22] In reality though, studies offer mixed results. Overall, there is fine interplay of normal chemicals and hormones that manipulate IGF-1, block it from exerting too much growth potential, and ensure that the body uses available IGF-1 to support itself and repair damage. While also vital for normal function, insulin still incriminates itself by its stimulation of cellular growth by binding both the insulin and IGF-1 receptor, while IGF-1 binds mostly to the IGF-1 receptor. Furthermore, insulin more often finds itself binding and signaling growth in our fat cells, whereas IGF-1 generally promotes muscle fuel and growth.

At this point, you may be asking yourself if this nuanced discussion of insulin and IGF-1 is really important. The significant amount of research implicating the issues with overconsuming foods that increase insulin and IGF-1 has become a de facto weapon of mass destruction, frequently deployed by each side of the recent diet wars. Those that promote a ketogenic or low-carbohydrate diet often tout their ability to channel innate cellular mechanisms that have been hardwired into our physiology after millions of years of periods of famine and inaccessibility to carbohydrate-heavy sources of foods, which can drastically lower insulin and blood sugar levels, particularly in those followers who are overweight.[23] Vegan and vegetarian groups, which often promote lowering dietary fat, tend to rely on IGF-1 as a reason to avoid all animal foods, due to the tendency of high-protein foods to increase IGF-1. Both sides use frequent scare tactics comparing sugar, carbohydrates, and animal foods to smoking, while several vegan sources go as far as telling readers "how not to die" and refer to otherwise normal physiologic processes, like IGF-1, as a "one stop cancer shop." Common readers are horrified at such claims, while others have become spooked at the thought of even eating fruit. It appeared that the initial dismissal of the role diet plays in cancer, voiced to me loudly during the publication of my *Nutrition and Cancer* article, had morphed into an all-out frenzy, rife with unsubstantiated, fearmongering claims.

Low-carbohydrate advocates have taken a reactionary stance on bread, pasta and other foods heavy in carbohydrates, as promotion of these items within the food pyramid and other governmental agencies helped to catapult the obesity epidemic to unimaginable levels. Vegan and vegetarian dietary groups often promoting "plant-based" diets have had difficulty deviating from recommending higher carbohydrate diets, as this would eventually lead followers towards higher fat foods like animal and dairy sources. As each side's weapons of mass destruction continue to be deployed, the collateral damage continues to be felt by the general public caught in the middle as confused victims who simply want to know what to eat to thrive and stay healthy.

٭

Over a decade before the FBI created their infamous Weapons of Mass Destruction Database, I sat on my couch wrapped in my *Tom and Jerry* sleeping bag watching one the most memorable cinema characters ever, Senior Drill Instructor Gunnery Sergeant Hartman, fire off a barrage of degrading insults to the Army platoon he had been placed in charge of training. At the time, I was on a road trip training in Virginia with several members of my traveling basketball team, and one of my teammates brought out a VHS tape of the movie *Full Metal Jacket* during a sleepover. Gunny Hartman's four-minute long drill speech to open the movie was nothing short of epic: hilarious, clever, scathing, and foul-mouthed; it put to shame any of the risqué adolescent school bus talk that I had grown accustomed to hearing at that tender age. Equal parts comedic genius and cringeworthy verbal abuse, the infamous scene made an enduring legend out of actor R. Lee Ermey and is arguably the most memorable scene in any of director Stanley Kubrick's catalogue of blockbuster films. Surely, the scene remains one of the most famous movie clips ever involving insults hurled, due to the sharp content and machine-gun swiftness with which the sergeant berates everyone in sight. Yet throughout the insults, one thing is abundantly clear: despite the foul treatment, the sergeant's intention is to ultimately benefit the troops. He intensely trains them, prepares them for war, and sends them off as a coordinated platoon to work together to beat the enemy regardless of, and in the face of, severe emotional and physical stress. Kubrick used humor and shock value to provide a clear message: to achieve success on the battlefield, troops must be pushed to their absolute limits during training.

While it seems odd to associate vegetables with Gunnery Sergeant Hartman's verbal jousts, the Gunny's technique for training his troops is present in an unexpected place when it comes to our immune system. Strangely enough, recent data reveal that the impact many vegetables have on our body is not unlike Hartman's vulgar rant. These leafy sources of nutrition are often viewed as a harmless and innocuous retreat from the violent minefield of the dietary world and its constant battle over which foods are healthy, fueled by the conveyor belt of population studies – a rare armistice between both sides of the dietary battle. Yet, this was not always the case. Vegetables were even viewed as controversial during some of the earliest creations of dietary dogma. In fact, in Judeo-Christian religions, the original diet of man (and woman) was that of Adam and Eve. They consumed only that which fell to the earth. Known as fruitarianism, this diet avoided the killing of all plants and animals. Even pulling a plant from the ground would cause death. As God commanded in Genesis, "*I give you every seed-bearing plant on the face of the whole earth and every tree that has fruit with seed in it. They will be yours for food.*" The King James version even translates the latter part as "*in the which is the fruit of a tree yielding seed; to you it shall be for meat.*"

Modern fruitarians have several reasons for continuing this diet. Staunch Christians translate the above verse from Genesis as a strict instruction to eat only fruit. Others view it as difficult and – following in the footsteps of the Platonic and Stoic calorie restrictors – enjoy the restrictive nature and challenge of the diet. Recalling once more Steve Jobs, he was apparently following a fruitarian diet that at one point was even limited to apples – thus the name of his company, Apple. (Unfortunately, he was also following this prescription as a treatment for his pancreatic cancer, the effectiveness of which is uncertain.) Oddly enough, when actor Ashton Kutcher, attempted to mimic this diet in preparation for his role as the protagonist in the biopic film Jobs, he had to be hospitalized. According to Kutcher, his pancreas was "all out of whack," and it was felt that the large elevations of his blood sugar from the all-fruit diet likely led to elevated stress on his pancreas as it was being forced to produce large amounts of insulin to lower his blood sugar to a safe level.

Apart from fruitarians, the rest of the modern world views vegetables as a safe and healthy part of the diet. They make up a fourth of the government's "ChooseMyPlate," recommended guidelines, and most dietary recommendations advocate vegetables at every meal. Like all of our current dietary recommendations, the consistent endorsement of vegetables relies on population studies. The reasons for this are plenty, but largely because funding is sparse when it comes to food studies in general – while billion dollar pharmaceutical and device companies have the capital to support massive randomized studies, scant funds are in place for many of our struggling farmers. On the cellular level, however, the effect of vegetables is less well-known.

From the original Food Pyramid to the more recent ChooseMyPlate, the overwhelming consensus of these population-based epidemiologic studies has been the long-standing recommendation of vegetables as part of a healthy diet. Other recommendations come and go, but the endorsement of vegetables has held strong. The consistency provides some issues from a scientific research point of view: it is nearly impossible to extract reliable attributions from any assessment of health benefits of different foods consumed by large groups of individuals that have already been repeatedly advised to eat fruits and vegetables, do not smoke, exercise regularly, avoid fat, and engage in several other physician-prescribed healthy activities. Statisticians attempt to separate these behaviors to the best of their ability, but these mathematical experts are not miracle workers. Much like with the hormone replacement therapy debacle, these studies often end up simply selecting for people that follow directions better than others, a factor that is difficult to account for with the most powerful mathematical models. In other words, people that eat sufficient vegetables (and fruits) also exercise, avoid smoking, and engage in many other generally healthy activities, leaving us with a potential "chicken or egg" quandary when we study them (remembering that hormone replacement therapy was the egg in this case, not the chicken as initially thought).

Plenty of studies exist supporting this notion that smokers, heavy drinkers, and those deviants that avoid exercise tend to eat less vegetables and fruit than their healthier counterparts.[24] Studies on the diets of over 120,000 men and women reveal that dietary fruits and vegetables may help them with – or are at least associated with – weight loss.[25] Similarly, heavy fruit and vegetable consumption is linked to a lower risk of dying from any health issue in general, and from heart disease in particular.[26] Yet – in a progression that seems to closely resemble the evolution from Doll and Armstrong's initial study to modern attempts to link fat and cancer – the closer we look, the more the benefits of fruits begin to disappear. The benefits of vegetables, however, are slightly more stubborn, refusing to budge as we focus in. While at times it is difficult to differentiate the two, as they are commonly viewed together, studies generally associate a larger health benefit from vegetables, and especially cruciferous,[27] green, and leafy vegetables.[28]

As the data continue to diverge from Adam and Eve's original fruitarian diet, those basing their diet on Biblical verse can find comfort in the fact that in Genesis, God also commanded us that *"Every moving thing that is alive shall be food for you; I give all to you, as I gave the green plant."* Who vegetables benefit, on the other hand, may be more telling as to why they are healthy. Studies reveal that those same deviants who rarely eat them – the smokers and heavy drinkers, already at a higher risk of cancer – seem to derive the largest anti-cancer benefit from eating vegetables.[29] These findings strongly suggest that some element of vegetables may offset the excess cellular damage that accompanies smoking and heavy drinking, and, as we will discuss in a moment, this protection from damage was confirmed in other studies utilizing cancerous chemicals.

Returning to breast cancer, the most common non-cutaneous cancer in women, the benefits of fruits are also less pronounced than vegetables, as women eating their leafy greens may have a 25% lower risk of cancer, at least according to 26 studies spanning 15 years.[30] While all of the typical limitations plague these studies, additional research in premenopausal and younger women do reinforce the findings.[31] For prostate cancer – breast cancer's equivalent in men – studies reveal similar findings, but specifically point to potential benefits from cruciferous vegetables.[32] In fairness, other massive analyses reveal no benefit of either fruit or vegetable intake in reducing breast cancer risk,[33] or the risk of any cancer.[28] Others have argued that the benefit is present when women consume vegetables earlier in life, thus protecting them from future sequela of damage,[34] but the mixed findings should come as no surprise at this point.

Moving past these roadblocks and instead examining vegetables on a cellular level may enable us to navigate through the potential smoke and mirrors. Focusing in on the bitter chemicals found in green, leafy, and cruciferous vegetables, their effect on our cells may question their traditionally innocent reputation. Studies reveal that, similar to the offensive drill instructor, these chemicals can stress our cells into lethal combatants to wage the future fight against cancer, without actually harming them. Vegetables have rightly been praised for their hefty dose of vitamins, nutrients, minerals, and fiber, but there is much more to the story. For instance, while fiber has been celebrated for its ability to regulate our bowel habits, in actuality its largest benefit may be its ability to feed our bowel bacteria to produce short chain fatty acids like butyrate.[35] The hundreds of trillions of critters that reside within our gastrointestinal tract help to support our immune system and fight inflammation,[36] ensure the integrity of our bowel lining,[37] and detoxify and metabolize potentially cancerous chemicals.[38] The vitamins, minerals, and nutrients found in vegetables are also present in many other foods. For instance, traditional foods like the liver and organ meats cherished and consumed by Leonardo also contain a massive spread of nutrients and vitamins. However, is there something else inherently healthy about vegetables, or has their presumed benefit mainly been an artifact of the data?

While population studies will never be able to answer this question, the cellular impact of the chemistry lab of compounds within these plants provides a better answer. Several chemicals within plants – the same chemicals that impart an unpleasant taste and smell – were the last place scientists would have expected to find vegetables' health-promoting secrets. However, their benefit may have been right under our noses. Sulfur, for instance, has taken its fair share of shots in the past several decades, but recent studies are providing this chemical well-deserved vindication. As the paramount agent in mustard gas chemical warfare during World War II and the chemical culprit behind the unmistakably unpleasant odor of rotten eggs, sulfur harbors a negative connotation among the general public. However, for plants, our pain is their gain as they have capitalized on the volatile elements of sulfur to utilize it as part of their defense mechanism; they may lack claws and teeth and the ability to run away, and they may be easily plucked from the ground and eaten, but they still have some methods to defend themselves. Plants may not have had to defend themselves from the fruitarians Adam and Eve, but this freedom was short-lived as future predators were soon lurking thanks to Darwinist evolution.

We rarely contemplate the often-invisible defense mechanisms of plant warfare that have been waged upon us throughout our post-Eve history. While vegetables are usually considered benign, they are often far from harmless. Plants contain many hazardous and lethal chemicals, from hemlock, Shakespeare's favorite deadly poison, to large doses of amygdalin from apple seeds. Pet owners know of these dangers, as dogs and other animals are often exquisitely sensitive to the chemicals in plants. Grapes, for example, can be fatal to dogs, even in small doses.

While there is an array of plant-based toxins poisonous to humans and dogs alike, sulfur may be the one we encounter most frequently and is easily recognizable when eating several typical vegetables. Pungent cruciferous vegetables contain substantial amounts of sulfur, and some of the most common sources are:

- Broccoli

- Bok choy

- Cauliflower

- Kale

- Cabbage

- Mustard leaves

- Horseradish

- Turnips

- Radish

- Kohlrabi

- Watercress

Other sources of sulfur include nuts, garlic, onions, and animal sources like meats, fish, eggs, and dairy. The animal versus plant sources of sulfur nudge our cells in slightly different directions when it comes to our health, given that plants use it for defense. For instance, proteins contain sulfur, often in the form of the amino acids cysteine and methionine. This "structural" form of sulfur plays a role in several important processes, including detoxification of potentially cancerous and harmful chemicals, supporting the energy-producing mitochondria of our cells and metabolism, and acting as the brick-and-mortar for the synthesis of important enzymes like the free radical-fighting glutathione. Building block amino acids containing sulfur support protein synthesis and function, protein structure, and enzyme function. Major sources of structural sulfur include:

- Eggs

- Beef and lamb

- Chicken

- Fish

- Cheese

- Pork

- Soy Products

- Legumes

- Nuts and seeds (lesser amounts)

The structural benefits of proteins and sulfur-containing proteins are well-established; however, the major anti-cancer benefits of plant-derived "chemical weapons" such as sulfur are only recently becoming recognized. The organosulfur compounds in many of these vegetables – the chemical that gives them their often-pungent taste – supports health in ways that are exclusive of the brick-and-mortar benefits of sulfur from other foods. Several different organosulfur chemicals provide the potent and often volatile smell and taste of some common plant foods; however, two main sulfurous vegetable groups exist, as described below.

Brassicaceae or Cruciferae:

Known to most as the cruciferous vegetable food group, these herbaceous plants give rise to crucifers, cabbages, and mustards. Broccoli, cabbage, turnips, and the exotic wasabi are all crucifers known for their pungent taste and smell. Glucosinolates are the strong-smelling sulfurous chemicals found in these plants; the chemical found in some of the most common vegetable sources of sulfur, including broccoli, mustard greens, and cauliflower, is called glucoraphanin. Sprouts, the younger forms of these vegetables, contain larger amounts of glucoraphanin than the adult plants. Upon cutting, chewing, or crushing these plants, a stored chemical called myrosinase is released and mixes with glucoraphanin, transforming it into sulforaphane. The word soup here can surely get confusing, but the important thing to remember is that organosulfur is an isothiocyanate, and provides the bulk of health benefits.

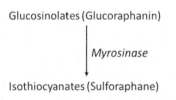

Glucosinolates (Glucoraphanin)

Myrosinase

Isothiocyanates (Sulforaphane)

Wasabi, for example, contains thioglucosides within its stem. The thioglucosides contain sulfur (thiol means "replaced by sulfur"). Much like a futuristic bomb in a James Bond movie containing two cartridges of chemicals which when combined will cause a massive explosion, myrosinase and glucosinolates are stored in separate areas to avoid any interaction. Upon grating wasabi or damage to the stem from a hungry animal or insect, myrosinase is released from its containment. It is now free to interact with the thioglucosides, leading to their breakdown and release of the volatile and pungent allyl isothiocyanate along with several other chemicals (the allyl is notable, as some researchers feel that more allyls mean more cancer-fighting potential). The release of this chemical is what produces the burning sensation in our nostrils experienced after placing a tad too much wasabi on our sushi.[39] The burning feeling is unattractive to predators like insects and animals, and the chemical provides the plant with antibacterial defense, further supporting its role in chemical warfare. Wasabi's caustic chemicals are not oil based, which allows it to expand and fill the air, explaining why it intensely interacts with our nostrils but dissipates rapidly (unlike the burn from oil-based irritants in chili peppers, which persists for minutes or longer in our mouth).

Allium Vegetables:

Another infamous and recognizable vegetable with pungent organosulfur compounds is garlic. Like garlic, allium vegetables have aromas that can fill a room, and most people have experienced this aroma after slicing chives, leeks, and scallions, with a harshness that can make the eyes tear. Garlic is perhaps one of the most common vegetables anecdotally linked with longevity. Within my family, garlic is often attributed as one of the major reasons my grandfather lived just shy of 97 – he used to eat multiple cloves of raw garlic per day. Regardless of its impact on his lifespan, it certainly made him, his house, his clothes, and our house smell like freshly-chopped garlic year-round.

When garlic is sliced, the severing of its outer membranes releases a stored chemical similar to myrosinase in wasabi and cruciferous vegetables that transforms a sulfur-based chemical into allicin. Allicin, which is analogous to isothiocyanate, contains plenty of sulfur, which explains why my grandfather smelled pungent for most days of his 97-year life. These chemicals are subsequently converted to sulfur-containing byproducts present in the urine and breath, thus explaining the phenomenon of garlic breath. (As a side note, the distinct odor of garlic can be avoided by slicing it into small pieces, swirling it in a cup of water, and swallowing it like a pill; allicin coming into contact with the lining of the mouth while chewing stains our breath with the typical garlic smell).

The sulfur-based chemicals in garlic, wasabi, and many similar plants provide more than a foul smell; they can kill harmful fungi on contact, which has earned them the title of "world's oldest fungicide."[40] Exposure to these chemicals can also prove fatal to insects, especially when digested. While excessive sulfur contact causes its fair share of problems in humans – skin and eye irritation, gastrointestinal upset, lung irritation, and coughing are side effects – serious toxicity from sulfur exposure is rare. These potent plant poisons might kill fungi and repel insects, but within human cells the damaging effects are certainly harsh but not lethal; one might say they resemble the infamous Senior Drill Instructor Gunnery Sergeant Hartman. When plants wage chemical warfare on potential predators, the effect on our cells is a beneficial process called chemoprevention. By definition, chemoprevention is the "use of natural, synthetic, or biologic chemical agents to reverse, suppress, or prevent carcinogenic progression to invasive cancer."[41] In other words, chemoprevention threatens our cells, and during this process trains and arms them to defend against cancer formation or to defeat already present cancer cells. Population studies may have failed to explain why certain vegetables are healthy, but laboratory and chemistry experiments may provide the answers that have eluded us for years.

8

FOOD QUALITY OR QUANTITY?

"Every moving thing that is alive shall be food for you; I give all to you, as I gave the green plant."

- Genesis 9:3

"As long as Man continues to be the ruthless destroyer of lower living beings, he will never know health or peace. For as long as men massacre animals, they will kill each other. Indeed, he who sows the seed of murder and pain cannot reap joy and love."

- Attributed to Pythagoras

Takeaways:

Food-activated cellular mechanisms are explored at the chemical and gene-regulated level, identifying beneficial and harmful effects of different macronutrients, while taking a deeper dive into the benefits of specific foods like green, leafy vegetables and spices.

Due to the limited amount of research focused on women up to this point, three large and costly studies were embarked upon, including the Women's Health Initiative (WHI), the Women's Healthy Eating and Living Randomized Trial (WHEL), and the Women's Intervention Nutrition Study (WINS). Each were plagued by Plato's lasting influence and the potentially misleading direction of earlier population studies that were unsupported by subsequent studies. While all three massive efforts sought to establish the benefits of a low-fat diet on overall health and reduction in breast cancer incidence, each became lost in its methods and findings.

In the fall of 2011, a sold-out room in Edinburgh, Scotland was filled with an anxious crowd waiting for Cynthia Kenyon to take the stage. Kenyon, a Herbert Boyer Distinguished Professor of Biochemistry and Biophysics at the University of California, San Francisco, was preparing to wow the crowd on a very unusual topic: worms. But these were not just any worms, and Dr. Kenyon's research was anything but ordinary. Shortly after receiving her Ph.D. studying DNA damage and repair at the Massachusetts Institute of Technology, Hanahan's alma mater and Weinberg's current employer, Kenyon decided to move to San Francisco to pursue her studies – with her precious *Caenorhabditis elegans* worms in tow – after a brief pit stop in Cambridge, England. Now, the crowd eagerly awaited her appearance to present some of her novel research just several hundred miles away. Gone were the days of crowding into sports stadiums for concerts starring the Beatles – with the advent of TED Talks, participants were nowadays scurrying to listen to lectures on worms.

Kenyon's research specialized in aging – specifically, methods to combat aging. She had become an overnight celebrity within the research world when she discovered that, within her focus group of invertebrate nematodes, the mutation of a certain gene could nearly double their lifespan. The gene, known as daf-2, serves as an intracellular gatekeeper guarding the nucleus, which is the important cellular structure that houses the cell's genetic material. Like a surly nightclub bouncer, daf-2 acts to prohibit entry of a transcription factor known as daf-16. Transcription factors turn genes on and off, allowing their DNA to be read and translated to RNA and eventually proteins that control important processes like cellular growth, division, and death. Kenyon and her group found that when they disabled the bouncer through a genetic mutation, longevity was enhanced in the worms.[1] They eventually discovered that when daf-16 entered the nucleus, it triggered the activation of several distinct longevity-promoting genes and proteins that enable the cell to repair and offset oxidative damage from free radicals. By blocking daf-16 access, daf-2 shortens the worm's life by hindering promotion of its longevity genes; Kenyon has even gone so far to refer to daf-2 as the grim reaper.[2]

While Kenyon's worms are the only species known to have the daf-2 "bouncer gene," the implications of her work translate to humans, as similar genes exist in our DNA. Perhaps more importantly, in times of nutrient and energy overabundance – or a cellular feast, so to speak – the bouncer strictly refuses admission to daf-16. Kenyon and her group found that simply inactivating the bouncer through a mutation would allow daf-16 to bypass him, enter the nucleus, and activate the longevity genes. These longevity genes do not directly increase lifespan, but rather battle aging by creating proteins that produce antioxidants, instead enabling the cells to fight oxidative stress and free radical damage, thwarting DNA and cellular damage and thus providing the worms with double the typical lifespan.

In 1993, Kenyon's research awarded her a spot in the coveted journal *Nature*, yet her follow-up research was equally impressive and perhaps of larger importance for advancing methods of cancer prevention. During times of famine, nutrient restriction (or calorie restriction), and other cellular stresses like heat and oxidative damage from free radical overload, daf-16 is permitted entry into the nucleus.[3] Calling to mind Moreschi and Tannenbaum's original studies, calorically restricting the worms promoted translation of the anti-aging genes that promote longevity. More importantly, these same genes thwarted the cancer-producing rust of oxidative damage. Kenyon's research team pushed things further – paying homage to Van Alstyne and Beebe's studies – when they found that feeding sugar to the longevity-prone daf-2 mutated worms eliminated their newfound genetically-induced longevity. Furthermore, a diet with an added 2% glucose reduced their lifespan by a whopping 20%. Kenyon found that dietary glucose keeps the bouncer in check, daf-16 out of the nucleus, and the several genes that protect our cells from oxidative damage deactivated.[4] These genes, when active, create superoxide dismutase, catalase, and glutathione s-transferase, all of which safeguard our cells from the oxidative damage of rust and free radicals. Daf-2, the cellular roadblock of antioxidant production, is sustained by insulin and therefore those foods that promote insulin's release by the pancreas. Counter to this, inactivating daf-2 through nutrient or carbohydrate restriction activates these genes and promotes cellular autophagy, reversing a hallmark of cancer. Faulty and precancerous cells are then commanded to fall on their swords and undergo programmed death – the cellular seppuku described in previous chapters. Their parts are then digested and recycled during the process of autophagy.[5]

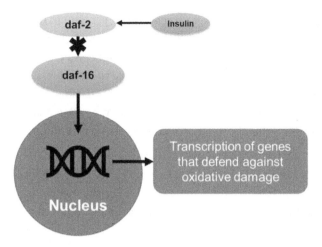

Figure 14: Insulin sustains daf-2, which stops daf-16 from entering the nucleus and engaging several genes that promote longevity by arming our cells to fight against oxidative damage.

Despite the exciting results of Kenyon's multiple studies, the fact that they took place in worms begs the classic question of whether these findings can translate to humans. If mice provide their share of concerns, we can expect more from the less elegant *C. elegans*. However, these worms are more similar to humans than their tiny size would lead us to believe; research in long-lived humans often reveals a similar mutation in the nematode "bouncer" gene.[6,7] Studies in centenarians – those individuals living past the age of 100 – reveal a genetic mutation in the equivalent human gene. In surveying the population of Italy, a country with a hefty supply of prosciutto, wine, and centenarians, the exact same mutation occurs with frequency in those individuals with extraordinary longevity.[8] Ashkenazi Jewish centenarians also regularly exhibit the same mutation.[9] So it appears the worms are not alone in their remarkable lifespan – the same condition is playing out within the human race.

Furthermore, human centenarians appear to exhibit double the insulin sensitivity in comparison to non-centenarians.[10] In keeping with Kenyon's sugar study, these individuals need less (approximately half) as much insulin to retain their blood sugar at a safe level compared to the rest of the population. Their decreased reliance on insulin leads to the promotion of several of the anti-aging genes within the cell's nucleus, not to mention less circulating blood sugar and IGF-1 and more binding proteins to inactive excess IGF-1.

The longevity in these worms and humans is not coincidental. Fascinating additional research on *C. elegans* reveals that the bouncer gene that inhibits the transcription of anti-aging genes is the same gene that is coded for the IGF-1 receptor. Furthermore, it is the worm equivalent of the insulin receptor in humans, and the proteins it produces are remarkably close to the IGF-1 and insulin receptor. Blocking the insulin/IGF-1 pathway by inactivating the landing pad for IGF-1, the double-edged sword in humans, was increasing the longevity of Kenyon's worms. A similar mutation in the IGF-1 receptor has revealed an equally heralded increase in the lifespans of human subjects as well. While Kenyon was able to decrease insulin in her worms by providing less stimulus to the insulin/IGF-1 axis, a mutation in the IGF-1 receptor in long-lived humans and their increased insulin sensitivity provided a similar physiologic consequence. The blood of many of these humans contains higher amounts of IGF-1 circulating throughout the body. However, their dysfunctional IGF-1 receptor leaves this IGF-1 unable to be pulled into the cell, similar to when it is inactivated by binding proteins. As a result, the insulin/IGF-1 pathway in these individuals is unable to keep the human equivalent of daf-16 out of the nucleus,[11] and transcription of the anti-aging, anti-rusting genes occurs, spurring their remarkable longevity.

Besides offering some clues on how to enhance human longevity, the strongest conclusion that can be made from Kenyon's work and other similar studies is that the stimulation of the insulin/IGF-1 pathway by various lifestyle and dietary activities will cause cells to rust and age prematurely and expose them to increased risks of cancer. Methods to slow down this progression may provide our cells protection from damage, aging, disease, and cancer. The insulin/IGF-1 pathway has proven itself as the proverbial "bigger, faster, stronger" light switch that allows children to grow into adults, pushes athletes to perform at higher levels, and – according to those internet advertisements – magically transforms elderly men into stallions feeling decades younger. Yet from Baserga's studies in mice to Kenyon's work in worms to the multiple population studies in human centenarians, the common thread is that if that switch is kept on too long, the lights can burn out prematurely. Old age, disease, and cancer follow.

IGF-1 is not alone in its role, and the overlap with insulin has led to the coinage of the term "insulin/IGF-1 axis." In other words, promoting this axis fosters growth and repair of the body's cells and parts, but eventually this process runs out of steam and aging ensues. Blocking the pathway in animals can increase their longevity, and removing the insulin receptor from fat cells in mice has been shown to increase their longevity.[12] Consistent with Kenyon's studies, sugar and yeast restriction increases the lifespan of fruit flies irrespective of calories,[13] and glucose restriction increases the lifespan of roundworms[14] and yeast.[15] While excessive IGF-1 and insulin promotion can harm our normal cells by hindering their repair, it can also assist already formed cancer cells; high carbohydrate intake by women with IGF-1 receptor-positive breast cancer is associated with an almost six fold increased risk of their cancer recurring after treatment.[16] Finally, exposing cells to continuously high levels of IGF-1 can damage mitochondria and interfere with their function, leading to premature aging.[17]

Other versions of Kenyon's studies have taken place; in these studies, when protein and amino acids are restricted in the diet of fruit flies a similar increase in longevity occurs.[18] Both restrictions decrease IGF-1, thus these results are hardly surprising; withholding dietary protein in mice – and specifically the amino acid methionine – modestly increases longevity. Both dietary carbohydrates and protein act to increase the insulin/IGF-1 axis in animal studies; in humans, however, the pathway is more sensitive to dietary carbohydrates.[19] Unexpectedly, the "odd man out" nutrient appears to be fat. While multiple studies across species reveal longevity benefits with the reduction of carbohydrates and protein, fat restriction has not provided such benefits.[20] Unlike dietary protein and carbohydrates, fat has a minimal effect on the insulin/IGF-1 axis. Furthermore, unlike with Kenyon's sugar-fed worms, when mice with a mutated insulin receptor are fed a high-fat diet, they continue to live significantly longer than their control group counterparts.[21] Finally, while reducing IGF-1 may enhance longevity, low levels may increase our risk of developing diabetes, cardiovascular disease, osteoporosis, and neurodegenerative diseases earlier in life.[22] Some have even questioned using growth hormone to stimulate the production of IGF-1 as a method to combat aging.[23] Successfully balancing the double-edged nature of IGF-1 is a difficult task to master, but research over the past century has begun to more consistently implicate certain dietary patterns in the quest for an optimal anti-cancer lifestyle.

·⦂·

Armstrong and Doll knocked over the initial massive domino decades before Kenyon's groundbreaking work on longevity; as a result of this push, interest in the interaction between our diets and our health began to grow. While Willett's attempts to implicate dietary fat with cancer risk had failed, this failure was a mere speedbump in the race to implicate dietary fat, a focus that left many other aspects of the link between lifestyle and health unexplored. While Kenyon and other scientists' data would implicate glucose and carbohydrates – and to a much lesser extent, protein – for disengaging our DNA defense mechanisms, population-wide measures continued to focus on dietary fat, ignoring these tangential studies that were not providing scientists the answers they wanted. As Willett would later describe, the dogma was sowing seeds of strong bias among the nutrition world. Furthermore, Armstrong and Doll's potential link between dietary fat and breast cancer left many individuals like my great-grandfather Leonardo Pesce with some difficult information to chew on: the same foods that were cherished as symbols of their culture were suddenly recast as harmful.

With no signs of slowing down, the momentum of this dietary domino effect appeared to accelerate throughout the 1990s, culminating in the decision to allocate hundreds of millions of taxpayers' dollars to fund a series of studies promoting and measuring the effects of a low-fat diet on several health markers and outcomes, including cancer. Willett's work, among others, was cast aside in a strange series of events, as funds were used to support several studies that encouraged women to follow a diet that was entirely unproven by modern scientific studies. In addition to the anti-fat dogmas of the 80's and 90's, several other noticeable issues were coming to light within the nutrition research world.

Around the time of Willett's initial studies, most of the available medical research, and especially lifestyle and disease prevention research, had focused on Caucasian males. The realization that women were being underrepresented within the research world provided the U.S. National Institutes of Health ample reason to support efforts to level the research playing field. Establishing links between lifestyle habits and the most common cancer in women in the US provided the impetus for the establishment of the Women's Health Initiative in 1991, known as the WHI.

Further emphasizing the strong push for female research, the National Institutes of Health required the inclusion of women in clinical research during the same year. The WHI was composed of several clinical trials and an observational study, designed with the goal of studying the three most common causes of death and illness in women: cancer, cardiovascular disease, and osteoporosis. At a price tag of $625 million, this first massive study of its kind enrolled over 160,000 postmenopausal women from the ages 50-79, signaling to the medical world that massive prospective population studies were no longer an idea of the future.

For more than a decade the WHI accrued women and progressed as planned. By 2006, the study data had matured, and results of the several arms assessing the low-fat diet were reported in the *Journal of the American Medical Association*. These studies randomized over 48,000 women to one of two arms. The first group of women, known as the control arm, remained on their normal diet, though they received the diet-related educational material *Dietary Guidelines for Americans*, and kept a food diary. Furthermore, they filled out forms every 6 months to help track their food intake. The other group, known as the intensive behavior modification group, followed Plato-approved recommendations in the hopes that they would reduce their total fat intake to less than 20% of total calories. Furthermore, they were advised to increase their fruit and vegetable consumption to five or more servings per day and grains to at least six servings per day. To increase adherence, they attended frequent meetings with dieticians and nutritionists to discuss their food choices and to motivate them to make healthy changes. Physical activity levels were assessed at each visit as well.

The trial was not testing a low-fat diet per se, but rather a low-fat, high fruit and vegetable, and very high grain diet. The Platonists within the intervention group decreased their fat intake by over 8% while increasing their fruit, vegetable, and grain consumption. Not surprisingly, overall carbohydrate consumption increased significantly within the intervention group. Yet somewhat surprisingly, measurements of the group's health indicators failed to change in line with their behavior changes. The initial reports on the intervention's impact on cardiovascular disease were somber: no significant reduction in the risk of coronary heart disease, stroke, or a combination of both was achieved from the dietary changes.[24] At this time it was felt that a high-fat diet was largely responsible for obesity, and the merits of a low-fat diet would extend to weight loss as well. Yet, another study reported similarly negative results; the weight of women in the intervention arm remained similar to the weight of those women in the control. These results were published in the *Journal of the American Medical Association*, where the authors concluded that, "the results of this long-term trial of diverse postmenopausal women demonstrate that long-term recommendations to achieve a diet lower in total and saturated fat with increased consumption of fruits, vegetables, and whole grains, and without focus on weight loss, do not cause weight gain."[25] An ironic twist within the conclusions – perhaps an attempt to soften the blow of a $625 million effort largely gone to waste – was the touting that the study diet did not cause weight gain. These attempts at a silver lining, remarkably reminiscent of the conclusions from the earlier breast cancer studies by the group at Harvard, further revealed the bias still deeply woven within the fabric of the medical establishment.

Regardless of whether this result was foreshadowing just how deeply ingrained the bias was or simply an attempt at doubling down to ensure taxpayers that their money was not misused, the conclusions morphed from testing the low-fat diet's ability to provide weight loss to ensuring that the diet did not cause it. Regardless of the failures of the $625 million-dollar study, questions still remained as to whether the diet could benefit more than just the pockets of the low-fat snack food industry over the past several decades. One in eight women were being diagnosed with breast cancer, and proponents remained hopeful that these dietary changes could help lower the most common non-cutaneous malignancy in women. Breast cancer, much like cardiovascular disease and weight, was also unaffected by the dietary intervention.[26] In keeping with past trends, the authors suggested in their conclusions that perhaps a longer follow-up of these women would yield significant findings. Additionally, colorectal cancer was also assessed within the WHI and was consistent with other findings, as no reduction in incidence was seen in the intervention group.[27] In a similar study known as the Women's Health Study, no link was found between dietary fat and colorectal cancer. However, the same researchers did find a potential link between fried foods and colorectal cancer, again implicating the role of free radicals and polyunsaturated fat in cancer development.[28]

The negative results of the WHI were surprising on several accounts. At the time of the study, many felt that these changes in isolation would positively affect multiple health markers. Yet, the intervention group was undergoing a barrage of changes, and many assumed the benefit would be additive, but at the very least one modification would benefit their health. Finally, the intervention group was being followed intensely and counseled on healthy lifestyle changes, so many felt that this counseling alone would provide the participants with motivation to follow a healthy lifestyle, regardless of what they were being counseled.

Due in large part to the negative findings and high price tag, the study has rightfully garnered its share of vocal critics. A major concern that surfaced at the outset of the study, prior to any results, was that the study's design might limit any tangible conclusions. The intervention included several control factor changes; although the goal was to reduce fat, this fat was instead replaced with fruits and vegetables and carbohydrate-heavy grains, in effect manufacturing an insulin-simulating diet to inhibit the ability of the subjects to lose weight amidst the study's other lifestyle changes. Furthermore, this study, like others before it, was plagued by intervention bias, or the potential ability of participants to derive benefit simply because they are contributing as part of a health intervention group. How much do monthly meetings with healthcare providers affect our motivations to be healthy? Additionally, how much does simply being part of the healthy diet intervention arm motivate us to change our behaviors, exercise more, or stop smoking? Weight loss can reduce a woman's risk of breast cancer, thus if these women lost weight and experienced a reduced risk of breast cancer, how would we know which factor was responsible – the lifestyle change or the weight loss? Critics argued that these issues begged the question of whether any benefit could be attributed to the actual intervention, or whether the trial was simply stacking the deck against the control arm at the cost of $625 million. This common criticism continues to haunt lifestyle intervention studies, since unlike randomized drug studies, providing a placebo is nearly impossible; participants are well aware of which arm of the study they are part of.

Be that as it may, in an area of scientific research fraught with controversy, strong opinions, and beliefs that are ingrained into our politics and religion since the dawn of agriculture – rightfully referred to as the dietary minefield – large prospective trials remain a financially feasible method of testing the impact of lifestyle changes in massive groups of people. One cost effectiveness study even went so far to suggest that the WHI has SAVED taxpayers billions of dollars.[29] Following in the footsteps of the behemoth WHI, two additional studies were established to analyze the impact of dietary fat reduction in women already diagnosed with breast cancer. One of these, the Women's Healthy Eating and Living (WHEL) Randomized Trial, placed women into a control and intervention arm. The latter group received intensive dietary counseling, including telephone calls, cooking classes, and newsletters promoting five servings of vegetables per day with 16 oz. of vegetable juice, three servings of daily fruit, 30 grams of daily fiber, and the reduction of dietary fat to 15-20% of total energy intake. And similar to the WHI study, the control group of the WHEL study was given print materials explaining the "5-A-Day" dietary recommendations, which promoted five servings of fruits and vegetables daily.

Echoing the issues within the dietary and lifestyle research world, the study was apparently funded by a challenge grant from a private philanthropist who strongly supported the study of diet and its role in cancer outcomes, since cancer survivors instead relied on "folklore, rumor, and hearsay."[30] Just like with the WHI, WHEL opponents cried intervention bias even before the study commenced; this time around, nutritional counseling for the WHEL intervention group was more frequent and more intense than during the WHI, providing additional fuel to the opposition's fire. The counseling was likely more intense to placate those supporters who felt that the WHI was unsuccessful due to its lack of extremeness regarding lowering dietary fat. Despite the pushback, the study launched across seven clinical sites within the US from 1995 to 2000. In total, it included 3,088 women previously diagnosed and treated for early stage breast cancer.

About half of the study subjects were placed into the intervention group, receiving the intense lifestyle counseling. The efficacy of counseling was improved from the WHI: during the six years of the study adherence rates and dietary changes between the groups diverged significantly. The control group increased their fat intake by 13%, while the intervention group far exceeded expectations, increasing their average vegetable and fruit intake to 12 servings per day. Increased vegetable consumption was even confirmed through blood tests measuring carotenoids, the pigmented chemicals that give vegetables their color and accumulate in our blood after vegetable and fruit consumption. Perhaps most importantly, weight changes were similar between the two groups, avoiding a major confounding factor. If the intervention group had lost more weight, this change could have skewed data, as overweight women have a much higher risk of breast cancer recurrence, and weight loss can offset this risk and allow these women to live longer.[31]

Yet, in line with the WHI study, no difference was observed between the two WHEL groups after seven-plus years of follow-up. The rates of breast cancer recurrence, new breast cancer diagnosis, and death were similar in each.[30]

After the failures of the WHI and WHEL, the low-fat diet advocates decided to give one last-ditch attempt to win over the medical world. The next of these massive studies following up WHI was the Women's Intervention Nutrition Study, known as WINS. As with its contemporaries, WINS promoted a low-fat eating pattern. Furthermore, it continued to follow the stepwise increase in intensity of the intervention arms. WINS represented what may have been the final effort at a massive costly endeavor to prove the anti-cancer benefits of a low-fat diet. Women within the intervention arm found themselves bombarded with methods utilizing social cognitive theory, goal setting, modeling, self-monitoring (fat gram counting and recording), social support, and relapse prevention and management. Instead of simple telephone calls, women were individually counseled during eight hourly biweekly sessions followed by sessions every three months and optional monthly group sessions. Following in the footsteps of the WHEL study, WINS emphasized that the point of the intervention was not necessarily to achieve weight loss, as this again could confound any benefits of the low-fat diet. The WINS control subjects, on the other hand, received a single baseline dietician visit and were contacted by a dietician every third month afterwards. They also were given written information on general dietary guidelines, including information on vitamins and minerals.

Similar to the WHEL study, the intense dietary intervention of WINS was effective, as these subjects decreased their fat intake by 19 grams per day at the five-year point, or to about 9% of total calories. Despite the intensive intervention, fat decrease results mirrored the results of the WHI study. Unfortunately for the researchers, this time around women in the intervention group reduced their overall caloric consumption, providing worries that the intensity of the intervention was generating significant intervention bias. When interim analysis revealed that these women lost significantly more weight than the control group, these worries were confirmed.[32] Furthermore, the interim analysis also hinted that the intervention was associated with a decrease in local recurrence, however, this suggestion was contested due to weight loss also observed in the intervention arm, along with several other issues.[33] While the authors did state that these results "could also be the result of chance," they concluded that a "lifestyle intervention reducing dietary fat intake with modest body weight loss may improve the relapse-free survival of postmenopausal breast cancer patients." To wrap up these massively funded public studies, the WHI published its long-term results in 2017, revealing that women within the intervention arm did lose more weight than the control arm after 16 years of the study. No difference was seen in deaths from breast cancer between the two groups.[34] Women within the intervention arm did experience a slightly reduced risk of succumbing to their breast cancer, further touting the benefits of weight loss on breast cancer recurrence.

The medical world now has three colossal, costly studies testing the hypothesis that dietary fat is associated with breast cancer; unfortunately, in their wake we are left with more questions than answers. Vegetable consumption was unfortunately consistently shackled to the low-fat diet, eliminating the possibility of assessing its effect on breast cancer diagnosis and recurrence. A low-fat diet seemed to have little or no effect on breast cancer occurrence and recurrence, consistent with Willett's data and Doll's concerns with his own data. Perhaps what these three massive studies signified – more so than all their medical findings combined – was the refusal to accept a lack of data supporting benefits to lowering dietary fat to reduce the risk of breast cancer. The anti-fat dominoes continue to fall in the opposite direction of the data, yet this has somehow not kept the sentiment from lingering throughout the halls of our hallowed medical institutions.

With the ability to analyze massive groups of individuals, their lifestyle habits, and their health statuses came the means to produce a continuous conveyor belt machine of studies linking foods and behaviors with health and disease at a rapid pace that quickly buried Armstrong and Doll's data and initial warnings. The WHI alone has produced almost 1500 publications, a previously unheard-of number of reports. The reports range from lukewarm to evangelical in their demonization of certain foods and activities. They have even been criticized for the melodramatic tone, which was felt to elicit "shock, terror, and controversy." Quite a few follow-up studies from the WHI even contradicted earlier reports, providing a "U-turn" sign and kindling inflammatory and contradictory media reports leaving the public fatigued, confused, and dissatisfied.[35] Over the last couple of decades, reporting by news sources on the contradictory nature of the studies has become commonplace, promulgating outrage enriched by the consistent production of inconsistent studies, causing many frustrated individuals to throw their hands into the air in resignation. The competing factors leading to these recommendations helps to provide further insight into the inconsistent, and often absent dietary recommendations that we observed in Doll's initial controversial study attempting to shed light on the root of the problem.[36] Methods to prevent cancer and the associated studies to support these methods remain perhaps the most inconsistent area within modern medicine.

⁘

Benjamin Franklin once said "An ounce of prevention is worth a pound of cure." His adage has been used to support everything from vaccines to exercise. In reality, Franklin was referring to fire safety; he used this line in an anonymous letter that he wrote to his own newspaper *The Pennsylvania Gazette* to rouse support for a volunteer fireman group, an idea that he invented. That being said, Franklin's words may be in their truest form when it comes to cancer. The war on cancer has been waged steadily since president Richard Nixon signed the National Cancer Act of 1971. After almost five decades and billions of dollars spent, countless lives have been taken by this dreaded disease. Both diagnosis rates and survival rates have improved, yet research has consistently reminded us that cancer is a far more complicated process than we originally thought. Furthermore, since cancer forms within our body – potentially from our own rogue cells – we might never be able to find a cure for the disease that is an innate part of humanity.

Like Franklin, we can aim to prevent the fire before it starts. In *Poor Richard's Almanac*, Franklin also told us "many dishes many diseases, many medicines few cures" and "the best doctor gives the least medicines." Needless to say, he did not particularly care for doctors. However, most contemporary depictions of Franklin reveal a rotund belly, questioning how much he followed his own advice when it came to health. Within the cancer world, his proverbial views on prevention are clearly appropriate, as cancer treatment is often difficult if not flat-out impossible. It comes as no surprise that researchers are always searching for better methods of prevention, and chemoprevention – or reducing the risk of cancer through medicinal compounds – has been an attractive area of research for the past several decades.

Chemopreventive sources occurring naturally within our food have immense potential to safely and effectively support the fight against cancer. Unlike the pills, potions, and radiation therapy used to fight cancer, food is necessary for survival, and methods to exploit those foods providing chemicals to help fight cancer are worth their weight in gold. Sulforaphane, the isothiocyanate and chemical in cruciferous vegetables, may be one of the most powerful of these chemicals. When our cells encounter this potential threat, a cellular process called nuclear factor erythroid 2-related factor 2, or Nrf2 for short, is activated.[37] Nrf2 then creates a chain reaction that – like Sergeant Hartman vociferously rallying his green charges – triggers the activation of a plethora of cancer-fighting genes and pathways, including regulating the body's response to oxidative stress and damage. The specifics are not too important, but we can think of Nrf2 as the alarm that sounds to wake the troops for battle – in this case warfare against free radical damage and oxidative stress – by activating what is known as the human antioxidant response system. This alarm bell engages several antioxidant genes to thwart oxidative damage and additionally activates several cellular mechanisms that detoxify harmful chemicals in our food and around our cells.[38]

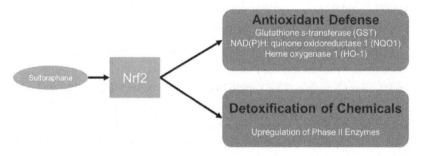

Figure 15: Sulforaphane signals to Nrf2 that danger may be coming. As a result, Nrf2 supports detoxification of chemicals and activates the antioxidant defense system via GST, NQO1, and HO-1 to disarm free radicals before causing any damage.

Besides enhancing the immune system, sulfur-based activation of Nrf2 also aids in the detoxification and removal of potentially harmful and cancerous chemicals, by increasing their ability to mix with water and then be discarded. In other words, Nrf2 is activated by oxidative stress and chemicals (harmful or not) to disarm them and alleviate any potential damage. Normally, Nrf2 acts as a patrolman floating around in the fluid-like cytoplasm within our cells and upon sensing danger jumps to action and relocates to the nucleus to activate several defense genes, similar to Kenyon's daf-16. Sulfur, a lethal chemical to insects, may pose little tangible threat to our cells, but it directly triggers Nrf2 activation as though it were a risk.

Glucoraphanin, the glucosinolate precursor of sulforaphane, blocks the initiation and progression of breast cancer in animal studies.[39] These findings are encouraging for humans, as studies reveal that a single dose of broccoli sprout preparation given to women prior to breast reduction surgery significantly increases sulforaphane within the urine and blood. Perhaps most notably in regards to breast cancer prevention, the sulforaphane also accumulated within their breast tissue.[40] Studies performed by the same group of scientists revealed similar findings in mice, confirming the uptick of the sulfur within their breast tissue. However, the sulforaphane within the breast tissue triggered several genes known to protect cells from cancer, including NQO1 and HO-1, two major components of the antioxidant defense system. While both enzymes work to halt oxidative damage, NQO1 forms NAD(P)H to protect our cells from harmful mutations that can promote cancer.[41] Such studies further illustrate that the benefits of these chemicals may directly influence organs most affected by cancer.

The key consideration with cruciferous and other sulfur-containing vegetables is the "false-alarm" signal that our cells receive from organosulfur and similar chemicals. This signal, like the grating Sergeant Hartman, alarms our cellular machinery to produce and train more troops for antioxidant defense and the disarmament of harmful chemicals – the proverbial battle against cancer that awaits us all. The difference between this false alarm and a real threat is that the sulfur merely acts to train the cells – realistically posing a minimal threat – to allow them to be better equipped to fight material threats like cancerous chemicals, heavy metals, and DNA-damaging free radicals.

Fascinating research points to the impact of these vegetables as slightly toxic and stressful to our cells, which results in a form of hormesis to upregulate pathways which can eventually fight cancer. Hormesis is our cellular equivalent of the phrase "what doesn't kill us only makes us stronger," and sulforaphane is effectively a hormetic chemicals. It acts as an oxidant, which provides the stimulus and activation of Nrf2 and several antioxidant pathways within our cells. Other similar stresses include exercise, extreme carbohydrate restriction and ketosis, fasting, and general food restriction; all are activities that stress our body to make it "stronger" in the long run. These stresses can upregulate the mitochondria, the organelle within our cells that is famous for its ability to provide us with energy but has also recently been lauded for its vital role in the fight against cancer.[42] Isocyothianates and similar chemicals appear to push the mitochondria into action, initiating an array of lethal defense mechanisms that may prevent or even help treat cancer by blocking the growth, proliferation, and survival of cancer cells.[43]

Similar to the physical and cellular burn of exercise that creates some oxidizing free radicals, the "stress" from cruciferous vegetables stimulates our mitochondria to produce homemade antioxidants to counterbalance the oxidation and protect our vital DNA.[44] Even cancer cells have caught on to this central role of our mitochondria; the stubborn bastards can amplify their own levels of some of these same pathways, further stressing their importance for survival.[41] However, our cells still seem to have the upper hand: multiple studies indicate that the organosulfur chemicals found in many of these vegetables can severely stress cancer cells, leading to oxidative damage and ultimately their death.[45] In addition to pungent vegetables, spices like turmeric[46] and bitter foods like coffee,[47] olive oil, and bold red wines also appear[48,49] to upregulate these cancer-fighting cellular mechanisms. Perhaps Galen was right all along when he referred to them as medicine two millennia ago.

Other vegetables contain an array of defense chemicals that can provide similar healthful stresses to our cells. Germicidal chemicals known as phenols are produced by many plants due to environmental stresses and insect attack. For instance, spinach grown throughout the cold winter contains more phenolic chemicals and higher antioxidant capacity compared to similar spinach grown in the milder spring.[50] Organic bok choy left to fend for itself against flea beetle attacks produces significantly more phenolic compounds in its defense as opposed to conventionally grown bok choy.[51] These chemicals are stored in their leaves, exposing anyone who consumes them to the higher antioxidant-producing chemicals.

The presence of potential chemopreventive properties of plant derivatives exemplifies the power of food, in this specific case, cruciferous vegetables. Studies even suggest that sprouts from cruciferous vegetables provide greater chemoprevention than mature vegetables.[52] While vegetables and their defensive chemicals may stimulate our cancer-fighting machinery through cellular stress, their ability to disarm carcinogens before they strike may be just as important. Mark Twain once said, "The secret of success in life is to eat what you like and let the food fight it out inside." The chemicals found in many of these vegetables certainly battle it out with our cells inside; however, this may be more of a war game exercise than an actual battle. Regardless, Benjamin Franklin can rest easy knowing that an ounce of cruciferous vegetables may be worth a pound of cure.

⁙

Looking out the windows of the laboratory, it seemed like a typical day in Jena, Germany. Inside of the laboratory, however, the experiments taking place were anything but ordinary. The chemical 2-deoxyglucose, known as 2DG, was being fed to the slithering *C. elegans* worms, the same worms that would experience a doubled lifespan when Cynthia Kenyon inactivated their insulin/IGF axis. 2-DG, a chemical familiar to veterinarians for its use as a nasal antifungal treatment in the past, works through its similarities and polar opposites to sugar. Just like glucose, 2-DG is pulled from the blood by our cells. However, unlike glucose, 2-DG is not broken down by our cells for energy, but rather, it plugs up cellular sugar inlets, blocking additional glucose from entering. We can decrease glucose in our diet to attempt to lower our blood sugar levels, but 2-DG all but ensures that sugar will be unavailable for the cell.

When Ristow fed his nematodes 2-DG, he likely had a "Eureka!" moment similar to Kenyon as he watched their maximal lifespan increase by 25%. He also began to notice that with a blocked glucose pathway, the worms began to utilize their fatty adipose tissue for energy.[14] The switch from burning sugar to burning fat within our cells is an important one; whereas glucose can be broken down in the fluid portion of the cell known as the cytosol, fat must enter a specific organelle within the cell to be broken down and metabolized. This organelle is the mitochondria, which serves as the powerhouse of our cells, burning through fats and other substances like coal in a power plant. Like the requirement of oxygen to stoke the fires in a coal power plant, our mitochondria draw in oxygen as a prerequisite for them to churn out ATP, the energy currency of our of cells. Metabolizing glucose to ATP in the cytoplasm, however, does not require oxygen.

When Ristow gradually added more glucose back into the diets of his mice, he observed their mitochondrial activity decrease like Kenyon's worms. Ristow discovered that blocking glucose uptake signaled an energy deficit to the cell. Without glucose present, the ability to generate energy is in jeopardy, and ATP begins to drop. AMPK, a de facto accountant tallying cellular energy, senses this drop and, like Nrf2, sounds the cellular alarm. Our cells require a constant supply of ATP to function properly and AMPK is constantly monitoring its levels. Any drop in quantity signals that other methods are required to increase its levels, and AMPK turns to a tried-and-true bag of tricks: it then commands the cell to burn glucose for energy, pulling it from the blood stream. Cholesterol and fat are broken down for energy as well, and these energy sources are shuttled into our mitochondrial furnace to be burned as fuel. The breakdown of fatty acids for fuel is known as beta-oxidation – fats are broken down in the presence of oxygen, creating surplus ATP to replenish the cell's energy supply. Ristow observed that by artificially depleting available cellular glucose, 2-DG directly engaged AMPK, so its activation was required to enhance the longevity of the nematodes in his experiments.

As the mitochondria of Ristow's worms churned through and metabolized more and more fat in the presence of oxygen, cellular rust began to accumulate. The formation of free radicals, or reactive oxygen species (ROS), would have been expected to drastically shorten the lifespan of the worms. Like the vegetable-oil laced free radicals of Pearce and Dayton's study, as well as the multiple mouse studies in the former half of the twentieth century, the ROS, which are highly reactive intermediaries, were expected to tear apart the cells, damage their DNA, and promote cancer. However, these free radicals were produced by the cell and within the cell, as opposed to the external sources often used to cause cancer. This difference may seem subtle yet is extremely important with respect to our cellular health.

Cynthia Kenyon may have revealed in 2009 that feeding sugar to worms can reduce their lifespan, but Michael Ristow showed two years prior that restricting sugar can increase it. While seemingly disparate in both method and conclusion, a deeper look at the two studies reveals uncanny similarities between their work. Dietary glucose restriction, glucose blockade with 2-DG, and genetic mutation of the bodyguard gene, daf-2, all activated mechanisms that informed that cell that energy was scarce. The effect from this alarm included the activation of several cellular mechanisms that help protect the cell from stress and damage, including free radical damage. The combined work of Kenyon and Ristow suggests that metabolic stresses from energy deficiency – or hormesis, as Ristow termed it – activates cellular processes that improve longevity. Ristow's work surprisingly showed that the same reactive substances that can encourage cancer and aging can unexpectedly produce the exact opposite. According to Ristow, "it works like a vaccination – repeated low doses of free radicals will increase stress resistance."[53]

To confirm his own hypothesis that the ROS formation was responsible for the impact on longevity, Ristow performed a similar experiment providing the worms with the antioxidant N-acetylcysteine, or NAC. NAC was given beforehand to scavenge and disarm any ROS produced during energy production and after glucose uptake was blocked with 2-DG. Consistent with Ristow's hormetic theory, ROS were no longer produced. To further confirm the theory, Ristow gave the worms a chemical which directly stressed their mitochondria to overproduce ROS, similar to the act of shoveling excessively large amounts of coal into the furnace of a power plant; once again, the worms lived significantly longer. Coming full circle, he repeated his initial experiment of blocking glucose uptake with 2-DG; only this time, he first gave the worms one of three antioxidants – vitamin C, vitamin E, or NAC – which effectively eliminated ROS production. The longevity witnessed in the original worms was blocked by the antioxidants.

Turning our attention back to Kenyon's studies, when she inactivated the daf-2 gene there was a similar increase in mitochondrial ROS. However, while Ristow revealed that blocking glucose uptake and stressing the mitochondria led to this outcome, Kenyon's data seemed to put the onus on decreasing or blocking the insulin and IGF-1 receptor. The end point, however, was the same: free radical fighting and stress response genes were activated, and the worms lived longer. Ristow exposed the worms to antioxidants in his trials, whereas Kenyon fed them glucose; in both cases, the longevity benefit of blocking or reducing the insulin/IGF-1 pathway was eliminated.[4] Ristow and Kenyon's studies have been confirmed in multiple different animal species, but the ability to increase longevity by simply blocking glucose uptake with 2-DG seems to be less pronounced in animals. Regardless, health-related improvements from reducing the insulin/IGF-1 pathway are indeed observed in animals and humans. Largely increasing insulin and IGF-1, on the other hand, may diminish healthy aging in all walks of life, from worms to humans.[54]

Ristow hypothesized that overworking the mitochondria for energy production and the subsequent cellular effects allowed his worms to better repair free radical damage and live longer. He had orchestrated a series of experiments that supported this theory, including perhaps most notably when he directly stimulated the mitochondria and increased their energy production simply by adding a protein called frataxin.[55] The exact mechanisms of frataxin remain elusive, but when supplied to cells it is transported to the mitochondria where it signals that ATP is running low; similar to when glucose is restricted, frataxin turns on the mitochondrial boiler to produce energy, in effect shoveling coal into the blast furnace to create ATPs. Ristow's earlier studies revealed that frataxin activates oxidative phosphorylation within the mitochondria, producing a hefty amount of ATP through the burning of fats as opposed to sugar. When the mitochondria are placed in overdrive, cells turn towards fats for energy; Ristow's mitochondria were on overdrive to such a degree that they began using over double the amount of oxygen during the process.

Ristow's results were groundbreaking in their ability to explain the several consequences experienced by patients with insufficient frataxin, a debilitating disease known as Friedreich's Ataxia. Individuals stricken with this disease have an average lifespan of 38 years and experience high rates of several types of cancer. Cells deficient in frataxin experience significantly higher levels of free radicals and a decreased antioxidant defense system, especially as these afflicted cells begin to rust.[56] With this information in hand, and on the heels of his initial study, Ristow next utilized frataxin to overheat the mitochondrial furnaces in colon cancer cells, observing several fortuitous changes in the cellular pathways that activated Weinberg's cancerous gene *ras*. The change seemed to block a potential Hallmark of Cancer, which was further emphasized when Ristow observed that the colon cancer cell growth was inhibited with the increase in mitochondrial energy derivation.[42]

What do Kenyon's experiments in worms and Ristow's subsequent experiments in worms and mice tell us about cancer in humans? While the studies are limited almost entirely to nonhuman subjects, there is clearly a trend towards several health benefits by avoiding a reliance on glucose for energy production within our cells and avoiding oversaturation of the insulin/IGF-1 pathway. Instead, turning towards the coal furnaces within our mitochondria to burn fat for ATP production seems to provide a more desirable outcome. While these two consumption processes are not mutually exclusive, their experimental findings suggest that lifestyle interventions leading to similar cellular changes are potently effective methods to reduce the risk of cancer. Furthermore, while we are unable to ramp up our mitochondria with frataxin or block glucose uptake in our cells by providing them 2-DG, we can still engage in several activities and dietary habits that replicate these processes and metabolically stress our cells, albeit to a lesser extent.

The issues that arise in individuals afflicted with Friedreich's Ataxia shed some light on approaches to apply the results of these studies to humans. Again, these individuals experience elevated levels of oxidative damage and free radical accumulation within their cells. On the surface, it is illogical that revving up the oxidative capacity of these cells – in essence creating more free radicals – would actually end up lowering their accumulation. Ristow's work however indicates otherwise, suggesting that a reliance on the mitochondria for energy lowers the levels of ROS – the same ROS than can damage our DNA and promote the Hallmarks of Cancer – within our cells. Ristow bylined his work with the phrase "Otto Warburg Revisited" paying homage to the cancer researcher who surmised that cancer cells had faulty mitochondria. Warburg, may have posited that cancer was caused by an overreliance on sugar uptake for energy derivation, but Ristow's work suggests that inefficient mitochondria may be largely to blame. In other words, methods to support mitochondrial function for energy production may provide the additional benefit of aiding in defending our cells against cancer.

While the differences between Kenyon and Ristow's research are superficially apparent, the similarities lie in the finer details including downstream effects. IGF-1 derives its ability to stimulate cellular growth and support our bones and muscles via several cellular pathways, including one known as mTOR that has achieved more mainstream popularity in recent times. Through these signaling pathways, IGF-1 enables cells to evade the multiple checkpoints and engage in processes to advance in growth and development. It can even allow the cells to avoid apoptosis, the process of self-implosion through programmed cell death utilized to rid the body of potentially dangerous and even cancerous cells.

In other words, some potential danger accompanies these otherwise normal mechanisms. More simply put, IGF-1 fosters cellular growth, and as Hanahan and Weinberg described in their seminal paper, cancer is a manifestation of the process of unregulated growth. Cancer cells have learned to produce their own IGF-1R receptors, displaying it on their outer surface to attract IGF-1 and accelerate their malignant growth. This is where our cellular contradiction surfaces: even normal cells contain this receptor, and in these ordinary cells, the overactivation of IGF-1R has an uncanny ability to press down the gas pedal of uncontrolled growth and the conversion to cancer along with protection from apoptosis, thus circumventing the body's natural process of pruning suspicious cells.[57] Well-known cancer researchers like Renato Baserga have found that IGF-1R is so vital for cancer initiation and growth that cells without the receptor are nearly resistant to transformation to cancer.

If IGF-1R is needed for cancer growth, then blocking it should be a potent method of hindering cancer development and enabling our cells to engage in normal apoptosis. Initial enthusiasm for targeting IGF-1R as a potential cancer treatment was high, as it was felt that blocking it may be selectively lethal to cancer cells while sparing normal organ cells. Like many other metabolic cancer treatments for which there were high hopes, the study outcomes unfortunately have not lived up to the optimism. However, the connection between the IGF-1 and the insulin receptor has helped strengthen the view that blocking both, or at least limiting the amount of circulating IGF-1 and insulin, can decrease or prevent cancer.

This movement, right or wrong, has been at the forefront of several groups of extreme dieters. Groups of individuals have severely restricted calories in hopes that it would also restrict their blood levels of IGF-1. Vegetarians and vegans have made similar attempts through their avoidance of animal meat or all animal-based foods. Most vegan and animal rights groups often use the IGF-1 argument as a medical reason to avoid meat – a simple internet search returns hundreds of pages touting this argument. Vegans avoid all sources of animal products, often for both moral and health reasons; other non-vegan groups attempt to reduce protein as it has been related to IGF-1 levels. To date, however, most attempts to lower IGF-1 and impact health have been largely unsuccessful.

So how does our diet affect IGF-1? The amount of IGF-1 in our blood is largely related to both our overall dietary energy intake and protein consumption.[58] However, like most aspects of the interaction between our diet and our physiology, the connection is more complicated than simple calories or even macronutrients. For instance, calcium – the most abundant mineral in our body and arguably the most vital one – increases IGF-1 and decreases its binding proteins, signaling our cells to grow.[59] IGF-1 is also increased by several other vital nutrients and vitamins including zinc, selenium, and magnesium;[60] this explains why attempts to provide the body with adequate amounts of vitamins, minerals, and protein through a complete diet while reducing IGF-1 is often futile. Overeating, on the other hand, is a tried-and-true method to raise IGF-1 excessively.

Besides the multiple studies previously discussed illustrating the concern with a diet that relies heavily on carbohydrates, the crosshairs have also been placed upon protein for several reasons. Combined with the concerns that animal protein may have a larger tendency to increase IGF-1, dairy has become a natural target for the low-IGF-1 evangelists. Many animal rights and vegan groups have taken a particularly strong stance against dairy products; however, the precise effects of dairy consumption on IGF-1 are unclear. Dairy contains varying levels of IGF-1, which was voiced as a reasonable initial concern of many of these groups. That being said, as with soy or any type of protein, it is more likely that the high amount of protein in commonly consumed dairy products – e.g. low-fat milk, low-fat cheese – is simply a hefty source of protein, which like breast milk consumed during infancy, increases IGF-1 and signals our cells to grow. Studies support this view: milk intake in children is associated with higher levels of IGF-1, and boys that drink more milk have longer leg length, reiterating the growth factor properties of IGF-1.[61] Upon looking closer examination, higher IGF-1 seems to be related to the protein content of dairy and not the IGF-1 within the milk.

Some epidemiology studies, despite their limitations, do point towards animal protein as a stronger stimulus of IGF-1 than plant protein; as such, many people have contorted these studies to support their dietary views. Animal protein is a more complete protein source, which may account for the difference, recalling that IGF-1 functions as a normal hormone whose production is supported by a nutrient and mineral-rich diet. Of course, there are other studies that conflict with those studies and reveal that both male[62] and female[63] carnivores and vegetarians have similar IGF-1 levels. However, in comparison to the standard American diet, subjects on a vegan diet may experience a modestly lower IGF-1 level. Yet, the multiple unhealthy aspects of a standard American diet, most notably its relatively high number of calories, prevents any definitive conclusions from being made. Furthermore, other studies question the "plant versus animal" protein argument: soy protein isolate, a vegetarian source of protein, significantly increases IGF-1,[64] with some studies revealing a more drastic increase in IGF-1 from soy as opposed to milk protein.[65] Soy also reduces the major binding protein IGFBP3, which acts to offset high levels of IGF-1.[66]

Lastly, rBGH, a growth hormone that acts much like IGF-1, is often given to cows to stimulate their milk production. This hormone encourages cellular growth and replication and not surprisingly shows up downstream in the milk of these cows. While studies reveal that rBGH may be inactive in humans, it is certainly present in cows, which also have higher levels of IGF-1. The jury is still out on the immediate and long-term side effects from rBGH ingestion, but it is left best avoided – what we do know now is that cows given rBGH may experience higher rates of infections and require the frequent use of antibiotics, leading to multiple health issues and an increase in antibiotic-resistant infections.[67]

To summarize our musings upon a study area of considerable uncertainty and controversy – with studies ranging from worms to humans and strong, often religious-like sentiments on both sides of health crusader camps – a diet that activates the IGF-1 and insulin pathways may increase our risk of cancer. High-carbohydrate diets may be the biggest perpetrators, with high-protein diets trailing closely behind. Many weight loss strategies include limiting carbohydrates, but dietary protein is necessary to support our bones, organs, and cellular function. Furthermore, dietary protein is satiating, which helps individuals prone to overeating experience less hunger. A practical dietary strategy to impact IGF-1 and insulin, based on the available studies, may be to keep our carbohydrate levels reasonably low and protein intake moderate.

9

PHILOSOPHY, COLD FOODS, AND COLDER SCIENCE

"Nevertheless, the discoveries about the role of the insulin/IGF-1 pathway in ageing have had a profound impact on her own lifestyle, which includes a tendency to discard the bread from sandwiches and eat only the toppings of pizzas. 'I'm on a low-carb diet. I gave my worms glucose, and it shortened their lifespan. [The diet] makes sense because it keeps your insulin levels down.'

No desserts. No sweets. No potatoes. No rice. No bread. No pasta. 'When I say 'no,' I mean 'no, or not much,' she notes. 'Instead, eat green vegetables. Eat the fruits that aren't the sweet fruits, like melon.' Bananas? "Bananas are a little sweet.' Meat? 'Meat, yes, of course. Avocados. All vegetables. Nuts. Fish. Chicken. That's what I eat. Cheese. Eggs. And one glass of red wine a day."[1]

- Cynthia Kenyon, PhD

Socrates: Will you ask me, what sort of an art is cookery?

Polus: What sort of an art is cookery?

Socrates: Not an art at all, Polus.

- Gorgias by Plato

Takeaways:

Food is often considered in philosophical and religious context, and Plato's histrionic view of diet is further explored alongside Pythagorus' more tangible, but fairly myopic, views.

Traveling across time, diet and nutrition is evaluated in the context of Judaic, Christian, Aztec, Sumerian and other cultural and religious groups, helping to explain the myriad of current dietary views.

A staple in Leonardo's diet, cheese and milk are considered, citing the importance of food quality by illustrating the differences in dairy produced from grass-fed cows. Milk from grass-fed cows results in higher levels of several key vitamins, nutrients, and other compounds that improve our metabolism and shape our body's defense mechanisms.

In 2003, Ella Haddad and Jay Tanzman published results from a rather simple study they executed assessing the dietary habits of over 13,000 Americans.[2] As part of the array of questions study participants were asked within their survey, the simple question "Do you consider yourself to be a vegetarian?" provided perhaps the most insight. Haddad and Tanzman were both scientists at the Department of Nutrition at Loma Linda University in California. Loma Linda is home to a Protestant Christian group known as the Seventh-Day Adventist Church. Officially established in the latter half of the 19th century, the Seventh-Day Adventists are well-known for their strong views on diet and health as an integral component of their faith. As "an indivisible unity of body, mind, and spirit," the Adventist Church was founded upon a strong contempt for tobacco, alcohol, and drugs, and also upon the promotion of vegetarianism. One Seventh-Day Adventist physician named John Harvey Kellogg, with the aid of his brother William, created Corn Flakes® and several other breakfast cereals to support a vegetarian lifestyle, help followers avoid meat consumption, and (apparently) reduce sinful sexual behaviors that would result from eating what was believed to be more libido-stimulating foods.

Regardless of their beliefs, Seventh-Day Adventists do generally experience good health and better longevity compared to the general population of America; many have attributed this health to their vegetarian diet.[3] Haddad and Tanzman are part of the scientific effort to analyze the Adventists' dietary patterns to find its connections with their health. Haddad has published extensively on vegetarianism, a major component of their dietary beliefs; in her research, she set out to assess which of the Adventists actually follow a vegetarian diet. What she found, however, were major inconsistencies between the diet individuals claimed to follow and what they truly followed; two-thirds of self-proclaimed vegetarians had eaten meat during the previous week.

In total, only 0.9% of the study population did not actually record meat consumption and were essentially vegetarian. In other words, most self-proclaimed vegetarians were simply lying. Why did the majority of self-proclaimed vegetarians answer dishonestly in a study that had absolutely no repercussions? The answer goes back deeper than we may think, with platonic undertones deeply rooted within the foundations of civilization.

As the United States approached the end of the twentieth century, we as a population found ourselves more obese than anyone before us in the history of humanity;[4] yet at the same time, we were significantly malnourished when it came to vital nutrients, vitamins, and minerals. We were over-nourished, yet somehow malnourished at the same time. The western diet had left us failing to meet the recommended dietary allowance (RDA) for vitamin A and B-6, magnesium, calcium, and zinc.[5] To make matters worse, almost one-third of the population fell under the RDA for folate, the B vitamin required for the creation and repair of our DNA and cells and a vital player in the fight against cancer.

Just several decades prior, the Dietary Goals of the United States were released to help improve the diet of the American public. Known as the "McGovern Report," the policy was championed by Senator George McGovern of South Dakota. The American people were advised to increase their consumption of carbohydrates to account for approximately 55-60% of total energy intake. The increase in carbohydrates would be accompanied by a reduction in overall dietary fat from 40% to 30% of total energy intake. Dietary saturated fat, salt, and cholesterol were targeted as well, with a goal of reducing saturated fat to 10% of the diet. Sugar, on the other hand, was to be reduced to a slightly higher amount at 15% of total energy intake. Whether the group felt that saturated fat was more harmful than sugar remains unknown, though the recommendations would certainly suggest this. What the population was left with – viewed by many as not just coincidental with McGovern's role as senator of South Dakota, a wheat production powerhouse – was a grain-centric diet that provided a small fraction of the vitamins and minerals of traditional human diets.[6]

On the heels of these questionable recommendations came the birth of the USDA's Food Pyramid in 1992. The base of the infamous pyramid –

familiar to nearly all Americans from their grade-school years – recommended six to eleven daily servings of bread, cereal, rice, and pasta, a dosage amount with which Kenyon, Tannenbaum, and Kritchevsky would take umbrage. The quantification and treatment of food more as a mathematical equation and less as a nutritious substance that supports life, however, would have been quite agreeable to Plato. Furthermore, the Pyramid recommended the reduction and counting of calories, with its accompanying information pamphlet mentioning the word "calorie" a total of 50 times.[7] Food was no longer a device of nourishment and sustenance, but was instead meticulously quantified via this novel currency known as the calorie.

Agreement that the creation of the Food Pyramid was the culmination of a set of massive missteps is one of the few common grounds between both sides of the current high-fat/low-fat dietary battlefield. The negative impacts of this dietary death triangle were covered ad nauseum throughout my earlier book *Misguided Medicine*. The Food Pyramid did precede – and for all intents and purposes, fuel – the massive obesity epidemic, the rise of diabetes to previously unimagined proportions, and the ushering in of a period of threatened health that humanity had never heretofore experienced. That being said, I was dead wrong in its degree of importance in shaping the role of diet in health. It turns out that a certain well-known philosopher and his work on triangles – to be named later – would have a far larger impact over the next 2,500 years than that of the short-lived Food Pyramid; the latter would be replaced in 2005 by the even shorter-lived MyPyramid Food Guidance System, and then once more with MyPlate in 2005. Sadly though, the tangible recommendations changed very little as we progressed from pyramid to plate.

The creation of the Food Pyramid, the inconsistency of Plato's teachings on food, and the blurred lines between religion and philosophy and the actual impact of food on health have more in common than one would have guessed. On one hand, Plato tells us that food nourishes the body; on the other, caution must be provided as it can quickly careen downhill into gluttonous behavior if not quantified properly. The Dietary Goals of the United Stated were released in 1977, chastising those nutrient-dense *opsa* foods that Plato felt "turned flesh into flesh and bone into bone." Yet, following Plato's later views and his reliance on nutrient-sparse foods, the USDA watched as vitamin deficiency skyrocketed. The promotion of their triangular guide further condoned these foods, with the base of the guide including the promotion of foods that are so naturally devoid of vitamins, nutrients, and minerals that these elements must be added to them via factory-produced chemicals. The adoption of the mathematical pyramid paved the way for counting calories, avoiding dense foods, and instead relying on often flavorless and nutrient-sparse sources of food. And so, Plato's conflict, after perseverating throughout history, has blossomed to full fruition; if not kept under check, food – a necessity for maintaining our most important physical being, the body – could quickly cause rotting of our most important metaphysical being, the soul.

While Plato's work provides no solution to the conflict, an understanding of his past and impact on the future provides valuable insight into how strong beliefs and the current dietary dogma has come into existence. Furthermore, it provides insight into why almost all discussions regarding a healthy lifestyle and diet, and their implications for preventing cancer, must at the very least include a cursory consideration of Platonic philosophy. Founder of the Academy in Athens, Plato was a philosopher trained in Classical Greece. While Socrates was his well-known and most immediate mentor, Plato was also heavily influenced by earlier philosophers, one of whom was Pythagoras.

Pythagoras is most famous in modern times for his mathematical and scientific deductions – we all learned in our high school geometry classes about the Pythagorean theorem, which relates the sides of a triangle to each other through a mathematical equation. Born on the Greek Island of Camos, Pythagoras would eventually leave his hometown to establish his philosophy school in the Greek colony of Crotone, 2,400 years before Leonardo Pesce would leave the same Mediterranean region for America. While Leonardo left on his own accord for a better life, the Pythagoreans were actually forced out of Calabria – their influence was so great that local politicians became fearful and responded violently. Nowadays, Crotone, like many other of its neighboring Calabrian subregions, is perhaps best known for its famous Crotonese cheese and flavorful red wines.

In ancient Calabria, Pythagoras and his supporters followed a strict set of lifestyle guidelines, many of which were designed to foster an immensely disciplined and modest life. They detested modern luxuries and espoused a lifestyle that remained pure through abstention. Their depiction of a simple life, however, would differ drastically from the 19th-century Calabresi when it came to food. According to Greek historians, Pythagoras was even-tempered, humorless, and avoided the "pleasures of love, all in an effort to remain grounded."[8] His even-keeled nature was reflected in his diet: apparently, he was a strict vegetarian and demanded the same of his students. For unknown reasons, he also avoided beans, and his followers were advised to abstain from them, along with fish and meat. Some historians even claim that Pythagoras believed that part of the soul would be expelled when passing gas, thus explaining his legume-phobia.[9]

Strangely, the earlier followers of Pythagoras apparently knew him to eat meat, while the later followers such as Plato believed he was a vegetarian. In paralleling the inconsistencies seen with Plato's advice versus his actions, according to the student Porphyry, Pythagoras had recommended that he nourish his body by consuming meat, since after all, he was an athlete.[10] The exact origins of the vegetarian Pythagorean view are unknown but are likely related to his belief in metempsychosis, or the transmigration of the soul between physical bodies – more simply known as reincarnation. Some have even suggested that Pythagoras claimed he could remember his past lives.[11] Regardless of the contrasting historical views on this subject, it was highly likely that much of the Pythagorean diet did not consist of meat, not on account of philosophical and religious views, but rather on account of his geographical confines – his town was surrounded by "irrigated fields" and "desert wasteland." To no one's surprise, meat in Ancient Greece was a luxury.

Regardless of the source, the attribution of vegetarianism to Pythagoras has persisted throughout time, correct or not. The famous Roman poet Ovid relayed a story of Pythagoras pleading abstention of meat to his followers in the famous epic *Metamorphoses*, furthering the philosopher's vegetarian reputation. Several subsequent English translations of the document strengthened the relationship, eventually leading to its introduction into Shakespeare's works, most notably in *The Merchant of Venice* in 1596. The character Gratiano proclaimed that according to Pythagoras, "souls of animals infuse themselves into the trunks of men." Even Leo Tolstoy, the famous Russian novelist and author of *Anna Karenina*, would partake in the "Pythagorean Diet," abstaining from meat.

A numerical mystic by nature, Pythagoras was also credited with the view that the planets rotated in harmony and under the laws of several mathematical equations. Like the later famous mathematician and noted vegetarian Leonardo Da Vinci, Pythagoras firmly believed in a harmony between math, science, and nature; he surmised that there was a mathematical equation to describe most relationships in nature. This view was surely rooted in his singular discovery of the groundbreaking namesake equation that predicts the lengths of triangle edges consistently throughout the eternity of nature. His interlacing theories on mathematics and nature heavily influenced Plato and the many philosophers that followed him; this unification of mathematics, philosophy, and religion is perhaps best illustrated by *The Vitruvian Man,* da Vinci's seminal drawing illustrating the perfect human body sketched by precise observations and mathematical calculations. Even da Vinci's other famous paintings, like *The Last Supper* and *Mona Lisa* can be broken into symmetric triangles hinting at his reliance on mathematical symmetry, even within his art.

So, what do Pythagoras and his mathematical equation concerning triangles have to do with Plato or the pursuit of achieving optimal health to prevent cancer? Everything, according to Plato's most famous student Aristotle. According to Aristotle, Plato's viewpoints, philosophies, and teachings were based heavily on the beliefs of Pythagoras. Furthermore, such views were further expanded when Plato's beliefs heavily influenced the formation of many modern religions, including Judaism and Islam. His work also left a massive imprint upon Christianity, which grew exponentially under the auspices of the Roman Empire as it expanded throughout Western Europe. This influence is widely accepted and even taken for granted in these modern times. Saint Augustine (354-430 AD) for instance was considered a Christian Neoplatonist during his era, due to the large impact of Plato on his religious views. A fervent theologian, Augustine created a total of 13 books as part of his famous work *Confessions*, influencing countless Christian writers throughout the Middle Ages ergo widely promulgating Pythagorean views.

While the far-reaching influence of Plato's views on modern philosophy and religion are well acknowledged, the impact of Plato's views on food – quantifying calories and avoiding meat – remains relatively unexplored, as little discussion to date has broached the topic. Pythagoras' vegetarian diet, regardless of the specifics, was supposedly further influenced by his following of asceticism. Asceticism was a philosophy that shunned all sensual pleasures; it was characteristic of many philosophers and religious figures of antiquity, from Plato to the Christian Apostle Paul to the aforementioned Saint Augustine. Finally, perhaps the most famous Catholic philosopher Saint Thomas Aquinas was an ascetic who blended the philosophies of Plato's prized pupil, Aristotle, with the ideologies of Christianity. Pythagorean views – which eventually became Platonic views – intertwined the role of discipline with diet well beyond vegetarianism. According to Panagiotis Skiadas and John Lascaratos of the Department of History of Medicine in Athens, Greece, "As opposed to the limitless desire for food and drink, self-restraint is considered by the philosopher to be the power with logic," and the Pythagorean School "had enforced a series of dietary restrictions for consolidation of the spirit of self-restraint and healthy living."[11] Food nourished the body, but lack of food, according to these philosophers, nourished the soul.

The former act of utilizing the diet as a means of nutrition and survival was replaced by the act of limiting the overall content of the diet along with the amount of meat and *opsa* as a means of displaying self-restraint. Power over food signified power over mind. Indeed, the inconsistencies within the actions and philosophy of Pythagoras and Plato signal a deeper issue: it appears the differences between their views on science and philosophy deeply conflict when it comes to food. They fully acknowledge that animal products are vitamin- and nutrient-rich and required to most adequately nourish the body, so much that they recommend them at times. Yet, their religious views on reincarnation and philosophical views on asceticism lead them to an entirely different conclusion that emerges within their philosophical works.

And so, the reasons for the inconsistencies in Plato's message become clearer. His attempt to merge the earlier Greek philosophies, including Pythagorean theory, with his own views and metaphors on health is a difficult task, even for the world's expert on philosophy and intellectual discourse. In a progression that becomes all too common when dietary science overlaps with philosophy and religion, incongruent topics promote incongruent theories. Plato, however, even begins to recommend milk and cheese products, acknowledging the importance of animal fat and protein for vitamins and proper nutrients. In his words, dairy "should hold a prominent position in the dietetic preferences." Indeed, cheese and dairy to this day remain a significant component of some vegetarian diets, along with the ever-popular Mediterranean diet; proponents who see the latter as a low-fat diet seem to frequently forget dairy's current and historic role throughout the area. Plato, however, will only go so far with animal food recommendations; the ghost of Pythagoras continues to haunt his thoughts, leaving him unable to fully recommend the consumption of animal flesh.

Plato's difficulties with the connection between food and health are perhaps best illustrated by his philosophical disdain for cooking, which he considers not an art but a habitude. Cooking, according to Plato, is clearly outside of the bounds of medicine and only serves the purpose of "satisfying the senses, ignoring what is really healthy." Current medical schools may disagree with Plato, as many have now added cooking classes to their curriculum. Cooking often enhances the taste of food, and in some instances, enhances its health benefits – a fact likely unknown to Plato. However, improving the senses only serves to adulterate the mind and soul in Plato's view. Though he consistently utilizes food in the philosophical metaphors of his writings, he still shuns cooking and instead claims physicians and trainers should provide insight into the nutritional values of food, and therefore health. Plato would seemingly disagree with those of us that believe that health begins in the kitchen and not at the doctor's office. Yet at other times, he does promote the medicinal benefits of a healthy diet, claiming "wherefore one ought to control all such diseases, so far as one has the time to spare, by means of dieting rather than irritate a fractious evil by drugging."[13] Plato's views on prevention hold to this day, and the physician's aim should be to reinforce the patient's body so that it can effectively fight disease and abate the hallmarks of cancer. This endorsement further exposes Plato's internal conflict, his notion that food is required to nurture the body, but any threat of harming the soul must be checked; food must be kept restricted, tasteless, and uncooked, with animal foods minimized and any semblance of pleasure from food removed. In other words, food, a necessity, must be counted and purposely made bland to ensure it will never threaten our mental and philosophical well-being.

Finally, it is likely that Plato, like many other Greek philosophers and dietary theorists preceding him, was heavily influenced by mythical legends and traditional religious stories that often revolved around the cultivation of grains and cereal foods as the source for life. A similar tendency can be seen in Western religious texts: Christians are familiar with the breaking of bread in the New Testament of the Bible, and both Christians and Jews refer to the many grain offerings as sacrifices in the Old Testament. In Islam, bread often refers to food in general. Overall, Plato's view of a temperate diet as most healthy was not uncommon in these bygone times.

Plato's disconnect regarding the importance of food is not unique; many cultures and religions – particularly those of western civilizations – are less focused on health, and more steeped in the supernatural when it comes to foods like grains. Many cultures utilize them to explain the origins and evolution of mankind and worship them for their role in helping man escape barbarism. For instance, in Mexican folklore, it took the Aztecs five generations to escape the savagery of hunting and gathering. Each generation marked an improvement over the previous one, with the third and fourth generation relying predominantly on *teosinte*, a maize native to Mesoamerica. The fifth and final generation was nurtured with traditional maize – an advanced grain helped man segue from a barbaric lifestyle to a more civilized one. According to the sacred Popol Vuh text, compiled further south in the Guatemalan Highlands, after several unsuccessful attempts by the Mayan gods to create man out of mud and wood, they tried again using yellow and white maize, finally finding success. Even further south – and more closely resembling the Biblical story of Jesus – the Incan sun god Inti sent his son and daughter – a married couple – to Earth to civilize humanity. How was this accomplished? He gave his son a golden stick, which eventually led to the cultivation and worship of maize. According to Tom Standage in *An Edible History of Humanity*, the Incas largely relied on potatoes for sustenance, but for some reason grains were worshipped as a sacred crop.[14]

Journeying eastward around the globe, similar traditional stories emerge. In Chinese legend, according to Standage, with the country on the brink of starvation the goddess of mercy and patron saint of Tibetan Buddhism, Guanyin, supplied milk from her breasts to feed the empty rice fields and create the grain that would become a staple throughout Asia. As the story goes, Guanyin squeezed her breasts so hard to nourish the crops that milk and blood were drawn, leading to white and red rice. Further south in the volcanic islands of Indonesia, oral tradition tells that when the slain goddess of the earth Sri was buried, rice grew from the corpse and was used to feed mankind.

Emerging from the cradle of human civilization – the modern-day Middle East – and reverberating throughout time and distance is a common chorus of humans progressing from barbarian hunter-gatherers to civilized farmers with the help of grains. While some of these tales incorporate the domestication of animals as a byproduct of this evolution, the majority seem to follow a Pythagorean view of grains and non-flesh sources that fueled the appetite of civilization. The flesh-eating barbarians are consistently left behind; a Sumerian hymn to the grain goddess, as described in Standage's anthology of humanity, pronounces the end of a barbaric age marked by the commencement of the grain goddess and the beginning of civilization.[14]

As fields continued to turn to gold while the dependence on farming and the production of grains became more prevalent across more human societies, nutrient deficiencies ensued and increased at an alarming rate. Tooth decay, scurvy, cavities, and infections became so rampant that Pulitzer Prize-winning anthropologist Jared Diamond has referred to the adoption of agriculture and dismissal of hunting and gathering as "the worst mistake in the history of the human race."[15] The exact reasons for the transformation are unknown, and the switch from hunting and gathering to a reliance on agriculture becomes more confusing as several studies have pinned farming as less productive and more laborious than hunter-gathering. Some scholars such as Professor Sam Bowles, who heads the Behavioral Sciences Program at the Santa Fe Institute, have surmised that the human desire of ownership – especially property ownership – has led man to overlook the additional work they experienced during farming and the cannibalization of their leisure time.[16] Some would even say that tendency carries on to today's times and is reflected in white-collar/corporate business culture across the globe.

So why the infatuation with grains and disdain for meat? Many theorize that government and religious leaders relied on the worship of grains, which paralleled civilization; a return to hunting and gathering would have threatened the continuance of modern society and the divide between the rich and poor that ensued. Governments required the worship of grains physically, philosophically, and religiously to keep society intact. Like Plato's philosophical motives, civilized societies' push for grains was anything but an issue of health.

Regardless of the myriad theories for our ascendance to a civilized society, one unifying theme continues throughout a multitude of cultures: civilization and religion overcome the savage and flesh-eating barbarian, thanks in a large part to grains. *Opsa* was overtaken by the grains it was once meant to improve upon. The threads of philosophy, religion, and dietary behaviors have been delicately woven into our culture and the medical practice since antiquity; this braided history continues to influence all aspects of dietary and lifestyle recommendations within current culture. Perhaps

Plato, the world's expert on philosophy, merely exemplifies the consequences that arise when political, philosophical, and religious figures elect to make dietary recommendations: we are left with dogmatic endorsements that have more to do with politics, ideologies, and beliefs than with actual health.

With 2,500 years of momentum building since Plato's era, it is unsurprising that the horrors of food restriction in the Minnesota Starvation Study went relatively unnoticed and dietary agencies still recommend similar caloric restriction for weight loss and maintenance. A review of Walford's multiple studies and reports on the calorie restriction that occurred in Biosphere 2 reveals an utter failure to characterize the misery that his colleagues experienced during the food shortage. Much like those individuals above who may have earnestly believed they were following a vegetarian diet while eating meat, it was as though an invisible hand, propelled by centuries of philosophical musings, had erased several realities of our diet: 1) Our body craves nutritious food sources that often include animal products based on their rich nutrient density; 2) As demonstrated in a barrage of studies, purposeful calorie restriction is miserable, which easily explains the massive failure rates of calorie-restricted diets for weight loss; and 3) As illustrated in Ludwig's work, many of the historically revered foods that are recommended instead leave us obese and hungrier. The ghost of Plato has continued to haunt the medical establishment, floating throughout history while biasing its victims to believe that we should be starving ourselves, turning food into a mathematical equation by counting calories, and relying on nutrient and vitamin-sparse foods, as if the misery that follows nourishes our souls.

While remaining in stark contrast to the science of a healthy diet, this view seemed to have eluded some of our greatest philosophers and medical researchers. If they had difficulty reuniting the physical and mental attributes of certain foods, or lack thereof, then Walford and others can be forgiven for their ascetic biases when it comes to calorie restriction and the antiquated recommendation of endorsing low-calorie foods. Food, however, is not a mathematical equation... and perhaps it is time to let go of this deeply ingrained ideology that accompanies Plato's invisible hand as it continues to exert its grip upon the modern medical world.

⁘

Leonardo Pesce had just finished unloading several wheels of cheese. The front door was ajar and the wind softly blew into the store, wafting to Leonardo's nostrils the floral, goaty scent of pecorino cheese. This pleasantly familiar scent now permeating the store led Leonardo to reminisce of his childhood in San Lorenzo – pecorino cheese is made from the milk of sheep, much like those that the Pesce clan and their neighbors chased around the hillsides of Calabria. As this cheese ages, it becomes ripened by the bacteria within its rind. Furthermore, the aging process gradually pulls moisture from the cheese, leaving it with a rough, hard surface texture poetically reflecting Leonardo's work ethic. It is the king of southern Italian cheeses, with a distinctly sharp taste that mirrors the jagged terrain of the Calabrese mountains and many other areas within Italy where the sheep climb to find and eat the scarce pockets of grass. The cheesemaking process had been passed down through the generations of many southern Italian families, and the taming of the bacteria within milk to yield the delicious cheesy final product gradually became a common knowledge trade secret among the villagers. However, with his limited understanding of science, Leonardo was unaware that the bacteria within his sheep ferment their grassy meal as it sits in their stomachs and this fermentation process provides the sheep with essential nutrients. This process, which also takes place in cows and other grazing animals, ultimately has profound effects on the nutritional value of the final cheese product.

As the grass churned within the multiple stomachs of Leonardo's sheep, it began to separate into liquid and a solid known as cud. The cud gets passed around and regurgitated within the animal, ensuring it is thoroughly mixed with saliva which helps to process the larger food components. The fermenting bacteria step in to gradually break down and digest the cellulose-based fibrous particles within the grass. Fueled by the carbohydrate and protein portion of the grass, the bacteria produce several short-chain fatty acids, including butyric acid, or butyrate. Proprionic acid, another short-chain fatty acid, is produced by a bacteria species found near our sweat glands and is responsible for the odor that often accompanies these areas. These fatty acids are then absorbed into the bloodstream throughout the gastrointestinal tract to provide nutrition to the ruminant animal. Throughout the process of the bacterial fermentation of grass, the significant production of conjugated linoleic acid, or CLA, occurs, along with butyrate and omega-3 fatty acids.[17]

Meat and dairy from grass-fed cows contain more of these fats, along with more vitamins, nutrients, and chemicals utilized by our antioxidant defense system. Pecorino cheese contains substantially more CLA when compared to typical cheese produced from grain-fed cows – CLA production requires the fermentation of grass within the rumen. CLA, butyrate, and omega-3s are anti-inflammatory fatty acids incorporated along our cellular membranes and within other fatty areas throughout the body to provide a mechanism to extinguish inflammation.

Besides the catastrophic health consequences for ruminating animals if their appropriate process of fermentation is disrupted, similar issues impact any human who consumes the meat or dairy products of these animals. For instance, when a hungry cheese lover eats grass-fed pecorino – as opposed to a typical cheese made from the milk of grain-fed cows – they will experience a reduction in several harmful inflammatory compounds within their blood. When scientists fed several fortunate clinical trial volunteers a weekly half-pound of mouth-watering pecorino cheese over several weeks, they experienced a slew of beneficial changes in their blood values; numerous inflammatory factors associated with cancer, like IL-6, IL-8, and TNF-α, were lessened from the cheese consumption.[18] Additionally, a protein that signals for blood vessel growth – an original hallmark of cancer – known as vascular endothelial factor (VEGF) decreased meaningfully in the study subjects. All these factors may increase the risk of cancer, and all are part of the original and newer hallmarks of cancer, including inflammation, accentuated blood vessel growth, and angiogenesis; the levels of all of these factors dropped on account of simply eating cheese. Targeting VEGF is currently a cancer treatment, as it is a potent angiogenic factor linking inflammation and cancer. Further illustrating its inherent danger, its overexpression is key in cancer initiation and progression.[19]

While the benefits of many of these anti-inflammatory components have come to light recently, CLA seems to be the most popular, and rightly so: studies reveal it supports and improves multiple physiologic processes including fat metabolism, atherosclerosis, blood pressure, immune system support, and cancer-fighting cellular properties.[20,21] By increasing the ability of our cells to take in fat and metabolize it for energy, it signals the cells to burn fat instead of storing it.[20] Furthermore, this improvement in metabolism helps leave the body better equipped to deal with fluctuations in blood sugar and more sensitive to insulin – in other words, the body requires less insulin than it typically would to eliminate the same amount of sugar.[22,23] Like Professor Ristow's frataxin protein, CLA increases the expression of several specific proteins known as uncoupling proteins within our mitochondria. These proteins act similarly to frataxin, shoveling coal into the metabolic furnace and signaling the mitochondria to increase energy expenditure and burn fat.[24]

These metabolic changes might eventually leave us leaner by programming our cells as fat-burning machines, which is why many companies have attempted – and failed, for the most part – to create synthetic CLA supplements. More importantly, these metabolic changes can prime our cells to be more potent cancer-fighting machines. Along these lines, a separate array of studies has suggested CLA possesses anticarcinogenic properties through its ability to improve cellular mechanisms to prune faulty and potentially precancerous cells through apoptosis; recall that apoptosis ensures cells progress through normal cell cycles, inhibits excessive cellular proliferation, and blocks unwarranted angiogenesis.[25] In animal studies, CLA-enriched butter decreases the growth of tumors and blocks their ability to spread throughout the body.[26,27]

Studies in humans, though limited, appear to reflect this data. Dietary consumption of CLA and high serum levels of CLA are associated with a lower risk of breast cancer.[28] Higher intakes of high-fat dairy have been associated with a decreased risk of colorectal cancer in a study of 60,000 Swedish women,[29] with every two additional servings of high-fat dairy associated with a 13% decreased risk. While such benefits may be coming from the butyrate in dairy – the same chemical produced by bacteria in our bowels – it is difficult to narrow down the potential benefit to one chemical. The same database, however, revealed no reduction in breast cancer risk.[30] Yet, a similar study from Finland provides evidence that higher serum CLA is associated with a lower risk of breast cancer.[28] The aforementioned issues with population studies are present in most of these reports, but the findings nevertheless are intriguing as we search for foods that can decrease the risk of cancer.

Revisiting the risks of overconsuming vegetable oils covered in the monumental study produced by Dayton and Pearce, the composition of cheese and butter produced from the milk of grass-fed cows further illustrates the drastic difference that might have occurred had they swapped out corn oil for some well-sourced dairy fat. Besides the considerable amount of the fat-soluble vitamins A and E, cheese and butter from grass-fed cow milk contain a 1:1 ratio of omega-6 to omega-3 fatty acids. While the amount of polyunsaturated fats in cheese and butter is low overall, both contain an optimal ratio of fatty acids to reduce inflammation. Such a ratio may be an additional reason why those study participants eating pecorino cheese experienced a significant drop in their levels of inflammatory markers. These dietary sources, along with fatty and oily fish and the fat in grass-fed beef, contain important fatty acids known as DHA and EPA that are not provided in plant-based fats.

Going back further than pecorino, the precise history of cheese remains elusive, particularly since humans began producing and mongering it way before civilizations reliably jotted down their histories. References to cheese were passed down by oral tradition and folklore but are littered throughout history. The Greeks take the lion's share of cheese lore, thanks to Homer and his multiple epic poems that remain some of the oldest historical documents of the modern world. As Homer writes in his famous *Odyssey*, the sorceress Circe presented cheese to Odysseus and his travelers. The cyclops Polyphemus tormented Odysseus and his men in the tale, but he also apparently had an eye for cheese, so much so that he hoarded it in his cave. Odysseus and his men later ransacked the cave, partaking in a cheese that per his description resembled feta in both texture and taste. Even Hippocrates, history's most famous physician, used cheese medicinally to treat disease. His recipe for the medicinal cheese concoction remains:[31] "Take a black grape, the inside of a sweet pomegranate, crush (together), and mix in dark wine, scrape in some goat's cheese, sprinkle with some flour from roasted wheat and, well mixed, give it to drink."

While the exact origins of cheese remain unknown, claims of its mainstream inception range from Europe to Asia and the Middle East. Some scholars have even pointed to Northern Africa as the birthplace, since cheese was a substantial part of the ancient Egyptian diet. In fact, rumor has it that a trader kept milk in a pouch, and during an uneven journey on horseback the bag bounced up and down through the warm climate of Northern Africa, steadily churning its way into a delicious sack of cheese. The true history of cheese's birth will remain elusive, but the horseman story arguably remains history's entertaining and fantastic placeholder. Regardless of the origins, evidence supports that cheese was being produced around Switzerland 8,000 years ago, with indications that even more cheese was produced around 4,000 years later in the Sahara, Greece, China, and eventually modern-day Italy.

Regardless of the veracity of the horseman's tall tale that churned its way through history, it nevertheless does illustrate the cheesemaking process well. As this culinary pioneer rode his horse throughout the Fertile Crescent, the milk sloshed around in his pouch. Fashioned out of the stomach of a cow, this ancient pouch contained an enzyme called rennet, which helps to digest food as it enters the acidic intestinal cavity. Within the horseman's pouch, the digestive enzymes began to coagulate, curdle, and separate the milk; the warm climate promoted the growth of lactic acid bacteria. The coagulation process solidifies the protein component of milk, leading to the gradual formation of cheese. The lactic acid and other bacteria eat away at the milk sugar, known as lactase, leaving a cheese with a higher fat and lower sugar content. While the sound of a bag of bacteria would scare most modern cheese consumers away, in actuality fermenting cheese is a hostile environment for harmful bacterial growth due to several reasons: 1) Most of the sugar is digested, leaving little fermentable food for the harmful bacteria; 2) The pH is low, a harmful state for some bacteria; 3) Little oxygen is present to support growth; and 4) The salt present creates an inhospitable environment for microorganism growth.[32] In addition, the low levels of oxygen promote anaerobic fermentation, which fuels the conversion of bacterial food to several substances, one of which is butyric acid.

Butyrate, the lesser known healthy fat produced during fermentation, is a short chain fatty acid named after butter, or the Latin term *butyrum*. The substance was discovered in the early 1800s by two French chemists, Henri Braconnot and Michel Eugène Chevreul, both of whom independently described the substance around the same time while experimenting with butter. Like its more famous cousin CLA, butyrate is produced from the fermentation of grass within the stomachs of cows, sheep, and other ruminant animals. Unlike CLA, butyric acid emits a foul odor that is often recognized in vomit, spoiled butter, and wet dogs. Despite its unpleasant smell, butyrate provides a sweet aftertaste and, as discussed previously, is assumed by many to be the secret ingredient in Milton Hershey's chocolate that yields the sweet taste that Americans prefer, as opposed to the darker, richer taste exhibited in European chocolate. Like the ruminants of cows, human colons contain bacteria that ferment indigestible fibers to butyrate through a similar process. Indigestible starches, plant cell walls, seeds, and several other plant components (like the skins and fibrous parts of plants) present in vegetables like onions, Brussels' sprouts, cabbage, and other greens are converted to butyric acid in the far end of the colon. The cells lining of the colon then use the butyrate as a potent energy source. As with the agents used in Dr. Ristow's studies, butyrate is utilized by the mitochondria as an energy source, resulting in improved metabolism, potent anti-inflammatory effects, and other multiple cellular effects that may help ward off cancer.[33,34] Cows produce butyrate from indigestible vegetable products entering their GI tracts; humans convert butyrate on the way out of theirs. Butyrate is like the rent check these bacteria pay us in return for allowing them to reside within our bowels, consummating our symbiotic relationship.

When cows ferment cellulose in grass, they produce CLA and butyrate a step ahead of our bowel bacteria. What we are left with is a cheese or butter with high levels of anti-inflammatory CLA, omega 3 fatty acids, and butyric acid, all of which have been shown to result in several physiologic and cellular changes that tip the scales to reduce the risk of cancer and improve our health. Furthermore, the bacteria-ridden cheese has several components that both feed our bowel bacteria and improve our health. These bacteria then help to breakdown and detoxify potentially harmful chemicals.[35] As described by Elaine Khosrova in *Butter: A Rich History:* "Indulged with a banquet of natural green grass to feed on between late spring and early fall, these roving cows give milk that contains a biochemical bounty. Compared to conventional butter derived from feedlot grain-fed cows, the pasture butter has as much as four times the amount of desirable fatty acids (CLA and omega-3s) as well as a greater pool of subtle flavors, aroma, and healthy nutrients."[36] Furthermore, the characteristic dark color of grass-fed butter results from the carotenoids digested in the grass, which provide the milkfat with beta-carotene, the precursor of vitamin A. Some nutritionists have even considered this a major reason why the French, who eat so much cheese, are so healthy.

Pecorino cheese, on the other hand, is a typical Italian cheese produced from 100% sheep's milk. Often called Pecorino Romano, it at one point served as an essential part of the diet of Roman soldiers due to its transportability and high nutritional density. While the Roman soldiers were merely following orders, recent studies confirm that when individuals follow a similar switch to higher fat foods within their diet, their hunger and cravings drop substantially,[37] a characteristic that would have been valued for a group often left with less than adequate sustenance during battle. This characteristic may be just as valuable for those modern-day individuals who have trouble with appetite control when attempting to lose weight. Furthermore, such a food seems perfect to achieve the Walfordian and Platonic goal of reducing one's overall food consumption for health of both the body and soul.

Various sources from ancient Roman times confirmed that cheesemaking had become a cultured profession to satisfy the expanding palates of the Roman elite. Recipes for cheesemaking can be found in various historical documents, including Cato's *De Agri Cultura* and several other historical cookbooks. Cheese graters were found in the tombs of the buried elite in the Campania area of southern Italy.[38] The Bronze Age ushered in an era when Leonardo's ancestors could grate the hard pecorino cheese to accent their meals. As described by Paul Kindstedt, author of *Cheese and Culture*, "culinary enthusiasts apparently came from all over the Mediterranean to train under the Sicilian masters like Archestratus, and Sicilian chefs were in demand all over the Greek world."[38] In this surging global enthusiasm for food, however, again came Plato and his recommendations for soul searching. This time, however, Plato was more agreeable, as "it was against this backdrop of culinary luxury and extravagance that Plato railed against the gastronomic excesses of Athens, and pined for a return to the simple *opson* (barley and wheat loaves and cake) and *sitos* (olives, cheese, roots, and vegetables, figs, peas, and beans) of the past in his masterpiece *The Republic*."[38] Cheese was not only a method for poor farmers to nourish themselves with nutrient-dense animal foods, but it was also a more philosophically and ethically approved food source for the philosophers and Platonists.

Ironically, cheese, despite its compositional simplicity, illustrates the intricacies when it comes to eating to improve health and to avoid cancer. Full-fat dairy and cheese is incredibly calorically dense, a feature of food that would lead many health professionals to balk at even the thought of promoting it. Yet at the same time, the rich foodstuff provides a plethora of health benefits, including anti-cancer fats that decrease inflammation and comprise many of the building blocks of our cellular structures. Furthermore, full-fat dairy includes a hefty supply of fat-soluble vitamins like A, D, E, and K, which further arm our cells for optimal health, repair, and defense against infections and cancer. Additionally, unlike refined carbohydrates full-fat cheese has low amounts of insulin-stimulating sugar, likely satisfying the criteria of Dr. Ludwig and others whose research is based on the insulin theory of obesity. And to top it off, full-fat cheese tastes exceptional and alleviates hunger, allowing those who partake in it to spontaneously eat less and maximize their metabolism.

Beyond the health benefits of well-sourced dairy, its ecclesiastic promotion is more aligned with a more global worldview, as opposed to the western worship of bread. For example, while Jesus fasted for 40 days in the desert, Zoroaster, according to Pliny the Elder, was claimed to have survived in the Persian desert for twenty years on cheese alone. This sustenance on cheese apparently allowed Zoroaster to avoid overindulgence and remain young. One sect of Christianity known as the Artotyrites even offered cheese along with the standard bread during the holy Eucharist in mass; their actions came from the belief that the first humans offered food products from both the earth and sheep.

In ancient Sumerian culture, the goddess Inanna held many important positions of power to oversee humanity, including governing the natural cycle of the seasons and enforcing divine justice. The Sumerian equivalent of the Greek Aphrodite, Inanna was the goddess of love, beauty, war, and several other ingredients in the recipe of impassioned living. When Inanna had to choose a human spouse, she passed on the grain farmer Enkimdu and instead chose Dumuzi, after he offered her a life filled with cream, ghee (clarified butter), fermented milk, butter, and cheese. Bread may have won over the west, but the east was beholden to butter. Not far away in ancient India, the Vedic texts were littered with references to cheese and ghee regarding their importance in both health and religion.

While bread – the "soul food" of antiquity and western philosophical thought – was promoted for its philosophical and physical emptiness, numerous instances of cheese references are scattered throughout both eastern and western historical and religious texts. For instance, the Bible reports that while serving in his father King Saul's army, David – who would eventually slay Goliath – would receive grains and bread from his father to snack on and share with his brothers. To the commander of David's army, however, Saul would send ten cheeses – a far greater gesture. More dense foods like properly formed butter and cheese contain several key ingredients for a sturdy, healthy, and nutritious source of sustenance; many cultures understood this potential and modern science now backs these views.

Poor Southern Italians like Leonardo relied on nutrient-dense and calorically-dense foods to provide them with the largest bang for their buck. Eating empty foods, while surely promoted by Plato for strengthening the soul, was illogical for those individuals that were barely getting by. Lard, for instance, served as a major source of fat for Leonardo. Cheese, on the other hand, provided an artisanal source of nutrients and flavor. For example, Leonardo's pecorino, like cheeses of other Southern Italian locales often contained black peppercorn and thus came to be known as Pecorino Pepato; nowadays, pecorino from Calabria is referred to as Pecorino Crotonese, and is now even certified by the *Denominazione di Origine Protetta* and carries the mark "DOP" on its label.

Throughout history, cheese and dairy have literally and figuratively remained a soft spot for philosophers and physicians alike. When Plato recommended the avoidance of meat in pursuit of a lower fat, non-nutrient-dense diet, he hedged his bets when it came to cheese and dairy. Even the modern Mediterranean diet, often touted as a low-fat diet, contains a long list of dairy fat and cheese sources numbering in the hundreds and containing many of the same products that filled the shelves of Leonardo's shop.[39] From a health perspective, cheese has typically been viewed as a simple mixture of protein and calcium, yet the health benefits of cheese could not be further from those two subcomponents. Cheese also contains medium chain triglycerides (MCTs), the mid-sized fats that improve metabolism, enhance energy expenditure, decrease hunger, and increase the metabolism of adipose tissue to reduce obesity.[40] Conjugated linoleic acid, butyric acid, and omega-3s comprise dairy's trifecta of anti-inflammatory fats, and cheese also contains several other components that work as building blocks for cellular growth and recovery. Calcium may have a well-known reputation as the building block of our bones, but without vitamin D and vitamin K2 – both found heavily in dairy fat – this calcium would simply float around in our arteries and cause damage; Vitamin D and K2 extract calcium to help ensure it ends up in our bones, instead of collecting in our arteries and increasing the risk of atherosclerosis. While K2 can be found in all forms of butter, studies suggest that the butter from grass-fed cows contains significantly larger amounts. As with butyric acid and CLA, vitamin K2 is produced during bacterial fermentation, so aged cheese is imparted with a significant amount of K2 as well. Other foods containing ample K2 include egg yolks, organ meats, and fermented soybeans, known as *nattō*.

Properly made cheese and full-fat dairy creates a healthy food product with benefits that Plato, Pythagoras, Kenyon, and Kritchevsky alike would all agree upon. Unknowingly, Leonardo was stocking his store's shelves with anti-cancer foods: products with low amounts of insulin-stimulating sugar, high levels of anti-inflammatory fats, and moderate levels of protein.

⁝

Like many other European immigrants, Leonardo continued his time-tested and cultural practices of producing homemade cheese, wine, and soppressata. To this day, the basement of Leonardo's former home still contains a massive concrete drum molded to the floor where he would place his crushed grapes every autumn to ferment into his homemade wine. Unbeknownst to Leonardo, his cheesemaking process would create a likely Kenyon-approved delicacy absent of nearly all sugar and carbohydrates and full of fat with minimal protein. The remainder of the cheese was comprised of about three-fourths fat and just a quarter protein. Other dairy products like milk and low-fat dairy can stimulate significant insulin release; fattier dairy sources like heavy cream and Leonardo's full-fat cheese elicit much less of an insulin response. The latter Calabrian cheese also contains high levels of anti-inflammatory fats like CLA and butyric acid, along with a hefty amount of calcium, zinc, phosphorous, and Vitamins A, B, and D. While these healthy components are not limited to pecorino cheese, the nutritive value herein helps to further explain why Roman soldiers would carry wheels of pecorino with them in their marches to battle. Unfortunately, other processed low-fat or no-fat cheese sources have most of these benefits removed, leaving a high-protein, high-carbohydrate caricature of cheese that would have been frowned upon by the Roman Legion and rebuked for its minimal health benefits. Consumption of this imposter version of cheese also results in a much higher insulin response by the pancreas and instead signals many of the pro-cancer pathways discussed previously.

The emasculation of butter, cheese, and full-fat dairy reached a zenith during the anti-fat crusades of the late 20th century, but this campaign is only a microcosm of the entire story of dairy. History is littered with similar instances of resistance to dairy fat, based more so on religious and financial motives than on tangible health rationale. For example, butter met substantial resistance in Italy – and especially in Leonardo's Southern Italy – during the Middle Ages, at the hands of the highly influential Roman Catholic Church. To promote olive oil – an often-unaffordable luxury at the time in the south – fats like butter and the mainstay lard were condoned by the Church. Centuries later, few foodstuffs like dairy products still ignite modern-day controversies when it comes to diet, health, and cancer. The controversial view of managing our insulin/IGF axis via our diet choices fully encompasses this longstanding controversy, along with several of the missteps encountered along the way.

Skim milk may provide the best example of these missteps taken over the past several decades, along with tendencies to be supported more by ideology than physiology. To produce skim milk, the original fatty cream is "skimmed" from the top. Nowadays however, this result is generally achieved by centrifugation, which spins the heavier fat globules out of the milk via a more time-efficient process. The fat-soluble vitamins are extricated along with the cream, leaving a liquid comprised of mostly protein and sugar in the form of lactose. This version has been recommended as a healthy alternative to full fat milk or cream for decades, yet it would end up on the losing cellular side when it comes to insulin/IGF-1 and several other cellular growth pathways. Furthermore, while dairy fat is associated with higher insulin sensitivity, less abdominal obesity, higher HDL cholesterol, lower triglycerides, and lower markers of inflammation like C-reactive protein,[41] it is unclear what benefit would accompany the fat-free liquid left behind after the skimming process. Much like with bread, pasta, and many other less-dense and nutrient-sparse foods, the low-fat version of this milk is less substantial and may lead to a Plato-disapproved overconsumption of more food afterwards.

As David Ludwig phrased it, "The substitution of sweetened reduced-fat milk for unsweetened whole milk — which lowers saturated fat by 3 g but increases sugar by 13 g per cup — clearly undermines diet quality, especially in a population with excessive sugar consumption."[42] Furthermore, "in the 1960s, children may have had a glass of whole milk and 2 cookies for an afternoon snack. But a kid today might have 3 or 4 cookies as part of the snack, because nonfat milk is less filling."[43] Ludwig's comments are not without scientific support and likely explain why children who consume considerable amounts of skim milk experience higher rates of obesity during adulthood.[44] The much more substantial full fat dairy, on the other hand, is associated with a lower risk of obesity.[45]

Besides its beneficial effects on mitigating hunger, dairy fat would also be expected to have a nontrivial impact on these "growth" effects of our cells and fatty tissue. Studies support this: dairy fat consumption is associated with a strong decrease in the risk of type 2 diabetes,[46] a metabolic state leading to elevated levels of both blood sugar and insulin along with inflammation.[47] While we must be careful when assessing these population studies, the general bias against fat renders these findings quite intriguing. Additionally, elevated serum markers of digested dairy fat are associated with a lower risk of heart attack.[48] Such findings are unsurprising, as the anti-inflammatory compounds of well-sourced dairy are stored within lipids throughout the body and, much like a fire hydrant, serve as a local source to smother inflammation.

When assessing the remainder of our diet, the slaying of several nutritional sacred cows that occurs while considering dairy provides critical lessons that can be applied to other foods. Relying on nutrient-sparse foods, or those with the nutrient density removed, often leaves us with a tendency to crave nourishment and then in the end leaves our cells starved with an appetite to grow. Attempting to follow a nutritious and healthy diet and somehow lower our body's desired levels of IGF-1 further demonstrates the complications that arise. That being said, the whirlwind of dietary studies over the past century coupled with Plato's dogmatic views provide us with clues on how to optimize the difficult balance while avoiding Walford's missteps and the misery in Minnesota. The calorie restriction that worked so well to reduce cancer in Tannenbaum's mice is also effective at reducing IGF-1 in overfed and obese mice. This benefit has translated to other animals as well, though any effect in humans other than the misery of hunger pangs has yet to be proven. Calorie restriction seems less effective at increasing those proteins that bind and inactivate IGF-1 to thwart its tendency to promote excessive cellular growth. The method of calorie restriction that may be effective at lowering IGF-1 in humans occurs during sickness: intestinal malabsorption syndromes, gastrointestinal issues, or severe malnourishment depresses IGF-1, with an impact so strong that low IGF-1 is actually a method to test for these disorders.[49,50] Recalling that IGF-1 is strongly affected by many vitamins and nutrients, this correlation is to be expected, and a nutritious diet complete with adequate vitamins and nutrients will avoid malnourishment, however, a normal elevation in IGF-1 will ensue.

This latter point is an important one – states that nourish the body will often eliminate the ability to manipulate and lower certain hormones, like IGF-1. While we can readily over-nourish a cancer cell, starving it while still nourishing our normal cells remains a daunting challenge. Yet, with the failure of caloric restriction to lower IGF-1 has come a measure of success, as it has led scientists to attempt other dietary and lifestyle methods of manipulation. These strategies include intermittent fasting or the isolated restriction of a macronutrient, like carbohydrates, fat, or protein.

While most of the benefits of calorie restriction in animals – improved longevity and decreased cancer risk – have failed to translate to humans, lowering IGF-1 is one of the items that can be added to the crossover list. Protein restriction or the avoidance of protein overconsumption, on the other hand, may be one of the more effective strategies observed in humans. For instance, when scientists place individuals on a lower protein diet as opposed to feeding them pecorino cheese in the previously mentioned study, serum IGF-1 levels fall. To be exact, switching from a daily protein average of 1.67 g/kg of body weight to 0.95 g/kg for 3 weeks causes a drop in serum IGF-1 from 194 ng/mL to 152 ng/mL.[51] The switch would equate to about 0.4 grams of daily protein per pound of bodyweight, or about 75 grams for a 175 pound person.

Reiterating our prior discussion, some have theorized that switching from animal to plant protein would lower IGF-1 due to the differing amino acid composition of each. Plant protein, excluding beans, is low in methionine, an essential amino acid that can increase IGF-1.[52] Population studies may support this theory, as vegans – who by definition consume no animal products – have lower levels of IGF-1 when compared to individuals that adhere to the standard American diet.[53] These findings are not that helpful, as most studies reveal that ANY switch away from the standard American diet improves health. Furthermore, studies have yet to directly compare a switch from an animal to plant-based protein diet to test changes in IGF-1 in a Bradford Hill-approved trial. So far, some data reveal the opposite metabolic effect: a switch from a plant-based protein diet to one based on animal proteins improves insulin sensitivity, insulin levels, and blood glucose in type 2 diabetics.[54] And of course, other studies show the opposite. In reality, any difference between the two is minimal.[55] As protein remains a vital requirement by the human body for growth and repair, data may suggest that we avoid overconsuming it, but keep it as part of a well-rounded diet. Promoting veganism as a method to lower IGF-1 is not supported by substantial data. Furthermore, the avoidance of all animal products should be considered with caution: vegetarian diets often result in malnourishment and deficiencies of several nutrients that are present in animal-based foods and vital for both optimal cellular function and repair and optimal brain function, including vitamins A, B12, and K2, iron, zinc, and the omega-3 fatty acids DHA and EPA.[56-58] Though controversial, low levels of these essential nutrients are felt by many to be contributing factors to the unusually high rates of depression, psychologic disorders, and suicides in vegan and vegetarian dieters.[59-63] Furthermore, some studies have linked vegetarian and vegan diets with higher incidences of cancer, allergies, mental health disorders, an elevated requirement for health care, and a poorer quality of life.[64]

In other words, vegetarians and vegan diets take considerable effort to ensure proper nutrients are acquired through the diet. While certainly achievable with some additional supplementation – for example, B12, a necessary vitamin, is found in animal products but may be ingested in pill form – many practicing individuals often miss the mark. Our body requires dense sources of nutrients to function optimally, and purposefully limiting them in an attempt to lower an isolated hormone like IGF-1 has severe health consequences. As the production of IGF-1 is increased by many required vitamins and nutrients like zinc, selenium, and magnesium,[65] malnourishment that often accompanies veganism may be at least partially responsible for any theoretical drop in IGF-1.

Since general calorie restriction has thus far failed to reduce IGF-1, some researchers have hypothesized that intermittent fasting could be more effective and more pleasant. If an overall reduction of calories is ineffective in eliciting these metabolic changes in humans, then perhaps a Spartanesque defined period without any food would be extreme enough to elicit the desired metabolic changes. Less miserable than overall fasting, intermittent fasting allows individuals to go without food for an extended period, ranging from eight hours to several days. A moderate fast would involve eating an early dinner and then abstaining from food until lunch the following day. Many fasters continue to drink their morning coffee and follow an otherwise normal morning routine; for them, shorter periods without any food are more pleasurable than the constant attempt to deprive the body of food. Furthermore, a diet and lifestyle that leaves blood sugar levels relatively stable and avoids peaks and valleys makes these fasts much easier – at least anecdotally – as appetite is less of a concern.

Calorie restriction and fasting successfully lower IGF-1 in animals.[66] In humans, however, IGF-1 does not drop during moderate periods without food. Prolonged periods of fasting,[67] reminiscent of the extreme dietary regimen in the Minnesota Starvation Study, may reduce IGF-1 levels. However, as with intestinal malabsorption syndromes and other nutritional deficiencies, this reduction is most likely from the malnutrition that accompanies the extended fast. Additionally, even in animals, levels normalize quickly when the fast ends.

Despite the failures, these negative studies have exposed some additional benefits of fasting. During the period without food, insulin levels plummet and the amount of the binding protein IGFBP-1 increases, helping to inactivate free IGF-1. Furthermore, during the fast, the body begins to break down its fatty tissue for energy, leaving fasters leaner and more metabolically fit.[68] As observed in Ristow's studies, the decrease in energy availability during the fast signals to AMPK to initiate mitochondrial fat burning to provide fuel for the cell. Blood sugar drops and the mitochondria turn toward our own fat for their energetic meal. During this process, the mitochondria churn away like a furnace, producing free radicals that engage the cell's defense system to produce antioxidants to counterbalance any potential damage. The insulin pathway decreases, activating many of the longevity mechanisms Kenyon described in her studies. Throughout this process, blood sugar continues to decrease, and eventually the body begins to rely on alternate energy sources known as ketones. A metabolic reliance on ketones, the energy substrates that improved cognition in Mattson's multiple studies, further reduce the insulin/IGF-1 pathway as the amount of glucose and insulin within the blood drops.[69] Lastly, the fast itself signals a low energy state to our cells, activating several mechanisms like DNA damage repair and autophagy that prompt our good cells to cannibalize potentially cancerous ones.[68] In other words, fasts may not directly lower IGF-1, but they result in a handful of advantageous global metabolic changes that leave the cellular environment more inhospitable to cancer growth. So, despite their often-misleading influence on diet and health, Plato and the ancient religious, philosophical, and cultural figures of history strongly endorsed fasting, which may have been their greatest contribution when it comes to modern health.

Beyond the metabolic benefits of intermittent periods of avoiding food, others have attempted to parse out which foods leave us the best equipped metabolically to fight cancer and achieve optimal health. Certain foods have a propensity to increase insulin, glucose, and IGF-1, creating a hospitable environment for the germination and growth of unwanted diseases; scientists have attempted a wide range of studies to test which foods are the most culpable. Initial studies paid homage to the days of the adoration of skim milk, attempting to lower IGF-1 with a low-fat, high-carbohydrate diet; running counter to the accessible scientific data at the time, such attempts predictably failed. If anything, they were a pyrrhic victory in that they revealed the strong prevailing bias within the nutritional world for even attempting a study of this nature. Other studies confirm further missteps – a low-fat diet in women increases IGF-1 and reduces binding proteins to offset IGF-1, yielding a double negative effect by promoting both the insulin/IGF axis and cancer.[69] Such attempts may pay homage to Plato, Pythagoras, and Kellogg, but in reality they are effective only at illustrating the bizarre strategies employed within the dietary world. Somewhere along way, the intimate connection between low-fat foods, carbohydrates – and especially simple carbohydrates – and their ability to increase blood sugar levels, promote insulin production, and stimulate the insulin/IGF pathway became obscured by bias. It was almost as if the settling dust from the Food Pyramid fiasco covered much of the data supporting a beneficial role of fat in the diet, especially when it came to cancer. Or perhaps was it Plato's invisible hand covering up the implicating role of insulin in cancer development, merely to divert people's attention away from those foods?

While carbohydrates have been intimately linked to insulin, reduction of dietary protein has been a major target for reducing IGF-1. There is some support for this rationale, and it is likely reasonable to avoid consistently overindulging in either of these macronutrients. The exact amount of protein to consume remains elusive; being that protein is a vital nutrient, recommending the general population to minimize it is a cause for concern. On average, Americans eat 1-1.3 grams of protein per kilogram of bodyweight per day (or 0.46-0.59 g per pound body weight, for those of us not on the metric system), according to the National Health and Nutrition Examination Survey from 2003-2004.[70] If you are a 185 pound male, this equates to about 85-109g of protein per day. The Institute of Medicine (IOM), which is tasked with the nearly impossible job of creating the Dietary

Reference Index, recommends 0.8 g per kg bodyweight, or 0.36 g per lb. For a 185-pound male, this would be about 67 g of protein per day, an amount much lower than what the average American is consuming. The IOM must consistently navigate the stormy seas of internal politics, dogma, science, and civic government pressure to compile one-size-fits-all dietary recommendations for the entire population. On account of that, it is unclear how much weight or importance we as individuals should place on certain subsets of the IOM's recommendations.

In other words, these protein amounts are for average Americans, of whom less than 20% achieve the daily recommended exercise amount. While for them it may be reasonable to consume between 0.8-1 g/kg of protein per day (0.36-0.59 g/lb),[51] most of us – especially if we are exercising and lifting weights – may not need to worry as much about protein, especially since the overall effect on IGF-1 may be minimal. For instance, when postmenopausal women eating 1.1 g/kg of protein per day – already higher than the values above – were given an additional 30 g of daily whey protein supplement to intentionally *increase* IGF-1, it only rose by 5% at year one and then decreased by year two.[71] Dr. Rainer Klement, who has extensively researched and reviewed the effects of protein and carbohydrate within the diet and the capacity of insulin and IGF-1 to promote cancer, has found that both humans and mice are sensitive to dietary carbohydrate and protein in regards to their effect on insulin and IGF-1.[72] However, mice seem to be exquisitely sensitive to protein, while humans are more sensitive to carbohydrates. This characteristic may be rooted in our past – humans have been omnivores for most of their evolution and consumed generally low-carbohydrate diets, while the diet of mice has been nearly the opposite.

Like most physiologic aspects of the human body, IGF-1 involves a fine interplay of countless factors that impact our risk of cancer but allow us to function optimally with the greatest overall health. The only conclusion we can make from the current state of the data is to avoid too much or too little. Protein overconsumption can enhance IGF-1, even to levels that may promote cancer. Lack of protein consumption can lead to muscle wasting, decreased bone strength, and cognitive decline. Striking a balance is the most sensible approach. Recommending the switch from animal to plant protein may make sense if we are eating protein in excess; for individuals not overindulging however – ones eating healthy greens and fats and properly selecting animal foods that provide a plethora of vital nutrients and vitamins

– this endorsement is not appreciably supported by any up-to-date scientific data.

On the other hand, breads, pastas, sugary sweets, skim milk, and even grains are digested to simpler forms of sugar, eventually finding their way into our blood stream and shuttled into our cells under the aid of insulin. These same "less dense" foods were responsible for cancer induction in Van Alstyne and Beebe's study as well as with several other groundbreaking studies by their peers. Tangible mechanisms, a major missing element of earlier calorie restriction studies, accounted for this environment conducive to cancerous growth as the increase in insulin and the subsequent growth mechanisms were to blame. Kritchevsky not only hinted at this instrument of cancer growth but also made a strong plea for further studies testing this and other mechanisms. There remains no tangible mechanism by which calorie restriction may improve these metabolic factors in an individual that is not overeating, yet for some reason this myopic view of calorie restriction as the solution continues to linger throughout the medical field, and foods that may be less calorically-dense but create metabolic mayhem regardless of calories continue to be promoted.

With the laundry list of the vital functions IGF-1 serves in our cells, muscles, bones, brains, and bodies, we should feel justified in questioning any recommendation to minimize its creation and presence in our bodies. Moreover, the potential anti-cancer and pro-longevity benefits of IGF-1 reduction remain unproven in humans. Even if successful methods to reduce IGF-1 in animals translated to humans, the potential downsides are plenty. Severe calorie restriction, for example, increases our risk for vitamin deficiency and malnutrition, and severe calorie restriction leads to muscle loss and a lifestyle that would be too miserable for most to endure. This realization that these difficult and often miserable lifestyle changes are ineffective should be celebrated. In other words, we can enjoy our delicious and nutrient-dense foods while remaining healthy and fostering a cellular environment inhospitable to disease and cancer. We do not need to torture ourselves to be healthy; it is unbearable for most people to comply with a nutrient-sparse diet, avoid meat, and abstain from all animal products. It is no surprise that Haddad and Tanzman found that less than 1% of vegetarians truly avoid meat. It is also unsurprising that 84% of vegans and vegetarians return to eating meat, with the vast majority attributing their switch back to the worsening of their health.[73] The majority of vegetarians cite concerns about the treatment of animals as their reason for attempting their diet, which is certainly a noble cause.[74] However, from a health point of view, it is good news that vegetarianism, veganism, extreme calorie restriction, counting calories, fat-restriction, and other misguided, unpleasant, and difficult diets are unsupported by the current science. So, we can more fully enjoy our food and the health it brings us.

10

WALKING THE BLUE ZONE

"Without a struggle, there can be no progress."

- Frederick Douglass

Takeaways:

Several previously discussed metabolic pathways, including IGF-1, are discussed, focusing on the double-edged sword and intricacies of each. Furthermore, they are explored in the context of exercise and physical activity to illustrate how these vital, but potentially negative, processes can be turned into mechanisms that make us stronger and more able to defend against cancer and other health risks.

Exercise and tangible lifestyle changes are also addressed, including their influence on Nrf2 and AMP-Kinase (AMPK). Both are activated from certain eating patterns and intense activities, and both aid in the repair of our cells and DNA.

As Leonardo Pesce unloaded the pungent Southern Italian cheese from his wagon, the perspiration formed an array of beads upon his forehead. At just over five feet tall, Leonardo was never a particularly imposing figure, nor had he ever harbored any false aspirations of being one. In fact, he was a typical vertically challenged Southern Italian managing to punch above his weight when it came to strength and stamina, particularly on days like this when he deftly and tirelessly unloaded hundreds of pounds of goods and brought them into his grocery store.

Today, however, Leonardo had taken extra measures to account for his non-menacing stature. As he was stocking the shelves, he heard a click behind him as the front door opened. A young man dressed in a pair of pleated pants with a matching suit coat and fedora hat slowly sauntered into the store. Leonardo caught a glimpse of the man in his peripheral vision, and his muscles tensed. With a smug tone in his voice, the mysterious man asked, "So... have you given our proposition some thought?" Leonardo, ignoring the question, quickly made a beeline for the back store wall, occupied with shelves stocked with various foods and jars. The time between each pounding beneath Leonardo's chest began to shorten as he moved a jar aside, exposing a revolver resting sideways. Leonardo abruptly placed the shiny metal pistol into his right palm; as the chrome shook violently in his hand, he eventually mustered up the courage to turn, point the object at the well-dressed man, and scream in his broken English, "You come back again, I shoot you!"

Leonardo's endeavors to provide the local Italian community with their traditional foodstuffs was proving itself successful. His daughter recalls spending Saturdays turning 40 or more pounds of pork into Italian sausage, only to watch it fly off the shelves of Leonardo's store days later. His namesake grocery store, Pesce's, had become a well-known staple and weekly destination for the community, and McKees Rocks had grown from a banana republic under the shackles of the Presston slaughterhouse to a thriving Italian suburban community. Unfortunately – as was the case in many Italian communities throughout the United States at the time – the prosperity also attracted a wave of nefarious characters who, through duplicity and intimidation, sought to strongarm their way into stealing rather than earning their share of the growing economic pie. Prohibition ushered in the era of gangsters, grifters, and bootleggers, and McKees Rocks – with its sizable population of wine-making Southern Italians – became a hotbed for illicit alcohol-related activities. Al Capone himself would make frequent liquor runs to the area with his crew and was once even spotted walking down the street in front of Pesce's. A gang known as the Black Hand targeted Italian immigrants like Leonardo in Pittsburgh at the same time the more infamous La Cosa Nostra terrorized larger cities like New York and Chicago, and small-time Mafia impersonators ran their rackets in smaller suburban towns like McKees Rocks. On the heels of Capone's success, these offshoot wannabes offered Leonardo a deal: if he provided them a percentage of his profits, they would ensure that no other competing grocery stores would be opened. To this, Leonardo had calmly but firmly responded: "Anyone can open any store they like... This is America!" Needless to say, the local mob was incensed by this insubordination and sought to ratchet up the intimidation; and so, Leonardo found himself here in this moment, the cold steel of his last resort violently trembling in his farm-weathered hands as he boldly threatened this faux mobster's life.

The mysterious man backed down, smirked, turned around in silence, and slowly ambled out the front door of the shop. Leonardo had won this showdown, but it was obvious to him that this would not be the last time he would have to draw his pistol at these newfound enemies.

Leonardo closed up shop for the day and took to the streets for his customary walk home. Walking was his preferred mode of transport as he walked to and from his shop nearly every day. In fact, much like his countrymen in Calabria and across the Mediterranean region, Leonardo walked nearly everywhere.

In the book *The Blue Zones: 9 Lessons for Living Longer from the People Who've Lived the Longest*, author Dan Buettner travels to towns near Leonardo's hometown of San Lorenzo – Ikaria, Greece, and several villages along the island of Sardinia – to analyze the habits of some of the longest-lived humans in the world. Furthermore, Buettner traveled to Okinawa, Japan and other global hotbeds of longevity to gather more comprehensive data to test his hypotheses. Several longevity-prone communities scattered around Italy could have been included, though a book entirely on Italy would likely have been less appealing to global readers. Regardless, the large number of centenarians throughout Italy would certainly have provided enough data points for an impactful study on longevity. For instance, in Acciaroli, a town near Leonardo's San Lorenzo, it is estimated that one in ten villagers lives past the age of 100.[1] In 2011, census data revealed that there are now more than 15,000 centenarians in Italy.

Throughout *The Blue Zones*, a general theme percolates: groups of people throughout the world who live the longest are ones who are also the most active. Buettner, a National Geographic Fellow, received a grant from the National Institute of Aging to travel the globe, interviewing members of those groups of people that are the longest lived in the world. He also founded a travel and exploration company that has voyaged through many areas that house the origins of Western Civilization. As such, he is arguably more qualified than anyone to tell the story of what makes the world's longest living people so long-lived.

Time and time again he encounters Leonardo-esque characters, such as 102-year-old Giuseppe Mura from Silanus, a small village in the Gennargentu Mountains of Sardinia. Buettner describes his interviews with Mura at length. For instance, upon suspicions that Buettner wants money from him, Mura tells his interviewer to "go to hell," shedding light on the realities of his life over the past century. Like Leonardo, a former shepherd by trade, Mura would spend 16 hours a day following his flock or tilling the earth. Then he would also spend much of the evenings socializing, eating pecorino cheese made from the milk of grass-fed sheep, and drinking up to a liter of wine per day (during the interview, Buettner and his subjects were served both wine and prosciutto). Later in the book, Buettner interviews Giovanni Sannai, a 103-year-old who beats Buettner in an arm-wrestling match and then gleefully explains that he "drank goat's milk for breakfast, walked at least six miles a day, and loved to work."

The colorful tidbits of information Buettner gathers across his numerous interviews consistently emphasize the importance of exercise and thus explain why he strongly promotes walking as a health-enhancing activity. And rightly so: studies reveal that women who are more active experience less breast cancer[2] and more broadly that exercise can help all humans to maintain a more normal weight and reduce excess body fat.[3,4]

It should be noted, however, that Buettner's views on exercise may be slightly biased – after all, he does hold three Guinness records for endurance cycling. Indeed, while many in the past have considered long-winded grueling exercise to be the key to health – with all due respect, it does NOT seem that Buettner subscribes to this – it appears that a mixture of low intensity activity (i.e. walking) intermixed with periods of more intense activity (i.e. walking up a steep mountain chasing your sheep or lifting hundreds of pounds of cheese wheels) might be most healthy and least detrimental to our joints.[5] In fact, the intensity of our activities and our exercise habits may lead to different benefits and results. During more intense exercise, including the type that requires sudden bursts of activity, sugar is pulled from our blood and into our cells, and glycogen within our muscle is burned for energy.[6] Less intense activity, on the other hand, gradually primes our cells to burn away at our fat tissue for use as fuel for our mitochondria. Simply following one of these shepherds around during a normal day's work provides an adequate glimpse across the spectrum of healthy activity levels. Studies reveal that we can expect benefits from intense activities like heavy lifting, walking up sharp inclines, and sprinting, along with other benefits from less intense activities like riding a bicycle, performing household chores, and especially, walking.[7]

Unbeknownst to Leonardo, Giuseppe, and Giovanni themselves, men like these are masters of the exercise research world, as their typical activities lead to several physiologic and metabolic changes that prime their bodies to be healthy, cancer-fighting machines. A single bout of high-intensity exercise begins to break down the small amount of sugar that is stored within our muscles and liver in the form of glycogen. The sugar in our blood is rapidly pulled into exercising muscle cells to be metabolized as fuel. Consequently, our bodies experience a substantial lowering of blood sugar levels and insulin sensitivity is enhanced.[8] In actuality, these effects may have little impact on weight loss, but instead provide our cells with marked improvements in their metabolic machinery, which fosters an inhospitable environment for cancer cells. Furthermore, low-intensity exercise like walking enhances our bodies' insulin sensitivity and begins to breakdown fatty acids for energy derivation, and, these metabolic changes even persist well into the following day after exercise.[9] In other words, significant low-level activity interspersed with bouts of more intense exercise and the lifting of heavy objects – resistance training, as it is known in the scientific world – provide similar metabolic changes that occur during fasting and other dietary habits that do not supply our body with an endless supply of sugar to fuel our dropping blood glucose. Much like in Kenyon and Ristow's studies, the falling blood sugar elicits several cellular changes that engage a metabolic switch, priming our cells to fight disease and cancer.

⁖

Prior to his death, Kritchevsky, on his way to becoming one of the most influential cancer and nutrition researchers in the 20th century, contributed to several notable publications on cancer and nutrition and innumerable research studies connecting diet and cancer. He sought to make sense of the jumbled alphabet soup that was prevailing within the research world by openly discussing blossoming studies on diet and cancer and the underlying mechanisms that were being elucidated by the new wave of interest in the field of nutrition. While awareness of the cancerous effects of excessive insulin and IGF-1 was gaining ground within the cancer world, several other mechanisms began to show promise in the fight against cancer. As Kritchevsky noted in his book *Cancer and Nutrition* and also in his scientific article *The Effect of Over- and Undernutrition on Cancer*,[10] simply reducing the amount of food that mice consumed led to the reduction of the many cancerous mechanisms that we have discussed, yet the *enhancement* of several mechanisms that offset cellular damage may have been even more important.

As Kritchevsky noted, the reduction of certain nutrients increases cellular ability to repair DNA damage and enhance antioxidant production. Furthermore, he noted that these dietary changes "may provide a simple and inexpensive approach to reducing the risk of cancer in man." However, the initial notion that by significantly reducing the amount of food provided to these mice scientists were "starving" their cancer, began to appear outdated. Like the decrease in tumor formation that accompanied reduced insulin availability, a mechanism was activated during these dietary changes that enabled cells to battle damage and initiate repairs when the fight was ineffective.

The work of many relatively unknown researchers before this time found that other altered environments could decrease spontaneous tumor development in mice. For instance, in 1949 Tannenbaum found that housing mice at temperatures well below normal conditions, from 45-55° F, suppressed the formation of breast tumors.[11] He also found that the potentially toxic chemicals 2,4 dinitrophenol and sodium fluoride decreased the development of lung tumors. Whereas chemicals like DMBA were causing cancer, other potentially toxic chemicals seemed to be preventing it.

Dinitrophenol, or DNP, was used as a dietary supplement in the 1920s and 30s, as flapper girls in speakeasies found that it resulted in accelerated weight loss. DNP works by uncoupling our mitochondria; in other words, it allows protons to leak through a portion of the mitochondria, bypassing their normal routes and leading to the production of heat instead of energy. At the elevated temperature, the mitochondria then burn more and more fuel as they press to produce additional ATP to replenish the energy supply of the cell. As they continue to rev up their production – rather inefficiently, it should be noted – cellular metabolic rate rapidly intensifies, ultimately leading to weight loss as fat is burned within the proverbial cellular furnace. Those '20s flapper girls taking DNP would experience significant weight loss, and in particular fat loss. That being said, the benefits of DNP were offset by the side effects: the excessive heat production could possibly lead to death. And actually, this happened far too often during this era, which prompted the removal of DNP from store shelves in 1938.

Fluoride – that same well-known chemical added to drinking water and toothpaste to help fight cavities – works similarly, albeit by a different mechanism. Instead of placing the mitochondria on overdrive like DNP, fluoride directly increases free radical damage within the mitochondria, resulting in the subsequent activation of counter mechanisms to offset this potential damage. For instance, fluoride promotes oxidative stress within our mitochondria and the production of superoxide, a free radical so potent that our own cells use it to kill invading microbes. Well aware of the lethal properties of superoxide, our cells produce an antagonist called superoxide dismutase to disarm the cellular terrorist. What Tannenbaum had discovered, knowingly or not, was that both chemicals stressed the energetic mechanisms of our cells, eliciting significant downstream effects.

Recent studies reveal that this potential detrimental increase in oxidative stress imparted on the mitochondria with chemicals – first done by Tannenbaum in 1949, and more recently through several other dietary and lifestyle "stresses" – rouses a compensatory response of antioxidants, arming the cell with an enhanced ability to fight potential cancer-promoting DNA-damage from free radicals. With the focus squarely on calories during Tannenbaum's time, the benefit from these ancillary chemicals was felt to be from their metabolic enhancement and propensity to mimic an energy and thus calorie deficit. However, what Tannenbaum did not realize was that his study had now bridged the data from the first half of the twentieth century with the future of dietary studies for the prevention of cancer.

While Leonardo had never even entered a speakeasy – let alone thought about taking DNP like the flappers years later – he certainly provided his cells a similar stress simply through the lifestyle he chose. Anyone who has traveled to Sardinia, Greece, or Southern Italy can attest that the locals' view of walking is quite different from what we are used to in America. As Leonardo scaled the mountains of San Lorenzo, his "walk" was far more like a traditional leg workout at today's gym, due to the requirement of intense muscular contraction to propel him up the hill. This muscular contraction is a key component of the benefits of exercise and physical activity. While fatty tissue on our body works like an endocrine organ secreting inflammatory hormones that can foster a hospitable environment for cancerous growth, our muscles work in opposition to adipose tissue by releasing anti-inflammatory hormones. Furthermore, when we contract our muscles during activities and lifting heavy objects, they burn ATP for energy, which provides similar benefits to those seen in Tannenbaum's DNP and fluoride studies.

Similar to the results of Ristow supplying his experimental cells with frataxin, when cells within our muscles consume ATP the cellular energy accountant AMPK is activated. ATP, when used for energy, is converted to AMP. As the ratio of ATP/AMP decreases, AMPK jumps to action to produce more ATP to fuel the cell and improve this ratio. The response to this change is key: during low energy states – for example, during fasting, a drop in insulin during carbohydrate restriction, or ketosis – AMPK activates several metabolic changes including: 1) The breakdown of glycogen and pulling of sugar from our blood and into our cells to be used as energy; 2) The breakdown of fat, cholesterol, and triglycerides for use as energy; 3) The increase in insulin sensitivity (i.e. less is needed); 4) The construction of more mitochondria to produce energy, known as mitochondrial biogenesis; 5) The increase in antioxidant mechanisms to offset the free radical production of our mitochondria; and 6) The decrease in the mTOR pathway.[12] The last of these processes inactivates another cellular growth mechanism known as mTOR, which has been implicated in the progression of several cancers including prostate cancer.[13] In fact, this mechanism is so vital to cancer initiation and progression that blocking mTOR is currently a widespread cancer treatment.[14] Increasing insulin levels on the other hand works to blunt the anti-cancer effects of decreasing mTOR.

Through the normal activities of his daily life, Leonardo may have been channeling ancient cellular mechanisms to improve his overall health. Other studies connect the benefits of exercise and similar dietary strategies to signal low energy states to our cells. Tannenbaum's experiments with DNP linked the two over a half century ago, unbeknownst to researchers at the time. The benefits of exercise, however, go far beyond improving our metabolism.

÷

As Leonardo scaled the cliffs of Calabria in pursuit of his sheep, his steps required little thought. Yet, with each lunge forward over the rocks his brain sent a continuous stream of lightning-fast electrical messages to his leg muscles, commanding intense contractions of the muscles located on the front of his leg. The quadriceps, named as such because it encompasses four large muscles, provides the lower extremities the ability to walk, jump, and lunge forward over uneven surfaces as the body prepares to take its next steps. With each push forward, the leg muscles contract violently, thrusting the body forward to overtake gravity during a mountainous ascent. In conjunction, the gluteus muscles located behind the leg are activated to complete the motion of climb. These same muscles are often withered and atrophied in white-collar office-dwelling citizens due to disuse and constant static pressure from the seated position. Additionally, these muscles are frequently associated with chronic back pain, a state that will plague 80% of Americans at some point in their lives.[15]

Perhaps seemingly more like a squat workout at the gym, Leonardo's typical journey as a shepherd loaded his quadriceps, gluteal muscles, and multiple other lower and upper extremity muscles as he traversed the steep and uneven countryside. A simple journey for Leonardo provided cumulative muscular force and fatigue that far surpasses what the typical American experiences in a week. Peering deep within the cells of Leonardo's muscles provides some insights as to why exercise may provide its largest health benefits, even independent of the preconceived notion that exercise promotes weight loss. Like the fuel injector in an eight-cylinder car engine, the brain signal reaches the muscle, sparking the transfer of several different ions and chemicals, including sodium, potassium, and calcium. This transfer – similar to the electrical charge emanating from a battery – creates a voltage that drives the contraction of the muscle fibers like a piston expanding, providing a force that ultimately propels the legs forward. ATP within the muscles is utilized to fuel the process, as one of the phosphates – the "P" in ATP – is torn off to create ADP.

As ATP levels drop, several changes provide a signal to the cell that an energy deficit is mounting, a process reminiscent of the cellular changes elicited from fasting and ketosis. During intense periods of activity, the muscles rely on the freely available glucose and glycogen within our liver and muscles as fuel for energy. This process of anaerobic glycolysis metabolizes sugar without the presence of oxygen. The process provides a quick source of energy but also produces lactic acid, the byproduct incorrectly blamed for the burn that we experience in rapidly contracting muscles. Less intense exercises can engage the mitochondria for energy when oxygen is present during the process of aerobic glycolysis. The latter process of energy derivation is substantially more efficient, while the former is faster in providing our muscles fuel.

When the mitochondria are activated to generate energy, the cellular furnace once again begins burning, producing free radical byproducts during the process. The antioxidant defense system is activated to offset these potentially damaging radicals, accompanied by their typical array of benefits. Consistent with Ristow's work, a large benefit of exercise may be from the creation of these free radicals, their ability to stress our cells, and the cellular response from enacting the antioxidant defense system. Furthermore, like AMPK activation, this stress improves our body's insulin sensitivity and leaves our cells metabolically healthier. Coming full circle, Ristow has also produced research revealing that antioxidant supplementation with vitamin C and E prior to exercise blocks the subsequent and beneficial antioxidant gene expression in muscle and blunts the improvement in insulin sensitivity.[16] Without the production of free radicals and activation of defense systems to offset them, there would be no benefits to exercise. Moreover, an additional benefit of exercise is the production of new mitochondria to aid in energy maintenance, providing the aforementioned array of benefits that accompany our mitochondria. Direct antioxidants like vitamin C and E interact with free radicals to diffuse them, whereas indirect free radicals like the chemicals in green vegetables, spices, berries, and red wine produce oxidative damage that indirectly stimulates cellular antioxidant production. Exercise, fasting, and periodic ketosis act as indirect antioxidants, explaining why direct antioxidant supplementation can offset this benefit and is not helpful.

However, several other local and systemic hormonal changes accompany the persistent contraction of our muscles, paralleling Ristow's findings. It is well known that repetitive contraction of a muscle will signal the body to increase its size, known as hypertrophy. These benefits of both muscle mass and muscle contraction bring the role of IGF-1 full circle as it is locally released to promote this growth. Systemically, however, levels of IGF-1 may remain unchanged; the stress on our muscles from heavy lifting and contraction, much like the stress on our cells from several sulfur and food-based chemicals, trains the muscles to prepare for more future contraction and IGF-1 release. The body releases IGF-1 locally to stimulate anabolic muscle growth, which follows the increases in IGF-1 production within Leonardo's contracting muscles as he ascended the cliffs.[17]

Paralleling the potentially harmful free radicals produced while our mitochondria churn out energy, exercise produces some potentially harmful chemicals as well. For instance, IL-6 is an inflammatory hormone released during infections or after trauma. The trauma to our muscles during exercise, while different from an infection, also signals the release of muscle-derived IL-6. On the surface, the rising levels of IL-6 may hint that exercise produces some unhealthy consequences. While Hippocrates had no knowledge of IL-6 itself, by 400 BC he was writing about the damage inflammation could cause to the body. One of the earliest documented physicians, and the one to whom all physicians pay homage to when they recite the Hippocratic Oath during medical school commencement, Hippocrates began treating patients with willow tree bark to alleviate their symptoms of pain and fever.[18] Hippocrates may not have realized that he was calming these patients' inflammatory symptoms with aspirin found in the bark of the willow tree. Still, he was aware that willow tree bark alleviated many of the signs of inflammation like pain, redness, and swelling. Over 2,000 years later, physicians continue to prescribe similar drugs including aspirin as a method to combat the symptoms of inflammation. While oftentimes these medications only blunt symptoms as opposed to treating the cause, they have broadened our knowledge of the connection between cancer and inflammation.

Chronic stress and inflammation wears at our cells and organs over time, and both have been linked to cancer in a plethora of studies. As one of the hallmarks of cancer, inflammation is often considered the match that ignites the flame of cancer,[19] but may more accurately be described as kindling for the fire or perhaps better yet the fertilizer that nurtures cancer's initiation and growth. Unsurprisingly, several diseases characterized by chronic inflammation often culminate in a cancer diagnosis. For instance, inflammatory bowel disease frequently leads to colon cancer,[20,21] while chronic pancreatitis is associated with a high risk of pancreatic cancer.[22] Cigarette smoke provides a constant source of lung inflammation in heavy smokers and chronically inflames the lungs; it directly produces free radicals, leading to DNA damage and lung scarring that eventually leads to chronic obstructive pulmonary disease and cancer.[23] During inflammation, several protein messengers can often be observed traversing the body, and elevated levels of these same inflammatory proteins – CRF, TNF, and IL-6 – often accompany a cancer diagnosis and can help fuel cancer progression.[24,25]

The thought of exercise, an activity typified as healthy, fueling the release of an inflammatory chemical should raise some eyebrows. The result is far from expected, however, as with IGF-1, viewing this chemical in isolation is medically nearsighted. Muscle-derived IL-6, squeezed from our muscles like the juice of a lemon during contraction, sensitizes the body to the inflammatory hormone IL-6. As with the various activities that increase free radicals within our cells, overall levels of IL-6 decline afterwards. In this regard, while fat secretes an array of detrimental inflammatory hormones, muscle acts in opposition as it lowers overall levels of inflammation. For instance, fat tissue secretes the inflammatory cytokine TNF-α, which stands for tumor necrosis factor as our immune cells release it in the presence of tumors, whereas muscles release anti-inflammatory myokines. Several points illustrate the beneficial hormonal barrage from our muscles versus adipose tissue:

- Adipose-derived TNF is inflammatory, while muscle-derived IL-6 is anti-inflammatory.

- Muscle-derived IL-6 signals to our body to break down lipids and burn fat.[26]

- Adipose-derived TNF causes insulin resistance and impairs glucose uptake by our cells (both leading to increased blood sugar).[27]

- While serious and often fatal events like septic shock cause a sudden release of TNF, excess adipose tissue causes the chronic release of TNF.

- Muscle-derived IL-6 helps regulate AMPK (while muscle contraction directly activates AMPK), which stimulates the breakdown of fat and cholesterol, kindles our mitochondria, and potentially fights cancer.[28]

Blood sugar and IL-6 have an analogous relationship; too much of either can be detrimental, but exercise sensitizes our cells to both, leaving them at lower levels when we are at rest. During activity, our muscles and liver mobilize their stores of glycogen, pouring it into the blood to help fuel our muscles. The increased blood glucose could in theory be concerning, as higher levels correlate with an increased risk of several cancers,[29] yet this rise in blood sugar is only transient with levels dipping 30 minutes afterwards.[30] Mirroring the internal production of free radicals and IL-6 within muscle, exercise and resistance training increase insulin sensitivity, and overall we are left with lower blood sugar and insulin levels.[31]

Muscles continuously secrete IL-6 even at rest, but exercise intensifies this release by up to 100 times.[32] Furthermore, frequent exercise and muscle contraction sensitizes our muscles to this release while at rest.[33] In other words, the science suggests that more muscle is beneficial to fight inflammation both during exercise and at rest. While excess body fat on the other hand produces inflammation, desensitizes cells to the action of insulin, and increases both insulin and excess blood sugar, contracting muscles can offset all these detrimental effects. The amount of IL-6 secreted by our muscles depends on several factors, including the intensity and duration of the exercise and the size of the muscle contracting.[34] More contractions of more muscles leads to more release, so focusing on resistance training as part of one's workout is a metabolically advantageous approach. Other factors such as diet come into play as well – for instance, carb loading before a workout may blunt IL-6 release.[35] Once again, it appears advantageous for our muscles to secrete their own fuel supply when stressed for energy.

The anti-inflammatory effects of exercise are far from subtle – muscle contracting exercise can even blunt the inflammatory response from *E. coli*.[36] *E. coli* would typically cause a tripling of levels of harmful TNF, and injection into healthy exercising volunteers is effectively stifled simply through exercise. Along these lines, trained athletes generally have lower levels of numerous inflammatory factors[37] while elevated background inflammation is frequently seen in inactive individuals.[38] Inflammation is the likely cause of or contributor to many diseases beyond cancer, including atherosclerosis and diabetes. Inflammation's effect parallels that of free radical damage, the other major cause of disease and cancer.[39] Much like inflammation, high levels of free radicals damage our cells, wreck our DNA, and expose us to a higher risk of cancer; yet when we increase our cellular supply of both through healthy activities, they decrease in the long run.

Any intensification of energy production by the mitochondria – including fasting, ketosis, carbohydrate restriction, intense activity, exposure to phenolic chemicals in wine, berries, and green tea, and sulfurous chemicals in cruciferous vegetables – produces free radicals and activates the antioxidant defense system. Our cells have spent millions of years fine-tuning an internal defense mechanism against this damage, and exercise, which is a stress on the body, activates this system. For example, when middle-aged men engage in muscle-contracting resistance training twice a week, glutathione peroxidase is activated, defusing the potential damage from free radicals that can become bound to the fatty wall around our cells. Another similar antioxidant enzyme, superoxide dismutase, is increased within our cells and mitochondria via muscle contraction during weightlifting, but not during endurance training.[40] The process of dismutation involves breaking a chemical apart, and superoxide dismutase tears apart the harmful free radical known as superoxide, rendering it no longer a threat. Just as AMPK signals to our cells the necessity to break down their components for energy, attuning our metabolism, these potentially harmful free radicals signal our cells to engage their defense mechanisms. Like the sulfur in some green vegetables and chemicals in several spices, these signals indicate potential harm, pushing our cells into action. Newer studies reveal the benefits of ordinary active aspects of daily life for laborers like Leonardo, as they were arming their cells to fight disease and cancer. The similarities between the physiological response to exercise and eating vegetables, fasting, and engaging in a diet and lifestyle that favors nutrient-dense and lower carbohydrate foods are nothing short of extraordinary.

⁘

As the front door opened, the brim of Leonardo's hat led the way across the threshold as he entered into his home. He hung his hat atop the coat rack as the scent of roasted Delmonico steaks filled the room. It was Tuesday, the one night of the week where dinner included a massive steak, which was Leonardo's favorite treat. Other weekly meals usually included soups made from boiled bones and marrow, garnished with leafy greens, eggs, and cheese. Sometimes they would add pastina, a tiny pasta cooked in butter. Simmered greens were a staple at the dinner table, but tonight was steak night and the fattiest cut would be saved for Leonardo. He had worked hard all day, spending part of it at the steel mill doing manual labor and the rest stocking shelves at his grocery store.

Throughout his otherwise routine day, Leonardo's muscles were activated during the intense contraction from lifting the large pieces of steel, heavy wheels of cheese, soppressata, and jugs of olive oil. The tears in his muscles released IL-6, which traveled throughout his body to extinguish what little inflammation lurked within. His muscles gradually exhausted their supplies of available energy or ATP. Unbeknownst to Leonardo, Dr. Ristow's experiments were taking place deep within his muscles, as his cells were breaking off the phosphates – the "P's" of the ATPs – to provide the sinewy fibers with energy. This left the cells with more ADPs, as ATP has three phosphate groups (T is for tri) and ADP has two (D is for di). In final desperation, Leonardo's muscle cell tears away another phosphate, leaving the original ATP as an AMP, the single remaining phosphate signified as an M for mono in AMP.

Like a bank being robbed, the theft of phosphates from the original ATP sounds several alarms, initiated by the security guard at the door after being signaled by the accountant, AMPK. AMPK, or AMP-activated protein kinase, is activated by the presence of AMPs, which signal to the cell that it is running low on phosphates due to the theft. AMPK is an enzyme extensively expressed in our muscle, liver, and brain. AMPK takes its job of supplying ATP very seriously, and after its activation all hell breaks loose within our cells as the mitochondria work overtime to provide them with energy. AMPK achieves this while orchestrating a change in cellular processes from those that favor growth to those that focus on breaking down sugar as fuel for energy, extracting glucose from the bloodstream and into cells, metabolizing the efficient energy sources of cholesterol and fat, and signaling the cells to build additional mitochondria for a greater yield of energy production and fat/cholesterol burning.

In other words, AMPK strongly signals to our cells and organs that they best avoid growth and building and instead focus on breaking down any surplus energy. Just as fat and muscle can be viewed as Jekyll and Hyde when it comes to our metabolic health, AMPK and cancer are similarly juxtaposed when it comes to cells functioning normally. If we view muscle as the opposite of fat when it comes to our health (and yes, we do need both), AMPK also functions as the opposite of growth, and therefore stands in the way of cancer. Cancer cells digest large quantities of glucose and nutrients to support their rapid proliferation, propagate the hallmarks of cancer, and eventually spread and kill their host. AMPK, on the other hand, shuts off the process of cancer growth, instead allocating these nutrients to sustain our own cells.[28,41] The same growth mechanisms channeled by the overconsumption of specific foods can be blocked by AMPK, including the downstream actions of IGF-1, insulin, glucose, and mTOR.[42] Other processes, like intermittent fasting, carbohydrate restriction, and ketosis, to reiterate, can lower these pathways as well, by signaling an energy deficit to AMPK.

Returning to Warburg's hypothesis regarding his mighty mitochondria, Warburg revealed that cancer cells generally prefer the utilization of glucose to support their growth and metabolism. Regardless of oxygen's presence, they tend to avoid the more energy efficient, but oxygen-required, process for producing energy within our mitochondria. Our normal cells, on the other hand, will gladly engage the mitochondria, as it provides them with significantly more ATPs than the breakdown of sugar, known as glycolysis. AMPK acts as the gatekeeper for this process – both the front desk worker by day, and back room accountant by night. Based on these principles, it may come as no surprise that AMPK can inhibit several pro-cancer pathways, and recent studies suggest it may directly block the Warburg Effect by hindering the ability of cancer cells to utilize sugar for energy.[43] AMPK is forced into action by several mechanisms, including: 1) Muscle contraction during exercise,[44,45] with more intense exercise resulting in increased expression of AMPK;[46] 2) Restriction of carbohydrates, potentially even when calories are increased;[47] 3) Intermittent fasting;[48] and 4) Periodic ketosis.[49]

The release of hormones from our contracting muscles signals a decrease in energy levels to other organs as well, promoting remote AMPK activation[50] and the breakdown of components for energy. These hormones also signal for the bones to grow and strengthen.[51,52] Similar to the release of IGF-1 after the consumption of certain foods, the way in which hormones crosstalk with other organs and cells throughout the body further illustrates the shortcomings of viewing them in isolation. Analogous to IL-6, IGF-1 produced by muscles seems to function as a separate entity. The body responds quite differently to growth hormone-stimulated IGF-1 – or in other words IGF-1 produced by the liver in response to growth hormone secreted by the pituitary gland – and the local production of muscle-derived IGF-1.

The liver, which produces IGF-1 in response to growth hormone, remains the major determinant of widespread IGF-1 levels within our blood. Increasing IGF-1 through exercise is a local phenomenon; in other words, increasing IGF-1 production in a specific muscle leads to the isolated growth of that muscle without the growth of other organs throughout the body.[53] Furthermore, the "burn" that we feel within our muscles during a workout, typified as the acidic environment surrounding the muscle, forces binding proteins to release IGF-1. As a result, more free and bioavailable IGF-1 is accessible to the muscle.[54] Both high and low-intensity exercise prompt the immediate rise in blood levels of IGF-1 by around 20-25%, which some scientists theorize is at least partially responsible for the benefits of exercise on brain function and bone strength.[55] However, much like the potentially harmful inflammatory hormone IL-6 that is increased during exercise, our muscles absorb this released IGF-1 to aid in their repair and growth,[56] sensitizing them to future elevated levels of IGF-1. Consistent with these findings, 12 weeks of strength and endurance training has been shown to decrease serum IGF-1 levels.[57] The transient increase in IGF-1 during exercise appears to be countered by a compensatory increase in the IGF binding proteins.[58] The increase in IGF-1 is short lasting, and levels drop within 20 minutes after completion of a workout. By the following morning, they are back to normal.[59] Despite these general trends in IGF-1, the exact influence of exercise seems to depend on the study – some show an increase, decrease, or no change in serum IGF-1 over the long term.[60]

While exercise signals to many IGFBPs to release their IGF-1 to promote muscle growth and repair, shortly thereafter binding proteins quickly bind to the remaining IGF-1 to inactivate it, helping to return levels back to normal. With further exercise, our body becomes more sensitized to the IGF-1, almost as though we can exercise away excess IGF-1. Much like the way in which exercise initially increases blood sugar but then pulls sugar from our blood and into our cells for fuel, improving our insulin sensitivity in the process, the same may be true of exercise and IGF-1. The harmless stress of exercise, similar to the aforementioned defense mechanisms of chemical-laden foods, activates several compensatory responses that leaves our cells healthier and more robust.

Regardless of the concerns toward IGF-1, founded or unfounded, many of the benefits of exercise are likely due to the release of IGF-1 from our muscles. The same hormone villainized for its "growth" effects is vital in maintaining our health. The brain has a proclivity for extracting IGF-1 from the blood, exploiting its reparative qualities to support brain function and improve cognition.[61] When scientists block the brain's ability to take in IGF-1 prior to exercise, animals no longer experience the cognitive and neuroprotective benefits of exercise.[62] Nature's experiment of decreasing IGF-1 has revealed other issues as well: IGF-1 levels naturally decrease in the elderly, leading to an array of health issues including muscle loss, weakness, and fatigue. These symptoms all not uncoincidentally resemble the issues that accompany malnutrition. Exercise[63] and increased dietary protein[64] in the elderly can increase their levels of IGF-1 to avoid these issues, improve their health, decrease their risk of cancer, improve cognition, strengthen their bones, and decrease muscle loss. With falling levels of this vital hormone, the elderly is a population that can benefit from increasing their protein consumption to stimulate production of IGF-1.

While excessive IGF-1 may have negative effects on the middle-aged, its ability to increase muscle mass while reducing adipose tissue must be appreciated. Regardless of the other issues with IGF-1, this dynamic – coupled with exercise – provides a cellular terrain inhospitable to cancer growth. The switch from inflammation-promoting fatty tissue to an increased volume of muscle mass encourages the production of anti-inflammatory hormones that further sensitize our cells to insulin, which provides a "triple threat" against cancer as it blunts inflammation, blood sugar, and insulin. In other words, IGF-1 may have its potential downsides, but it fosters a muscular and metabolic environment that optimizes the ratio of muscle to fat via secretion of beneficial hormones. Exercise and intense muscle contraction help to ensure that the IGF-1 is not used to promote unwanted cellular proliferation and instead is utilized for muscle growth and support.

For instance, the ability of exercise to pull nutrients from potentially harmful places and shuttle them to where they are beneficial is illustrated by the amino acid leucine. During exercise, leucine is used as a building block for skeletal muscle-derived IGF-1. While amino acids have many biological functions, they are often used as the building blocks for proteins and hormones. Leucine is a particularly popular amino acid as it helps to build muscle, but it also stimulates the cellular growth pathway mTOR. This complex connection has left many researchers questioning its relationship to cancer. Leucine may favor directly targeting our muscles,[65] and as with the other amino acids, blood sugar, IGF-1, and IL-6, our exercising muscles have a tendency to selfishly hoard leucine to assist in their repair and growth. Furthermore, as our muscles generate beneficial anti-inflammatory hormones during exercise, they utilize leucine to fuel the process. Once again, the bigger-picture view exposes the complex interplay of these vital sources and the potential dangers of viewing them in isolation.

Moreover, the metabolic changes that accompany exercise further illustrate the ability of the body to tilt the scales in its favor. During intense physical activity, skeletal muscle digests leucine at a high rate. Protein is broken down into several amino acids, which are then oxidized and catalyzed for energy. During this process, leucine, the amino acid that may fuel the cancerous pathway known as mTOR, is even pulled from non-muscular sources like the liver and gastrointestinal tract and shuttled to the muscles for fuel.[66] In other words, less is left for potential cancerous cells, as it has been pilfered by our own muscles. Paralleling IGF-1 and IL-6, this activity works to sensitize the body to these excess hormones, as if to deplete it of them. Both dietary leucine and foods that increase insulin like excess carbohydrates increase the mTOR pathway to enhance protein synthesis, especially after exercise. Such insights suggest that the best time of the day to consume carbohydrates would be after exercise or activity.

Yet when mice are supplemented with amino acids including leucine, they can paradoxically live longer.[67] Research would predict a faster burnout of their metabolic flame due to excessive promotion of the typical cellular growth pathways, like IGF-1 and mTOR; however, this does not happen. As AMPK is triggered into action during low energy states, so too is mitochondria triggered into overdrive by amino acids; muscles become exhausted of their ATP reserves,[68] and mitochondria ignite their oxidative furnaces for energy production. Rusting ensues, and the free radicals produced yet again trigger the many mechanisms in place to offset their potential damage. As our mitochondria run full throttle from exercise or an influx of amino acids, the excessive production of free radicals activates these antioxidant enzymes, along with several other mechanisms.

This leads to an enormous double-edged sword: our mitochondria are vital for life as they churn out energy like a hydroelectric dam, but with more power comes more potentially harmful free radical byproducts that can damage the mitochondria and its sensitive parts. The fix, which has been designed, built, and perfected over several million years, is the antioxidant defense system. It is not by coincidence that the more we "stress" our mitochondria with reactive oxygen species (ROS), the more they fight back. While the above activities may directly affect IGF-1 levels, turning on the regulator of our ROS defense system provides some valuable lessons. Fasting, carbohydrate restriction, ketosis, exercise, muscle contraction, and even cold weather deplete our cellular energy supplies. Furthermore, these spartan activities intensely activate AMPK, creating a chain reaction that signals the cell to produce more mitochondria and increase the expression of many processes and enzymes that disarm free radicals. The end result is the production of antioxidants to offset these ROS to levels lower than they were prior to the stressful event. In other words, a little stress to our cells generates a much larger amount of antioxidant defense.[69]

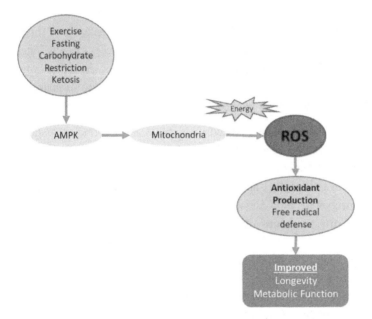

Figure 16: AMPK activation turns on the mitochondria to quickly replenish an energy deficit, creating reactive oxygen species (ROS) in the process. As a result, antioxidant mechanisms are activated, improving health and longevity.

Finally, several events occur during an intense bout of exercise that sound the cellular alarms. The bombardment of free radicals within our contracting muscles gestures to the other defense mechanism previously mentioned, known as Nrf2, to jump to action. Recall that Nrf2 normally floats around in the fluid of our cells, but it is pulled into the nucleus by cellular stress to spring to action, much like daf-16 in Kenyon's worms. Nrf2 triggers a handful of genes that disarm free radicals and repair DNA damage, stopping cancer in its tracks. Once again, an initial stress on our cells produces a manageable number of free radicals that signal multiple cellular responses, orchestrating an overall decrease in the amount of free radical damage. In other words, fasting, carbohydrate restriction, exercise and other Spartan-like activities engage a metabolic switch in our cells and instigate them to improve their robustness. The stress of these activities is where the benefit lies – without the production of rust-producing free radicals within our cells, the benefits of these activities would be limited. Providing direct antioxidants like vitamin C and E prior to exercise blunts the otherwise typical instigation of the antioxidant defense system and its anti-stress chemicals.[70] Our cells require the internal production of these free radicals to prompt them into action, and several behaviors are effective at engaging the process.

Insulin and IGF-1 counter this beneficial process by disengaging oxidative stress resistance mechanisms after overloading our cells with ATP and energy, signaling a state of abundance to the cell.[71] The foods that generally overwhelm the system happen to be many of the same ones that David Ludwig and other scientists have found to promote obesity. As a result, oxidative and free radical damage run rampant, cellular parts break down, hair turns grey, and we all age. But the fact that leucine – an amino acid that can increase IGF-1 and mTOR, which would potentially age us and increase our risk of cancer – improved muscular function in mice and allowed them to live longer merely illustrates the intricate relationships between these processes, and the shortcomings of focusing too closely on one element.

Returning to Tannenbaum, Rous, Kritchevsky, and the other trailblazing scientists of the 20th century, we begin to see through the smoke and mirrors. These original studies may have exposed a general benefit of calorie restriction in decreasing cancer. However, the diets of mice vary between studies; they were (and to this day still are) fed a general chow composed of significant amounts of the same foods that increase glucose, stimulate insulin, and shut off cellular defense mechanisms. Furthermore, the chow is often laced with vegetable oils, adding further insult to injury by bombarding the cells with an external source of free radical damage. Additionally, in many of the older studies, a high fat diet was often combined with a high carbohydrate diet – a metabolic cocktail providing these mice the perfect storm for cancer development and growth. Simply eating less of this cancerous cocktail might have been the largest benefit of the experimental diet groups in these studies. Finally, lab mice generally overeat this cocktail while crammed in a cage allowing no access to free movement and exercise. (Studies now reveal that simply placing mice in an enriched environment after injection with cancer cells can blunt tumor growth – something that does not occur with mice in a crowded cage.[72])

The control diets in most of these traditional studies were stimulating the same cellular pathways that shut off our cells' antioxidant and damage defense system, blunting AMPK, Nrf2, and the several other mechanisms that act to fight cancer and maintain our cell's health. In other words, the control diets were acting as anti-exercise by enacting the opposing cellular mechanisms from what the research of Ristow, Kenyon, and Mattson's research had indicated. Calorically restricting the mice was merely decreasing the amount of bad they were experiencing; as a result, tumors grew slower in the malnourished mice. Simply cutting calories in humans has not led to these benefits, but the cellular mechanism triggered throughout these studies has still provided priceless insight into how our bodies and cells respond to different activities, and how they are primed to fight cancer and disease.

There are multiple ways to stress our mitochondria to derive benefits for healthier cells and make them more adept at warding off cancer. Some of these methods may be easily implemented, while others may be more difficult. Plato may have been correct in his views of the many benefits of fasting, but a century of studies has indicated that humans do not need to starve themselves to stress their mitochondria into fighting cancer – rather, this can be accomplished via a handful of other activities, from intentional fasting to simply cutting carbohydrates. For those of us unwilling to undergo such spartan activities, simply eating foods with certain chemicals may spark the same mechanisms, as of course will engaging in regular exercise. Plato's invisible hand may have shunned many of the cultural dietary habits of Leonardo, but it was unable to hide the realization that numerous benefits accompany these activities. We cannot have one without the other.

11

THE MEAT OF THE ISSUES

"Good food that provides appropriate proportions of nutrients should not be regarded as a poison, a medicine, or a talisman. It should be eaten and enjoyed."

- Dr. David Kritchevsky and the National Research Council
Food and Nutrition Board

"The beef industry has contributed to more American deaths than all the wars of this century, all natural disasters, and all automobile accidents combined. If beef is your idea of "real food for real people" you'd better live real close to a real good hospital."

- Neal D. Barnard, M.D., President of Physicians Committee
for Responsible Medicine and animal rights activist

Takeaways:

Now that the research has been dissected and the cellular mechanisms explained, several evidence-based recommendations are provided on lifestyle modifications, physical fitness, and dietary regimens, all harkening back to the simple approaches protagonist Leonardo innately and routinely engaged in without any scientific knowledge.

The importance of preparation of food at home is noted, highlighting the significance of avoiding short-cuts, while focusing on the importance of food and treating mealtime as the vital social and cultural experience that it has been throughout our history.

A specific food type near and dear to Leonardo, that of cured meats, is used to exemplify the differences between quantity and quality and highlight the issues of viewing food in the same vein as harmful chemicals. Finally, focusing on certain foods and vegetables may differentially impact the many mechanisms and anti-cancer detoxification pathways within our bodies. These same pathways can be activated by vegetables and foods prepared with equal consideration.

It was a typical warm and humid July day in Maryland. As temperatures slowly advanced into the upper eighties, the sun baked the grounds at the Bethesda campus of the National Institutes of Health. About seven miles away in Washington D.C., Mitt Romney was engaged in an equally heated political campaign in an attempt to uproot the incumbent Barack Obama from a second term as President of the United States. Willett approached the microphone at the Lester Hill Center Auditorium to wax informatively and perhaps even poetically on a topic that few knew better than him. Decades into his own campaign to find the hidden links between food and health, Willett began his lecture, *Diet & Cancer: The Fourth Paradigm*, by describing the most recent paradigm linking diet and cancer – obesity. As Willett seamlessly dissected and explained study after study, he naturally segued to his old stalwart, a discussion on the link between dietary fat and cancer. This time around, however, Willett's conclusions were different. "There was never any strong evidence for this idea, but it was repeated so often that it became dogma in the 1980s and 1990s," Willett informed a likely perplexed audience. "The hypothesis that the percentage of calories from fat in the diet is an important determinant of cancer risk, at least during midlife and later, is not supported by the data." Willett's exoneration concluded emphatically: "I think we really did bury the low-fat paradigm."

After nearly a century of inconsistent dietary studies, the expectations of a low-fat diet exceeded the realities, the link between fat and cancer remains a weak one, and more than enough studies should have exonerated the wrongly accused fat. To Willett's credit, he has killed his darlings, publicly described the slaying, and remains open about the bias that permeated throughout the medical and research field during his time. Willett even suggested that we may have gone in the wrong direction, stating that "higher total dietary fat intake during midlife does not increase breast cancer incidence, and under some circumstances, low-fat/high-carbohydrate diets might contribute to higher risk."[1]

Unfortunately, as University of Toronto psychologist Lynn Hasher had found through her research in the 1970s, relentless repetition of an idea – true or not – will eventually lead the public to believe it.[2] According to Hasher, "Repetition makes things seem more plausible," and the link between fat and cancer had been repeated enough to leave the strongest of doubters believing it. By the time Willett claimed that "support for a major relationship between fat intake and breast cancer risk has weakened considerably as the findings from large prospective studies have become available,"[3] many views were already firmly established.

Willett's talk at Bethesda was a direct rejection of the often-repeated mantra of the 80s and 90s, as he took the audience on a start-to-finish tour of the history, rationale, and failures of the anti-fat movement to help prevent cancer. His presentation – at times resembling a confession testimony – was both a stepping stone and testament to his desire to further the field as opposed to furthering egos. Several other dietary "paradigms" had evolved over the last several decades, but the low-fat debacle seemed to have created a vacuum that pulled in even more dietary theories steeped upon scant research. Perhaps more collateral damage than wishful thinking, the fruit and vegetable paradigm followed. While fruits and more so vegetables have certain health benefits, Willett explained that these benefits were largely overstated. The benefits of these foods are likely modest, and Willett apologized for some of these recommendations that he felt were strongly biased in their overemphasis of the ability of these foods to reduce cancer risk. Many of the supporting studies were poorly executed population studies plagued with bias and error. If anything, vegetables may have never been given their fair assessment.

Yet by no means was Willett dismissing the benefits of vegetables and fruits; he was, however, explaining that their cancer-fighting benefits may have been shrouded with more Plato-esque propaganda than science. Willett advised that while there are certainly benefits to vegetable consumption, particularly in relation to specific cancers, they are modest and may not provide a substantial decrease in cancer risk as compared to other major lifestyle changes. In other words, the often-heard simplistic advice of increasing fruits and vegetables without several other lifestyle changes is unlikely to make a dent in current health issues.

Several years later I found myself thousands of miles away from Bethesda, suffering in equally sweltering summer heat. Sweat drenched my collar as I entered a modest shop; I was promptly greeted by swarming flies and the unmistakable humidity of an indoor space lacking air conditioning. Forty-pound wheels of cheese rested behind the glass and under the counter, extracting whatever cool air they could muster from their refrigerated enclosure. The strong smell of cheese permeated throughout the shop, a scent that immediately pulled me into a conversation with my grandfather, who always spoke fondly of the "stinky cheese shop" once run by Leonardo Pesce. My grandfather would later marry Leonardo's daughter, who he affectionately dubbed "the stinky cheese girl." We ordered a half pound of the comté, the golden yellow semi-hard cheese aged for up to 36 months and surrounded by a several inch-thick rind. Somewhat ironically, the cheese monger gestured to us that it was edible. Seeing the amusement on our faces, he immediately cut off a large piece, tossed it into his mouth, and after minimal chewing, swallowed it whole. We spoke little French and he spoke no English, but we were instantly united in our mutual love of cheese. Excited, he showed us several pictures of Eastern France, where the unpasteurized cow's milk was converted to cheese during its storage in the caves below the Franche-Comté region. Comté cheese is produced under strict rules, including one regulation that only 1.3 cows can occupy a hectare pasture, ensuring they get adequate grass for sustenance. Furthermore, fertilization of the pasture is limited, and the use of silage for feed is banned. The result is a deliciously decadent cheese, fortified with as much flavor as vitamins and nutrients.

As the monger was handing us the wrapped cheese, we spotted the cured duck links hanging from the ceiling. Below them was a sign with several words; one of them was *canard*, and another *saucisson*. With little French vocabulary, I knew what *canard* meant; I had eaten it daily for nine straight days to compare the different preparation techniques of duck throughout Southwest France. Besides its delicious flavor, duck fat contains around 50% oleic acid, the anti-inflammatory monounsaturated fat providing olive oil its fame as a healthy fat. It is a rarity on American menus, leaving it as an infrequent delicacy for those of us who enjoy it. I had never indulged in cured duck meat before, and after trying it later that night I realized I had been missing out.

Earlier in the day, I had indulged in a delicious ribeye from a grass-fed cow, washed down with a bold glass of red wine and a plate of mixed vegetables. Apart from the latter food, such a meal would make most modern dieticians grimace in shock, especially on the plate of a physician. However, meat from grass-fed cows has always held a soft spot in my heart. Its delicious flavor is matched by its plethora of vitamins and nutrients that help our cells build and repair damage, including iron, vitamins A, E, B3, B6, and B12, selenium, zinc, conjugated linoleic acid, and omega-3 fatty acids. Furthermore, it does little to impact our blood sugar and amply satisfies my appetite. Repeated studies reveal that happier and healthier grass-fed cows produce meat and fat with significantly more of these vitamins and nutrients.[4,5] I knew from my research, and perhaps from the genes inherited from Leonardo, that these nutrients were densely present in bone broths and organ meats which were often a part of my dinner table.

A discussion of red meat in the same breath of a healthy lifestyle conversation may seem absurd. This is certainly true, if we are viewing it through a Platonic lens of calories and the macronutrients that make up those calories. On the contrary though, red meat illustrates – or perhaps advises us – on the various issues of viewing food like Plato as opposed to Leonardo. On the surface, the issues with even considering red meat as a single food group are countless; the body responds quite differently to meat raised appropriately, and the methods of preparing the meat will produce almost incomparable sources of sustenance.[6] For instance, after a meal consisting of wild game meat such as kangaroo, the body responds differently than it does to beef from a hybridized cow breed raised on grains to marbleize its fat content to increase flavor. The grains form an acidic environment within the cow's rumen and increase its risk for infection, prompting antibiotic usage; they also eliminate the healthy and anti-inflammatory byproducts of grass fermentation. Considering these sources, a parallel metaphor would be replacing the engine in a Ferrari with one from a Mazda Miata yet still considering it the same vehicle. Recent research studies have exposed the differences, as kangaroo meat improves blood lipid levels[7] while marbleized beef in comparison significantly raises several markers of inflammation, including TNF-α and IL-6, within the serum of individuals 1-2 hours after a meal.[8] Even within the category of the meat, the cuts of meat largely dictate the nutritional value: fattier cuts and organ meats often contain significantly more nutrients.

Chicken Breast (no skin)   Sirloin Steak (fat trimmed)   Beef Kidneys

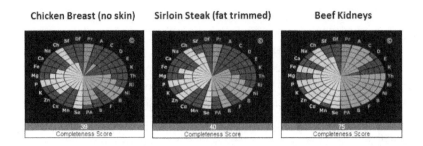

Figure 17: As we move from lean muscular meats to organ meats, the nutrient "completeness" score, which measures vital nutrients like magnesium and zinc, rises significantly. (Images created in nutritiondata.self.com)

All that being said, few foods have been as intimately associated with the harms of dietary fat than red and processed meat. While Willett's lecture at Bethesda excluded any discussion of red meat in its exoneration of dietary fat, other sources have further vilified the nutrient-dense food. According to a report from the International Agency for Research on Cancer (IARC) – a special arm of the World Health Organization tasked with identifying cancerous agents – my steak meal was apparently exposing my body to a cancer-promoting substance, as opposed to providing it with actual food. The near constant lambasting of red and processed meats occurs so ubiquitously within the health arena that many have merely opted to ignore the warnings, and the IARC warning was no different. Several years before my epicurean awakening blessed by duck prosciutto, the issues of processed meat were centrally thrust into the spotlight when the IARC classified it as a Group 1 carcinogen to humans, citing data linking it to colorectal cancer.

While red meat has taken a beating for years, it pales in comparison to the thrashing given to processed meats, including cured meats, hot dogs, sausage, pickled meats, and beef jerky, to name a few. The release of the report led to a media frenzy, with some outlets (and scientists) going as far as comparing meat to cigarettes. But are all processed meats the same? The report described a strong association in epidemiologic studies between processed meats and colon cancer, thus supporting its labeling as a Group 1 carcinogen. The association between red meat and colorectal cancer was found to be less consistent, thus red meat was demoted to Group 2A, or "probably" a carcinogenic food. While the report backed its views with controversial population studies, it also stressed that animal studies have yet to back up these claims; while several chemical and physiological mechanisms may connect red meat to cancer, this connection is less clear.

As expected, the controversial report was met with substantial controversy. While not the first of its kind, this did successfully cross the slippery slope of lumping foods and chemicals together; the placement of nutrient-dense foods alongside harmful chemicals was a rough pill for many to swallow. Processed meats were in the same category as car exhaust, arsenic, and tobacco smoke – quite the damning accusation as red meat joined the likes of petroleum and lead. I dedicated a long-winded chapter in my previous book *Misguided Medicine* as a thorough analysis of the report and likely health issues with meat, but even the fine print of the IARC report itself provided some caution with their use of epidemiologic studies: "Chance, bias, and confounding could not be ruled out with the same degree of confidence for the data on red meat consumption, since no clear association was seen in several of the high quality studies and residual confounding from other diet and lifestyle risk is difficult to exclude."

The multitude of issues with the report aside, its publication did portend several recent societal attitudes toward health, as well as the medical field's newfound approach to food. The grouping of food with chemicals (including car exhaust!) illustrates the demise of the cultural and historical view of food as nourishment and the rise of the more modern view of food as simply a combination of several chemicals – chemicals that, as we know, might all cause or prevent cancer depending on the particular study used to support one's position. Furthermore, the actual association with red meat and colorectal cancer, beyond all its shortcomings, revealed a potential overall increase in risk of less than 1%.[9] Contrasting this minute risk to Doll's original study renders the comparison of red meat and cigarettes all the more ridiculous, and also reveals the deeply rooted disdain for meat by many health leaders – a disdain so strong that one can only surmise it is based more on culture and conviction than on medical reasoning.

Some have simply dismissed this risk as too small to provide any tangible consequences, while others have viewed it as vital insight, particularly when considered on a population-wide level with subject numbers in the millions. Regardless of the polarizing views of meat's impact on our health, an analysis of red and processed meat provides valuable clues into the role food plays in the promotion and avoidance of cancer.

As with Willett's multiple studies assessing dietary fat and cancer, the associations between red meat and cancer are weakened when other factors are taken into consideration. Heavy meat-eaters generally engage in unhealthy activities like overconsuming alcohol, smoking, and avoiding exercise. Based on these unhealthy habits, heavy meat eaters unsurprisingly have worse overall health and are more obese. In a polar opposite twist from those studies that selected for healthy women asking their doctors for hormone replacement therapy, some of these studies select for the unhealthy smoking, meat-and-potatoes eating American that drinks heavily and rarely exercises.

While most foods provide some compositional element that may increase our risk of cancer, a more thorough assessment of meat provides insight into how to offset several of these chemicals. Leading the recent charge against the usual suspects when it comes to meat and colon cancer is a chemical known as trimethylamine-N-oxide, or TMAO. While TMAO is not present in red meat, it is produced by our bowel bacteria during their processing of carnitine. L-carnitine is found in muscle and heart tissue; its largest source is within red meat, followed by seafood, chicken, pork, nuts, and green vegetables. When bowel bacteria digest carnitine, they release TMAO.[10] As opposed to the potential anti-cancer effects of the fatty acids butyrate and CLA, TMAO has been linked to colorectal cancer and heart disease in humans.[11] While L-carnitine is utilized by our cells to function optimally – our mitochondria use carnitine to effectively burn fatty acids for fuel – TMAO is not, as it causes inflammation throughout the body.

TMAO speaks less to the issues with meat and fish – after all, carnitine is found in an array of healthy foods – and more to the importance of nourishing healthy bowel bacteria.[12] Many nutrient-dense foods are converted to TMAO by our bowel bacteria, so a prudent strategy would avoid throwing the baby out with the bathwater. More prudent would be hedging our bets with cruciferous and green leafy vegetables – the same vegetables that stimulate our cells to fight cancer – to feed different strains of bowel bacteria that produce less TMAO. While the exact dangers of TMAO remain unexplored due to limited research to date, the bowel bacteria of heavy vegetable consumers demonstrate another benefit of having them in our diet:

vegetarians seem to produce less TMAO after consuming the same amount of carnitine as nonvegetarians. In other words, their frequent consumption of greens and vegetables habitually nourishes the non-TMAO producing bowel bacteria, encouraging their growth and reproduction. So, to reiterate, meat, seafood, and carnitine consumption in isolation may not be the culprit, and the onus lies more on habitually feeding our healthy bowel bacteria. Fostering the growth of these bacteria within our bowels will not only produce less TMAO, but it will also leave more carnitine undigested and able to find its way to our cells to support their cancer-fighting mitochondria. Research continues to evolve and uncover which foods most efficiently feed the non-TMAO-producing bacteria. A recent study has even revealed that cheese intake can lower levels of TMAO.[13] Adding more confusion to an already confusing topic, a recent study of over one million subjects found absolutely no connection between red meat consumption and heart disease, strongly questioning the purported connection between TMAO and health issues.[14] Further muddying the waters was the analysis of the large European Prospective Investigation into Cancer and Nutrition – a study of 63,550 men and women – that revealed a 39% higher risk of colorectal cancer in vegetarians compared to meat eaters.[15] Pick your side, look for a study, and you will likely find some support.

While studies on TMAO are mixed, they illustrate the vital connection we have to the critters that reside within our gut. Eliminating the bowel bacteria of mice with antibiotics leaves them unable to produce TMAO after consuming carnitine. As bowel bacteria coat the gastrointestinal tract, protect its lining, and play a vital role in its repair and health, this is a less than optimal strategy.[18] Additionally, the lining of our bowels is constantly bombarded with bacteria, chemicals, viruses, and other threats, which further emphasizes the importance of nurturing these bacteria to maintain its structural integrity. Recalling the benefits of green grass to the health of fermenting bacteria within the rumens of cows provides several lessons on the importance of maintaining the health of fermenting microbes within our innards. In fact, feeding our cells with nutrient-dense foods while incorporating nourishment for the GI tract bacteria – like green, leafy, and fibrous vegetables, sweet potatoes, and fermented foods like kimchi, kefir, and sauerkraut – may provide the most well-rounded approach.[19] Instead of treating real food like chemicals and eliminating them out of fear, our best strategy is likely instead incorporating foods that nurture our cells and bowel bacteria to foster their symbiotic relationship.

In addition to TMAO, iron is the other villain found in muscle meat that some deem problematic. Like other double-edged swords in our diet, iron can form N-nitroso compounds (NOC) within our gastrointestinal tract. This iron, as we know from our earlier bridge studies, can then cause rusting, oxidation, and damage along the lining of our bowels. Yet, iron deficiency is one of the most prevalent nutrient deficiencies in the world,[16] and iron from red meat is an efficient source that is readily usable by the body to maintain properly functioning red blood cells to transfer oxygen to our cells. Other studies, reminiscent of Dayton and Pearce's, reveal that when iron is heated with vegetable oils and polyunsaturated fats, the oxidation and free radical production process is accelerated.[17] Like other foods, these studies suggest that perhaps moderation is key.

In my last book, I declared that while red meat is certainly no Superman, it is surely not the Lex Luthor that the public has been led to believe. Perhaps red meat is more like Iron Man – a flawed superhero that should be praised rather than vilified because at the end of the day he does more good than harm. Regardless of its reputation, the modern controversies of red meat fully illustrate just how far we have come from viewing food as food.

❖

A visit to the home of Leonardo and his wife Philomena on Highland Avenue in McKees Rocks reveals a giant concrete vat molded to the floor. The purple and red stains from the crushed grapes that filled the vat's belly have since been washed clean, but the passed-down family stories of Leonardo's homemade wine continue (with many family members in agreement on how bad it tasted). While crushed grapes found their home fermenting on the floor, the Pesce basement ceiling would be decorated with soppressata given their ample space to ferment as they dangled like ornaments on a tree. Leonardo would spend countless hours preparing and curing the meat according to his family recipe passed down through the generations, a meticulous yet calming natural process that – to the delight of

Cato and Cicero – would feed Leonardo's soul along with his physical appetite.

Processed foods – or the joining of chemicals and preservatives to naturally occurring foods that were grown or raised – has blurred the lines when it comes to viewing our food as food instead of a conglomeration of chemicals. Processed meat is a term used to describe one of the various sources of animal flesh that undergo any process to increase its shelf life or flavor, a method utilized and highly cherished by Leonardo and others who were not able to store their meat in a refrigerated setting. The curing of meats dates back far before Leonardo's time: salting and drying meat and fish was first recorded in Egypt around 3,500 BC. The Chinese first documented the use of salt to cure meat about 2,000 years later, and the Greeks followed around 200-300 BC. The Greeks' recipe – like many of their customs – eventually made its way into the Roman daily life, and one of the oldest recorded recipes is from the Roman senator and philosopher Cato the Elder. The recipe – which is a basic set of directions to add salt, let the meat sit, and then remove the salt – culminated with the meat hanging to dry, just as it did millennia later in Leonardo's basement. Curing was not limited to pork and red meats: the Greeks also produced salsamentum – which is purely salted fat – and mixed fermented fish with olive oil and wine to make œnogaros. Curing meat was not only local to the Mediterranean basin as Native Americans documented by the Jamestown settlement in Virginia had been salting their meat for centuries. From Europe to Asia and America, curing meat has been a long and integral part of human history and culture across the globe.

The elegance of curing meat lies in its simplicity and effectiveness; both are likely why recipes and methods have survived for thousands of years. The fundamental process involves adding salt to meat, poultry, or fish to extract water, dehydrate the flesh, and kill off any harmful bacteria. Leonardo and other curing aficionados often used a pastured, well-raised pig which generally contained healthier meat. They taste better too; according to home chef, food author, blogger, and charcuterie expert Michael Ruhman, "Grocery store pork is, typically, uniformly bad, but the dry-curing process magnifies the badness."[20] Spices may be added, and some meat sources are even cooked or smoked as part of the process. This cultural form of meat preservation was prized for thousands of years, until the industrialization of the process in the 18th century uprooted the traditional method to trade quality for mass production and profits. Critics of the movement, like Upton Sinclair in his seminal *The Jungle*, exposed the problems of mass production within the meat industry, many of which still exist today.

Regardless of any controversy surrounding cured meats, and particularly modern factory-produced meats, preservatives remain a familial tradition and heritage within the basements of many cultures around the world, from Spain to China and everywhere in between. Places like Parma, Italy – famous for Parma ham and parmesan cheese – still use the same ancient technique, which has been carried forward through the centuries along with the Adriatic Sea salt brought by sailors and used by locals to cure their meat as it swayed in the dry winds of Parma.

Ignoring the monumental cultural significance of cured meat, there are few foods that have received as bad a rap as processed meat. For instance, a recent study revealed a potential link between processed meat consumption and cancer when it found that the association between pancreatic cancer risk rose from 1.4% to 1.6% in those that ate more processed meat. (While the outcry from this study was heavily deliberated on the nightly news and many media sources, few actually considered the numbers.) Others have also pointed to salt as an issue with cured meat, but these concerns remain unsupported by research.

Despite all these inconsistencies, there are realistic concerns with modern processed meat consumption, especially when the IARC lists it as a carcinogen. Deli meat contains a laundry list of preservatives and chemicals, including monosodium glutamate (MSG), citric acid, corn syrup, butylated hydroxytoluene, butylated hydroxyanisole, gelatin, modified food starch, soy protein, sodium phosphate, sodium nitrite, sugar, dextrose, carrageenan, and sodium diacetate. This describes a food that clearly deviates significantly from the cultural food that hung from Leonardo's basement ceiling, and is even more dissimilar to the grass-fed unprocessed meat I savored along with a bottle of Cahors red wine in France. The chemicals that are put into these highly processed meats are done so for various reasons, the most prominent being to cut costs, increase shelf life, and avoid bacterial contamination.

While meats have been cured in unsanitary caves and the basements of old-school Italians like Leonardo for thousands of years, the risk of bacterial contamination, particularly from botulism is a real concern. In fact, sausage poison (the Latin word *botulus* means sausage) is why appropriately cured meat requires salt and the removal of moisture as *Clostridium* bacteria thrive in a moist, non-acidic environment without oxygen; like cancer cells, bacteria have their own hallmarks for growth, and a hospitable environment is required for proliferation.

Required methods to rid food of potential deadly microbes is at the core of this nuanced discussion on cured meats. The time-honored method of ridding foods – meats and vegetables – of potentially harmful pathogens and bacteria is of course to cook them. This introduces tradeoffs as well, as burning food infuses it with potentially harmful and even cancerous chemicals, as we will discuss momentarily.[21,22] Additionally, cooking already processed meats can lead to excessive production of these chemicals. It also raises several important points: 1) At what point, if ever, is it reasonable to consider a food as a chemical and not source of sustenance, cancerous or not? 2) If the manipulation of a food source results in a potentially harmful final product, is it appropriate to blame the initial food for this harm? and 3) Should our governing bodies cease from grouping different foods that vary tremendously in their composition, manufacture, and end effects into one overarching category for simplicity? I have heard point 3 here likened to considering plants carcinogenic because the tobacco plant, when burnt and inhaled, causes lung cancer and when placed in a pouch along our gumline causes oral cancer. This would of course be ridiculous, yet the same occurs quite often with meat.

The potential of burnt food to promote cancer has been known for decades, and scientists have long experimented with burnt food components to establish how and why they may promote cancer. In 1987, animal experiments with burnt meat first revealed the anti-cancer effect of conjugated linoleic acid; scientists were burning meat to create carcinogens and instead found that CLA cut cancer risk in half. TMAO and iron may provide theoretical health risks of consuming lean red meat, but evidence strongly suggests that the biggest potential threat from meat is its often-charred components from overcooking. Kritchevsky, Tannenbaum, and colleagues exposed mice to carcinogens like 7,12-Dimethylbenz[a]anthracene, known as DMBA. DMBA can promote cancer through mechanisms that are remarkably close to two chemicals known as heterocyclic aromatic amines (HAA) and polycyclic aromatic hydrocarbons (PAH).

Both HAA and PAH are found in petroleum, coal, and combustible products derived from fossil fuels, and are produced during the heating and processing of food.[23] High heat cooking can generate these chemicals, and using wood or charcoal to smoke foods can amplify this production. Leaner grilled meats, typically produce more TMAO when metabolized by bowel bacteria, but create less PAH than grilled fattier cuts (melted fat that drips onto fire and charcoal creating plumes of smoke). Smoked fish also contains substantial HAA and even cereals and vegetables have their fair share as well, with some research implicating them as a major dietary source of PAH.[24] Grilling vegetables produces similar chemicals that can damage our DNA,[22] further questioning how often we should grill any foods if our overall goal is to minimize our risk of cancer (I begrudgingly got rid of my grill years ago).[25] Finally, similar to those oils used in Dayton and Pierce's study, vegetable oils are laced with even higher levels of PAH than smoked meat, and cooking sprays add insult to injury as they also contain a hydrocarbon propellant. Even roasted coffee contains significant amounts of PAH[26] (if you want to continue drinking your daily cup of joe you can find some comfort in the multiple studies that reveal coffee's overwhelmingly positive influence on our health[27]).

Moving past the issues with burnt foods, the process provides us several opportunities to explore our body's defense response to carcinogens in cooked food and strategies to maximize this mechanism. For instance, while pan cooking can remove the charring that occurs with a grill, high-heat cooking can still damage our food and any cooking oil or fat. Cooking at lower temperatures, never smoking the pan, and using more stable fats – lard, tallow, ghee, coconut oil, etc. – can help further limit this damage. Low-temperature pan cooking at just over 200°F seems to create little to no HAA, while turning the heat up to 500°F will favor their formation.[28] In addition to avoiding open flame cooking and grilling altogether, limiting cooking temperatures to 350°F or lower seems to be a prudent cooking strategy until further information becomes available from future studies. Beyond the frying pan, even the acidic environment of our stomach and gastrointestinal tract can cause similar oxidative damage to both meat and vegetables.[29]

While the impact of curing meat on our health is less clear, it raises some important points on the effect of adding other ingredients to meat and vegetables during the cooking process. The ancient cookbooks are more than just interesting views of cooking throughout history; they provide important strategies to improve the health of our food. For instance, their oft-recommended strategy of dousing meat and vegetables alike in several concoctions works remarkably well to offset the formation of cancerous chemicals. The use of marinades dates back thousands of years; in an ancient Roman cookbook from 1 AD, Apicius describes marinating lamb liver with bay leaf, lovage seeds, black pepper, and fish sauce which often contained wine or vinegar.[30] Marinades are a process of tenderizing and flavoring meat, poultry, seafood, and vegetables by soaking them in a premade solution prior to cooking. Common ingredients in marinades include oil, vinegar, lemon juice, wine, spirits, herbs, and spices. On top of their colorfully distinct flavors and their ability to improve the texture of food, marinades offset the formation of harmful chemicals during cooking by 70-90%.[31-33]

The unstoppable creation of potentially harmful and cancerous chemicals within our food, particularly during cooking, leaves us with two conclusions: 1) Such chemicals may be largely responsible for that potential association – however miniscule – between red meat and colon cancer; and/or 2) If indeed these chemicals were carcinogens, the fact that only a small percentage of the overall population winds up contracting colon cancer reveals that we must have potent mechanisms within our GI tract to disarm these chemicals. Given that our cells are quite adept at fighting off this damage, at the very least, this latter conclusion must be true.

Indeed, several enzymes within our cells – notably CYP1A2 and NAT2 – are activated to aid in the metabolism of cancerous substances. Both are triggered from exposure to the burnt chemicals PAH and HAA; while NAT2 seems consistently elevated after cooked meat consumption, the increasing levels of CYP1A2 after consuming high-heat cooked food indicate that cells are pushed into overdrive to detoxify these chemicals. We will return to these important anti-cancer processes later, but for now keep them in the back of your mind.

As we round off this section, hopefully the in-depth description of the potential issues of cooking has not made you fearful of all foods. Rest assured, after most foods are consumed and enter our system, several other steps are equally concerning… Well before Apicius described marinating liver in his famous cookbook, the Romans had been curing meats with various salt concoctions. One such salt caused the reddening of meats; this particular salt contained nitrates, which worked incredibly effectively to kill off any bacteria that may have harmed the meat. When added, these nitrates are converted to nitrites by the bacteria within the meat. Issues arise when these nitrites further react with the muscle tissue, imparting the ruby red hue of the meats while also creating nitrosomyoglobin and amines. The process can also create compounds similar to those produced from high-heat cooking, known as nitrosamines. Nitrosamines are often confused with the heterocyclic chemicals described above, since both can occur during the chemical reaction with lean muscle meat.

Cooking these cured meats further facilitates the reaction between the nitrites and amines, and our stomach may foster the interaction as well. Adding insult to injury, our saliva is a large source of nitrites, vegetables are our largest source of dietary nitrates, nitrates are present in our drinking water, and the reaction occurs with protein.[34] These nitrates are also converted to nitrites by both our natural oral[35] and gut bacteria.[36] The ubiquitous nature of nitrates and nitrates will hopefully squelch some of your food fears, as if indeed these effects were as much of an issue as some in the modern nutrition community have made them out to be, we would be doomed as a species.

Returning to the conversation of TMAO, the same green leafy vegetables, sweet potatoes, and other fibrous vegetables that feed and support bowel bacteria help to metabolize nitrosamines before they cause any damage to the lining of our gut.[37] Broccoli, Brussels sprouts, and other cruciferous vegetables promote chemical metabolism and excretion before they cause any damage, while feeding our healthy bowel bacteria that also aid in detoxification.[38] However, the biggest benefit of these vegetables expands far beyond simply sustaining these bottom-feeding (literally!) bacteria.

While the judgment continues to be passed on a culturally-rich food that has been around for thousands of years, we can rest assured that evidence that such traditionally processed meats will cause cancer is lacking, at least when eaten in moderation. Furthermore, even in a worst-case scenario, the risk is small, risk indicators vary widely between studies, mechanisms point to burnt meat, and many studies do not account well for those other healthy lifestyle activities that offset the potential negative aspects of such "risky" foods. Ignoring the nutritional benefits of meat and other animal products based on shaky data is most certainly akin to throwing the baby out with the bathwater. However, burnt foods, charred meat and vegetables, cured meats, and the traditional foods added to them during the cooking process provide several valuable lessons. Regardless of their supposed negative impacts on our health, we can still count on them to build our cellular defense walls as large and sturdy as possible. However, the scaling of these walls by relentless invaders is all but inevitable… so as a backup plan to ensure victory, we must also train our cells and arm them with the appropriate weaponry to both withstand attack and repair damage.

·ː·

Leonardo arrived home, flung open and then slammed closed the front door in excitement, and ran into the kitchen. He had just walked his daughter home from the local movie theater, where she was watching *Steamboat Willie*. While this was the third Disney production featuring their new star Mickey Mouse, it was the first to be widely distributed to the public. The revolutionary black and white cartoon was also the first from Disney to have synchronized music and sound, an innovative feature when it first aired in 1928. Leonardo had caught the tail end as he met his daughter, Rose, at the theater to pick her up.

"In America, *anche i topi possono parlare!*" ("In America, even the mice are able to speak!") Leonardo excitedly exclaimed. Truthfully, Leonardo's excitement with America far surpassed its talking mice. Ever the optimist, the endlessly contented – and easily amused – Leonardo had somehow managed to compartmentalize the fact that he worked in a backbreaking, perilous steel mill that was averaging one employee fatality per day. Yet, Leonardo was not the only one to focus on the silver lining in his view of America, as many modern Americans tend to similarly view his back-breaking Mediterranean lifestyle through rose-colored glasses.

The Mediterranean diet is the Shangri-La of the contemporary diet world; its allure has taken global citizens by storm, and rightly so as many of its devotees thrive past their mid-nineties aging joyfully and gracefully with a daily glass of red wine in one hand and a plate of vegetables in the other. The diet and lifestyle of Leonardo and the ancient Mediterranean inhabitants may, on the other hand, be another story. As Dan Buettner describes during his travels through the "blue zones" of Sardinia and Greece, daily life was for the most part difficult and backbreaking, only lightly interspersed with periods of intense relaxation while enjoying good food and wine. Such steady and intense activity throughout the day certainly does not cater to snacking or overeating, as doing so makes a 45 degree climb up the side of a hill even more difficult than it already is. This lifestyle leads to longer periods without food; oftentimes, these longer fasts were undertaken by necessity and not by choice. Greek citizens, often held up as the standard-bearing constituents of the original Mediterranean diet, fast for up to 103 days per year; this provides them a plethora of health benefits, including improved heart health,[39-41] cognitive and brain health,[42] and potential anti-cancer effects.[43]

While the toggling between periods of intense activity and intense relaxation of the Mediterranean lifestyle is less of a challenge to emulate, assembling the actual "Mediterranean diet" is more elusive and remains in the eyes of the beholder. The popular media describes a spread of olives, vegetables, whole grain bread dipped in olive oil, and a small portion of fish. These definitions, perhaps not coincidentally, match up quite nicely with Plato's description of the optimal diet, and perhaps even better with modern dietary mantra that often advises us to avoid fat, cut calories, and exercise more. But as anyone who has ever savored bone broth or blood sausage or attended to a lamb's head party can attest, the Mediterranean diet varies widely based on which geographic subregion where you encounter it, which time period or era you are observing it, and who is describing it. While we will never know for sure just how much cheese, dairy, and meat in which the "real" Mediterranean diet followers indulged or how much bold red wine they imbibed, it is generally agreed upon that they sure did love their vegetables. In fact, when Leonardo was not in the basement making cheese, crushing grapes on the floor, or hanging meat on the ceiling, he was out back tending his garden next to the chicken coop.

As backbreaking and stressful as the required work was for those living in Southern Italy and other areas of the Mediterranean, the benefit from many of their vegetables may not have been too dissimilar from these activities. The lesson learned from the stressful benefits of cruciferous vegetables, their chemicals, and other agents of plant warfare is the prudent strategy to enhance our cellular mechanisms to fight both free radical and chemical damage. This also produces some answers as to why initial clinical trials assessing antioxidants have thus far revealed no benefit or even harm – we must be stressed to produce our own free-radical fighting machinery through some blood, sweat, and tears and no pills or shortcuts will replace this physiologic phenomenon.[44,45] Nature has stressed the bodies of our ancestors for millions of years, and the cells within have evolved to fight back for survival.

Tannenbaum, Rous, Kritchevsky, and dozens of others have revealed that cellular damage can occur from various sources ranging from excess adipose tissue, harmful chemicals, and free radical-laden vegetable oils to inflammation and diets that increase blood sugar. These same researchers have shown us that this damage can be mitigated with a healthy diet, exercise, and spartan-like activities like fasting and periodic ketosis. Yet again, this damage is impossible to avoid as countless other chemicals within the environment have an uncanny ability to provide us with unwanted injury. Sulfur-rich vegetables enable some mechanisms to lessen potential injury; however, research reveals that they have additional benefits in the war against cancer.

In the previous section, we asked the question of how potentially harmful carcinogens in our food could cause serious injury or cancer; vegetables, spices, and other chemicals and compounds in our food and wine provide some insights into this answer. Beyond repairing cellular damage to thwart the cancerous conversion of our cells, our body requires a mechanism to rid it of harmful chemicals and carcinogens. This is where we have evolved intricate detoxification mechanisms in several phases that are impacted by our foods and intimately linked to our lifestyles.

Phase I detoxification is the first step of our body's enzymatic system to counterbalance harm from toxic chemicals, pharmaceutical drugs and xenobiotics, and hormones within our foods (remembering hormones instruct our cells to growth, thus could be extremely dangerous when introduced from the outside). Part of this process includes CYP450, the notorious enzyme that helps our liver detoxify many common medications. Individuals prescribed medications are cautioned about combining substances such as grapefruit that interact with this mechanism, due to CYP450's prevalence in detoxification.

Within phase I detoxification, multiple subsets of enzymes are called to action to disarm toxins. During this process, enzymes metabolize or break down carcinogens, hormones, and pharmaceutical medications to less toxic intermediates prior to packaging them to be shipped out of the body. However, during this process some chemicals are converted to potentially more reactive and dangerous substances before they are handed over to other enzymes that prepare them for entry into phase II detoxification, which can rapidly lessen their harm. This is, however, assuming we have adequate support from a healthy and active phase II detoxification system – the support of which is another major benefit of eating those green leafy and cruciferous vegetables. Broccoli, supports phase II detoxification in conjunction with phase I detoxification, providing complete cellular detoxification of cancerous chemicals in both phases.[46]

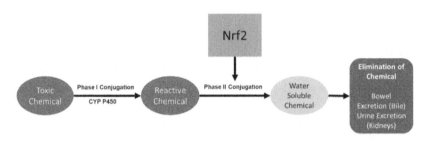

Figure 18: Toxic chemicals are disarmed via phase I and II conjugation (detoxification) and excreted through the bowels or kidneys. Nrf2 is intimately connected to the process.

Spices like curcumin, the bright yellow chemical found in turmeric, support phase I detoxification but can inhibit it at much higher doses – at least in petri dish and animal studies.[47,48] As is often the case with our physiology, it is far from straightforward, as some healthy sources of fruits and vegetables can also inhibit phase I, yet these same foods generally support detoxification by interacting with multiple enzymes embedded throughout the process. Overall, there is a fine interplay of chemicals from cruciferous vegetables, red wine, spices, teas, and other foods that impact multiple points throughout the phase I detoxification system. Some studies even suggest that cruciferous vegetables upregulate phase II detoxification while downregulating phase I, providing the perfect amount of push and pull to leave less cancerous chemicals present in our body.

Further closing the loop on our lifestyle and ability to defend against cancer, Nrf2, the cellular patrolman intimately linked to AMPK and metabolic stress, is activated during the detoxification process to utilize an array of substances to bind the reactive intermediate and allow the body to excrete it through the bowels or bladder. As an insurance policy, Nrf2 also upregulates the antioxidant defense system in case the toxic chemical causes any oxidative damage.

Foods that support our phase II detoxification system include: cruciferous vegetables, coffee, citrus fruits, tomatoes, teas, olives, rosemary, asparagus, berries, curcumin/turmeric, walnuts, curry powder, red wine, and salmon. Phytochemicals from cruciferous vegetables, blueberries, and even coffee interact with our cells, sounding the cellular alarm, pulling Nrf2 into the nucleus. In preparation for battle, Nrf2 activates an array of defense and antioxidant genes while promoting phase II detoxification of harmful chemicals. Nrf2's role is so vital to detoxification that when shut off in animal studies, mice lose many of the benefits from vegetable consumption and isocyothianate exposure.[49] Furthermore, Nrf2 serves as the cellular defense keystone, locking into place to support an array of ingrained defense mechanisms, intimately linking the benefits of exercise, fasting, periodic ketogenesis, and vegetable and spice consumption through the unification of these stressful, yet healthy cellular pressures.[50]

During the process of detoxification, the conjugation of harmful chemicals turns them into harmless substances that are dissolved in water and excreted from the body. This step overlaps with several other mechanisms that disarm free radicals, further providing redundancy within our cellular safety system. For instance, glutathione, one of our most important antioxidants, is produced during the process to sacrifice itself by binding to any reactive portions of chemicals during the intermediate phase of detoxification. With its selfless tendency to "jump on the grenade," glutathione is the most abundant antioxidant hero within our cells.

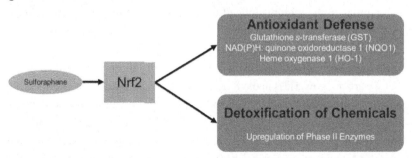

Figure 15: Sulforaphane signals to Nrf2 that danger may be coming. As a result, Nrf2 supports detoxification of chemicals and activates the

antioxidant defense system via GST, NQO1, and HO-1 to disarm free radicals before causing any damage.

These detoxification pathways overlap with several of the other dedicated antioxidant defense mechanisms listed in the picture above. Sulfur from garlic and onions, for example, supports phase II detoxification while increasing our cellular production of antioxidants.[51] Phase II enzymes rapidly clear toxic chemicals by utilizing the following pathways: 1) Glutathione S-transferase (GST), an antioxidant that disarms free radicals; 2) Glucuronyl transferase, which breaks down drugs and toxins; and 3) Sulfotransferases, which break down drugs and xenobiotics. However, the importance of glutathione extends far beyond detoxifying harmful chemicals and metabolites. Its ability to bind and offset reactive metabolites allows it to defuse free radicals before they bind to our DNA and damage it. Other plant chemicals like cinnamates (from cinnamon) and curcuminoids (from turmeric) act similarly to engage phase II enzymes to enhance detoxification, and they also have a seemingly large stimulus effect on antioxidant production.[52] Varying plant sources can have varying effects on different steps of the detoxification pathways, thus promoting a diet that includes an array of foods that activate these mechanisms, including, but not limited to: apiaceous vegetables like celery, turmeric, raspberries, blueberries, rosemary, green or black teas, purple sweet potatoes, fish oil, coffee, ginger, cruciferous vegetables, sources of CLA, allium vegetables, and some citrus fruits. Furthermore, as with their production of phenols and defense chemicals like sulfur, plants also have their own similar internal pathways to increase antioxidant production upon encountering toxins and stress, favoring sources grown without the use of large-scale pesticides.[53]

Similar to the aforementioned theoretically harmful chemicals in burnt food and meat, methods to avoid all dangerous environmental chemicals are mostly futile. While benzenes, parabens, heavy metals, hormones, irradiation, petrols, and exhaust bombard us daily, recent studies emphasize that we are not powerless in the fight against their chemical damage. We have the mechanisms previously discussed in place to prevent chemical damage either by disarming the toxins before they inflict any damage, or if all else fails, fixing the damage before it progresses to a more serious issue like cancer. Methods of supporting these damage control mechanisms mirror the ways in which we support the human body: through a healthy diet and lifestyle, coupled with exercise that stresses and trains our cells. The defensive chemicals from the vegetables listed above "exercise" these pathways by calling them to action, and, like Leonardo's intense work lifting dozens of pounds of cheese, stress our cells into a healthier state while posing little actual danger. These same foods contain many of the building blocks to support the repair of damage, providing an effective one-two punch when it comes to detoxification and cellular restoration. Moving away from the discouraging discussion that views nutritious food in the same vein as harmful substances like car emissions, these findings put us back into the driver's seat when it comes to impacting our health.

Returning to the scene of earlier chapters, the rusting bridges were not the only negative public safety byproduct of the steel industry in Pittsburgh: harmful pollution was poured into the air for centuries, barraging the lungs of its inhabitants. Similar chemicals entered the food and water supply, exposing other organs like the digestive tract to their damaging effects. While we could never purposely expose someone to a carcinogen in the name of a scientific study, both situations provided researcher opportunities to study the effect food may have on offsetting this already occurring damage.

Besides the skin, the lungs are perhaps the first organs to be exposed to harmful chemicals. As the muscles of the diaphragm contract and tighten, pulling downwards, air is inhaled into these spongy organs. It initially passes through the cartilaginous pipes, known as the bronchi, before entering the alveoli. Within these pouch-like alveoli, oxygen is extracted into the blood and transported to cells to aid in several other physiologic procedures including energy production within the mitochondria. During this process, air gets sucked through multiple sponge-like structures within our lungs, providing ample opportunities for toxic chemicals and foreign structures to lodge in the walls, or perhaps worse, enter the blood stream.

The chemicals that we breathe are eventually absorbed and metabolized within the body, yet ideally detoxified and excreted before inflicting any damage. Cigarette smokers are the group of people with perhaps the largest introduction of harmful and cancerous chemicals into their lungs, providing ample opportunity for research studies. The chemical levels within these individuals can be measured before and after they are provided foods and medicines to evaluate any effect on chemical absorption and breakdown. Studies confirm that when smokers ingest a blend made from cruciferous vegetable extract, harmful toxins from cigarette smoke are no longer absorbed and metabolized. Instead, they are simply broken down and detoxified into a water-soluble chemical and excreted in the urine, which effectively eliminates their ability to damage our cells and DNA. When the cruciferous compound is discontinued, the watered-down toxin is no longer found in the smoker's urine and is instead metabolized and absorbed within the body.[54] Progressive studies support these findings, revealing a decrease in free radical damage within the lung tissue after ingesting cruciferous-based compounds, along with a decrease in the occurrence of cancerous lesions that accompany this free radical damage.[55]

After the lungs, our gastrointestinal tract places second in the contest of carcinogen exposure. The esophagus, running down the middle of the lungs, is afforded similar protection from cancer after exposure to cruciferous vegetables. The cancer that typically occurs from exposing mice to Kritchevsky's often used DMBA is blocked within both the lungs and esophagus after cruciferous vegetable exposure.[56] The number of animal studies revealing the protective effects of cruciferous vegetables is so vast that the IARC has dedicated a large swath of their *Cancer Prevention Handbook* to their benefits. In total, dozens of animal studies illustrate the ability of isothiocyanates to offset cancerous damage in the esophagus, lung, breasts, and liver.[57]

Moving even further down the gastrointestinal tract, the bowels are perhaps the most commonly discussed area when it comes to cancer risk and food. Exposure to high levels of those chemicals from charred meat leads to deleterious changes throughout the colon in mouse experiments. Aberrant crypts, the prototypical abnormal cellular changes throughout the lining of the bowel, begin forming from this chemical exposure.[58] These crypts can lead to polyps – mushroom-like lesions often discovered, and then abruptly snipped off, during a colonoscopy – which can serve as a precursor to colon cancer. Brussels sprout and red cabbage extract, according to studies, can both detoxify these dangerous substances and protect the lining of the bowels from damage and crypt development. As in the lungs and esophagus, the formation of cancerous lesions in the bowels is greatly reduced, signifying an improvement in cellular damage defense and repair.[59] While these cruciferous vegetables provide a combination counteroffensive to cancer by both neutralizing and repairing damage, they can also provide a third benefit by helping to block the generation of the harmful chemical in the first place.

Returning to marinades, those containing allium vegetables like garlic and onions inhibit the formation of HAA during the cooking process.[60]

In an interesting twist of fate, CLA – the previously mentioned cancer-fighting wonder found in the fatty portions of meat and dairy produced from grass-fed cows – provides similar benefits when consumed alongside carcinogens.[61] Many of these unpasteurized dairy sources contain *lactobacillus*, the bacterial species camping within our bowels. While some of these vegetables provide sustenance for these bacteria, the bacteria themselves appear to play an additional role in binding and metabolizing carcinogens.[62] Nurturing these bowel bacteria helps to increase their presence in our gut, further potentiating the breakdown of harmful chemicals like HCAs, while in parallel converting organosulfur compounds in vegetables into their cancer-fighting byproducts.

The ability of onions, cruciferous vegetables, and leafy greens to support and promote our antioxidant and chemical defense systems is certainly not limited to these all-star vegetables. Tea, spices, red wine, and generally most foods with a bitter or tannic flavor contain chemicals with similar benefits via their ability to train and rouse our cellular defenses. Contact with chemicals in coffee, thyme, broccoli, rosemary, turmeric, red onions, and many other foods signals that imminent danger, springing Nrf2 into action to assess and address the threat.[63] It quickly relocates to the nucleus, binds to the cell's DNA, triggers the transcription of multiple antioxidant genes, and galvanizes the production of an array of damage defending proteins and enzymes. By the time Nrf2 realizes that these chemicals were in fact no threat, multiple anti-cancer mechanisms and repair genes are already primed and activated. Similar chemicals also increase the expression of the numerous detoxification enzymes, providing both training and proper defense of threats, along with mechanisms to defuse the threats before they pose a risk.[64]

Furthermore, defensive plant chemicals like tannins in red wine and terpenes in trees mirror the sulfur in cruciferous vegetables, inhibiting many inflammatory cellular pathways with uncanny similarity – some of the highest levels of tannins are found in the delicious Southern Italian wines made from the Aglianico grape.[65] While these chemicals calm inflammation in our normal cells,[66] they fiercely disrupt the function of cancer cells by interfering with their reproduction, often acting like the frataxin of Ristow's studies, triggering them to undergo apoptosis.[57] In other words, isocyothianates rewire cancer cells to self-implode while arming our cells with the wherewithal to stop cancer before it starts.

The science behind the benefits of eating pungent vegetables is beyond compelling, and while an ounce of daily pungent vegetables may already provide a pound of cure, there are additional methods to maximize the benefits achieved. Increasing the time that myrosinase interacts with the glucosinolates will maximize the production of sulphoraphane. Myrosinase is heat sensitive and becomes degraded during the cooking process, so cutting these vegetables ahead of time can facilitate its contact with the glucosinolates to increase the yield of sulfur. (Chewing raw vegetables can help release myrosinase, but it will be inactivated only a short time later when it descends into Dante's inferno, the acidic environment of the stomach.[67]) When it comes to raw veggie sources, young sprouts seem to contain more beneficial sulforaphane. While Brussels sprouts sautéed in butter are unquestionably more delectable, steaming vegetables is often the safest way to preserve and maximize their sulfur levels. In some instances, steaming may even increase the amount of sulfur, and it should be noted that freezing vegetables also tends to destroy myrosinase.[68]

As with most foods, it seems prudent to avoid the microwave when cooking sprouts and most vegetables. Finally, it should be mentioned that at least some degree of heat is advantageous, as it degrades a chemical that can convert glucosinolates to a sulforaphane-like byproduct without the many anti-cancer benefits of sulforaphane.

While cooked Brussels sprouts and other cruciferous vegetables still provide an ample amount of health benefits, there are methods to enhance the sulfur-based benefits. For instance, when cooking Brussels sprouts in butter in a the cast-iron skillet with sea salt and pepper, adding powder from mustard seeds, which contain a more durable form of myrosinase, can help offset some of these issues with cooking.[69] And to further enhance the stated benefits of marinades, lemon juice can be added to them to double the amount of available sulforaphane.[70] The final sulfur products are also heat sensitive, so adding spices like mustard seed powder after cooking may help to maximize the production of sulforaphane by breaking down the residual glucosinolates.

Garlic shares a similar fate: 60 seconds in the microwave or 45 minutes in the oven greatly weakens its anti-cancer benefits. Unfortunately, the pungency in garlic that leaves us with a potent breath is the same source of the beneficial chemical. Like with broccoli and Brussels sprouts, crushing garlic for ten minutes beforehand helps salvage some of its anti-cancer benefits that may be lost with cooking.[71] To derive all of the benefits of garlic while avoiding garlic breath, it can be cut ahead of time, then added to water and swallowed like pills.

Yet when all else fails, our trusty bowel bacteria are there to bail us out yet again. The residual glucosinolates in cruciferous vegetables are usually able to resist the damage from cooking, and by the time they reach our bowels, the local bacteria are often able to convert them to sulforaphane. Many of these bacteria include those found in raw cheese, and many are the same bacteria that feast on fibrous vegetables in our diet. Bacteria species like *Bacteroides*, lactic acid bacteria, *Enterobacteriaceae,* and *Bifidobaicterium* contain myrosinase and other enzymes that break down glucosinolates to sulforaphane. Feeding these bacteria is a prudent strategy to help increase yield of these beneficial compounds: animal studies reveal that just four days of a high broccoli diet significantly increases the number of those bacteria that thrive on cruciferous vegetables and create sulforaphane.[72]

Like our sacred cows raised on their heavenly optimal diet of grass and Leonardo's beloved sheep roaming the Calabrian mountainsides eating pasture, the quality and beneficial sulfur content of vegetables relies on their growing conditions.[57] Remembering that these chemicals serve as the plant's defense system, the ones that are subjected to harassment by insects – i.e. are not constantly sprayed with pesticides – tend to have higher amounts of these substances. Furthermore, just as cows and sheep convert their food into nutrients passed on in their meat and milk, nitrogen and sulfur-rich soil will impart healthier chemicals into the plants and enhance glucosinolate production. Plant stress parallels human stress; plants that undergo reasonable levels of natural stress generate more organosulfurs. In addition to insects, lack of water and higher temperatures are other stresses that increase levels of glucosinolates.[57]

Conversely, plants that are doused with pesticides and grown in soils depleted of minerals and nutrients are likely to contain less organosulfurs. Like their human "predators" higher up the food chain, plants need to struggle for optimal health so that they can pass that health onto us. Even the transportation of the vegetables is important; when Brussels sprouts are transported under cold storage, they can lose a majority of their glucosinolate content. While cooking broccoli for even several minutes meaningfully reduces isocyothianate content,[73] an optimal dose is unknown, nor is it known with certainty whether a "more is better" approach applies. All things considered, though, a cooked allium or cruciferous vegetable is better than none at all: it provides vitamins, minerals, nourishment for our bowel bacteria, and some residual beneficial chemicals. A pro tip I like to employ is to consume the garlic, onions, and other vegetables that cause bad breath at the start of the meal, then follow up with the other foods on my plate that mitigate the odor: foods high in water and fat seem to have the largest deodorizing effect. And of course, if all else fails, a little swish and swallow of baking soda seems to adequately lessen the intensity of garlic and onion breath.

Scientists are only beginning to scratch the surface on the plethora of anti-cancer benefits of allium and cruciferous vegetables, and so we still have much to learn. Defensive chemicals in other plants and spices may provide similar benefits. While growing conditions, storage, preparation, and cooking methods are important, the array of benefits that accompany these vegetables certainly provide us with a "more is better" preliminary strategy. The daily buttressing of our detoxification system to eliminate dangerous and cancerous chemicals and the deployment of the antioxidant defense system to disarm free radicals are both compelling reasons to make ingredients that activate both parts of our dietary armamentarium to fight disease and cancer and maximize our health and longevity. While the singular defense mechanism of plants involves waging chemical warfare on their predators, our human cells have evolved over millions of years to capitalize on their dire situation, turning potential poisons into anti-cancer potions as is our privilege perched atop the evolutionary food chain.

Throughout human evolution, the human body required dietary meat and fat containing vital nutrients like vitamin B12 and hefty amounts of omega-3 fats like alpha linoleic acid to fuel the development of our large and intricate brains. Fire and cooking served to kindle and accelerate the process – prior to the gift of Prometheus, our apelike predecessors relied on a primarily plant-based diet consisting of raw fruits and vegetables. The process of detoxification unites the two in perfect harmony, providing both cellular and historical justification for a well-rounded diet, dense with nutrient-rich and vitamin-rich foods to serve as cellular building blocks, coupled with chemical-rich plants to feed our bowel bacteria and stress our cells.

12

CLOSING THE DOOR ON CANCER

"You have to let them struggle – it is good for them. If you give them too much water, they will grow wildly but produce suboptimal fruit."

\- John Reichl at age 96

"Neither need you tell me," said Candide, "that we must take care of our garden."

\- Voltaire

Takeaways:

Our bodies are likened to a garden; the garden that receives too much fertilizer becomes overgrown with weeds while the garden that is given an ideal combination of nurturing nutrients and necessary drought to avoid overgrowth results in healthy and productive vegetation.

Tangible conclusions on living a healthy and cancer-free lifestyle are summarized.

L eonardo had just finished tucking his children into bed when he heard some rustling out back. His pulse began to thump rapidly, accelerating until it reached a rate that he had only once experienced, during his fateful encounter with the mysterious man at his grocery store. Was that pseudo-gangster back for revenge? He fumbled around in the cigar box buried deep in his closet until he found the shiny metal six-shooter. He slowly crept out of the back door with the pistol muzzle pointed forward leading the way, the moonlight reflecting brightly off his yellow brick house. Suddenly, a shadow darted from behind the chicken coop and caught Leonardo's eye, and his hands began to tremble from adrenaline – he had spotted his target. He steadied his hand, cocked back the hammer of his pistol, and with all his might squeezed his right pointer finger until it became numb. The disorienting clap pierced his ears moments later followed by a loud ringing and a plume of smoke emanating from the barrel.

The bullet had ripped through the backyard and terminated its flight with a sudden thump, indicating it had struck and lodged itself into an unknown target mass. Nervous heart palpitations sent shockwaves reverberating throughout Leonardo's chest; until today he had never fired a gun before, and he was still unsure if this pistol he had purchased years ago and brandished once upon a time to ward off a trespasser was even a functional weapon or just a decorative replica prop. Now his heart was beating so ferociously that he felt it was pushing through his ribs. He tiptoed closer and closer behind the chicken coop; the bright moonlight cast the silhouette of the building onto the area where his target lay slumped on the ground. Leonardo approached, leaned in, and squinted to focus his eyes on his victim. It was not a man in pleated pants, nor any man at all – instead, feathers were scattered around the crime scene... oh, and the chicken coop door was wide open. The identity of his victim suddenly dawned on Leonardo: It was not a revenge-seeking gangster but one of his own chickens that he had just shot. Leonardo laughed as he realized he had shot one of his hens, spraying its feathers over the backyard. Leonardo had just gotten a head start on preparing the evening's dinner. And in a more abstract sense, Leonardo's bullet was a metaphorical blow to the invisible hand of Plato.

÷

I stood sideways staring down along my extended left arm as my pointed hand pierced the banana tree through my line of vision. I slowly brought my backfoot inwards, and just as it approached my left leg, I violently twisted. My right arm extended backwards and then snapped forwards across my body like a rubber band, leaving my right shoulder no choice but to be yanked aggressively in the same direction. Just when my arm could extend no further forward, I let the spear go; it darted forward effortlessly, cutting straight through the wind like a needle until it ripped through the trunk of the banana tree, a mere inch above the prior spear I had thrown. I felt a rush of blood and endorphins coursing through my extremities, spilling over into my torso and eventually filling my head as I screamed in celebration. Mimicking a professional football player, I flexed at an imaginary television camera as I screamed.

Days before I was at an oncology conference on the other side of Maui, and my wife and I decided to make the winding drive along Hana Highway to spend a couple days in the middle of the jungle. Today, we were throwing handmade spears at banana trees. It was one of my greatest feats of athleticism in recent memory, to throw two spears in a row through a banana tree trunk measuring about 10 inches wide while on vacation. The primordial aftermath of flexing and screaming was unscripted and immediate – I had involuntarily channeled my inner evolutionary past. The immediate release of adrenaline occurred fully independent of my premeditated knowledge or willpower; it was merely a natural response to my actions. While the rapid heartbeat that accompanies the release of adrenaline is commonly experienced – an innate physiologic response to our surroundings – we are experiencing millions of these responses per day, and most occur without any awareness on our end. Oftentimes, we do have our suspicions – there is a reason our mood drops 30 minutes after consuming that pastry and we feel tired. Furthermore, these responses do not simply vanish afterwards – they cause a butterfly effect, impacting multiple cells and organs in the near vicinity and then further away throughout the body.

We have multiple cellular and physiological mechanisms that were forged and refined over the past million years. When we suddenly spot a lion, our bodies set off the following chain reaction: turn off your bowels, send all the blood to your brain and muscles as you navigate how to best escape, conduct synchronization of your fast-twitch muscle movements, and then run like hell in the direction opposite the lion. Eat some pungent garlic, cruciferous vegetables, or flavorful spices, and your cells are signaled to prepare for attack, the immune system is enhanced, you are left better able to fight infection, and you live a tiny bit longer to presumably consume some more spices. Times of fasting when food was not available, extensive periods of low carbohydrates throughout the winter, intense exercise while hunting and gathering, and downtime for relaxation were all plentiful throughout man's early history and evolution, so it is no surprise that the human body became accustomed to these activities and hence, channels the physiologic responses that accompany them. If we hedge too far from these normal activities and forget to ignite our primordial cellular imprint, then the body is often left in an unhealthy state prone to disease, the growth of fat cells, and ultimately, a higher risk of cancer.

In the hustle and bustle of modern society, activating those cellular mechanisms to prime our bodies to fight disease and cancer seems like more of a novelty these days. We often find ourselves going hours, days, or weeks without channeling our ingrained primordial past. Eating three meals a day plus snacks in between is a state foreign to our ancestors, who fasted for hours on end. We rarely go without insulin-stimulating foods like refined and simple carbohydrates – something our cells rarely encountered in the past, especially during the cold winter months inhospitable to plant life when we had scant access to fruits and other carbohydrate-rich foods. We consume prepackaged foods that take no more effort to "kill" than twisting our fingers to open; we no longer spend the time and effort to gather ingredients for a meal, nor experience the meditative-like downtime experienced from cooking a meal. We stay up late, wake up early, remain seated at a desk for most of the day, and then try to compensate for this by packing a lost day of activities into an hour at the gym.

All these activities may seem miniscule on an individual level when compared to the grand scheme of our lives, but rest assured they do add up. As a radiation oncologist, I use small doses of radiation to treat tumors. If these doses are kept small enough, it lengthens the overall treatment time but provides our normal cells ample time to fix the damage. I always caution patients that the individual treatments are so small that they are unrecognizable – there is no burning, warming, instant changes, nor do they leave the sessions radioactive from exposure. However, as with a simple x-ray, each treatment causes a small amount of damage that produces cascading effects, combining in number and eventually leading to treatment-related side effects, like a sunburn and suntan. Similarly, small and seemingly inconsequential behaviors and lifestyle habits leave an imprint on our cells, some for better and some for worse. Eventually, our cellular responses to such habits accumulate and then culminate in either side effects or the successful avoidance of cancer. While Tomasetti and Vogelstein informed us that oftentimes a little bad luck is involved, channeling our own innate cellular responses may help to shift luck in our favor.

We still have a lot to learn, but following nature's millennia-old blueprint while sidestepping modern dietary enigmas seems to fuel our body to perform to its fullest while channeling those mechanisms that help us prune the excesses within. Finding success at this is extremely difficult in a society of conveniences that often places focus on indulgences and material goods while leaving health and well-being on the backburner. Like laboratory mice, we sit in cages all day picking at food. The several lifestyle behaviors and eating habits discussed up to this point uniformly create a cellular environment nurtured to be vigorous at maintaining our health while warding off threats from cancer and other diseases. Many of these cellular changes are activated by channeling these ancient mechanisms that remain within us. Many of these spartan activities stress our cells, forcing them to rely on a phenomenon called metabolic flexibility – over millions of years our cells have acquired the skills to remain healthy during extreme conditions like feast and famine.

Perhaps rifling spears into a banana tree is a tad extreme for the average nine-to-fiver. However, channeling our innate metabolic flexibility by undergoing controlled stresses, frequent periods without food, and disciplined avoidance of snacking can provide our cells a frequent jumpstart to prune those unlucky, Manchurian candidate cells lurking within. Akin to Kenyon's worms, our ancestors of the past, and even more recently during winter months, avoiding simple carbohydrates and generally minimizing carbohydrates while engaging in intense exercise and the periodic lifting of heavy objects may enact these deeply buried, and often suppressed, mechanisms that can help us achieve our best health. This stress to our body also can be safely mimicked with pungent herbs and spices, green veggies, and yes, even bold red wines. Nutrient-dense foods, including fatty foods and animal products, and plant-based foods should not be viewed in isolation or as an arranged marriage between two unwilling partners, but rather as joyous nuptials consummated by good health and the avoidance of disease.

The quote to open this final chapter is from Leonardo's son-in-law and my grandfather John Reichl, who at the age of 96 remained a bastion of knowledge when it came to nurturing his garden. Producing consistently delicious and organic vegetables on a yearly basis takes decades of practice, and with almost ten decades under his belt Grandpa John was a seasoned veteran. At the time he dropped me this pearl of wisdom, little did I know I would be withdrawing medical care on him several months later. He had spent countless hours in his garden that summer, toiling away while temperatures around him pushed into the nineties. Pruning, feeding his plants compost that he had been producing for over half a century, and sometimes just walking around observing, John felt gardening was not just work or a hobby, it was an extension of him. His personality, calm nature, and meticulous Austrian upbringing intertwined with his wife's southern Italian culture took shape over most of the twentieth century, culminating in the ultimate balance of sufficient care and purposeful neglect.

Spending a large portion of my childhood observing my grandfather, I never truly understood the analogy between his garden, life, and our cellular health until after I watched him gasp for his last breaths before passing away on a cold night in January of 2014. As a cancer researcher looking for hints as to what foods and lifestyle activities help maximize our health and avoid the dreaded scourge of cancer, I only then realized just how closely John – a medical marvel – and his precious garden paralleled the field of cancer prevention research. Easy solutions were sparse: too little fertilizer, nutrition, or nurturing and the plants may live to produce fruit but are barely scraping by; too much fertilizer, water, or pesticides, and the plants may grow wildly, producing large vines with cancerous suckers sprouting from the sides yielding subpar or deformed fruit. Optimal strategies nurture and promote the ideal growth of the plant, while appropriate soil conditions can prevent the accumulation of weeds and other unwanted growth. Stressing the plants further builds up their immune system to fight potential threats like insects, fungus, bacteria, and other cancerous coercions within their environment. A balance must be met.

Achieving this balance requires no Ph.D., high school education, or instruction at the local community college. This balance is the art of gardening, passed down through generations and mastered through practice. It is a balance that keeps all gardeners amateur and professional observing, adjusting, and pruning our beloved plants for hours on end. This frustrating art carries a large learning curve, one that when finally mastered encompasses the joy of gardening. This art mirrors the balance within our lifestyle of maximizing our health and minimizing damage to our bodies while living a fulfilling life. Leonardo may have been a simple southern Italian shepherd and shop owner, but an analysis of his lifestyle provides many valuable lessons. He certainly engaged in some unhealthy behaviors, made whiskey during Prohibition, ate bread and pasta, and enjoyed his wife's delicious pies. However, even these were made of the highest quality ingredients and were a rare treat. His view of his traditional, cultural, and nutrient-dense foods as a vital component of his life – John's focus on the plants as opposed to the weeds – assured that consumption of these foods would never get the best of him.

Leonardo, like most of his family and friends from the Mediterranean and Southern Italy, ate meat and cheese and washed it down with homemade wine. His household used a lot of olive oil and cooked with lard. Leonardo made his own soppressata and heaps of sausage for his grocery store patrons. The irony that Leonardo, a shepherd, ran away when it was time to slaughter his sheep is not lost on our family. The ethical treatment of animals is not only better for them, but healthier for us. Consuming them as part of our diet should not be taken lightly, a major reason why people of many cultures and religions including Leonardo's direct descendants give thanks prior to each meal. Pythagoras, Plato, and many present-day philosophers know the ethical issues with consuming animals and raising them properly. Both meat eaters and vegetarians bring good arguments to the dinner table, but using religious, philosophical, and cultural beliefs to condemn the consumption of all meat and animal products, in essence wantonly ignoring their dense nutrition benefits in the process, is tenuous at best and dangerous, unhealthy, and deceiving at worst.

Food culture and culinary customs have not been passed down through millennia by accident. It is no surprise that the merits of the age-old traditions among inhabitants the Old World and Mediterranean regions have been recently appreciated, whereas the low-fat, calorie counting craze has left society more overweight and less healthy with a view of food as an unsolvable mathematical equation rather than a delicious part of our cultural identity and a basic component of daily life. The secret to a fulfilling and healthy lifestyle has more accurately been passed to us by our grandparents and great-grandparents than by pencil-pushing scientists and physicians who have never grown a garden, prepared a meal, or operated a grape press. The American infatuation with turning these easy solutions into complex calculations and processes only serves to convolute one of the true joys of life. As a result, highly educated individuals fail at a process that Leonardo easily mastered. He knew the importance of nutrient-dense, culturally cherished foods and needed no mathematical equation to quantify them. As a shepherd, he also knew the importance of caring for his animals, raising them appropriately, and feeding them the foods they were meant to eat. It is by no coincidence that when the innate cellular mechanisms of animals are supported, they are healthier and produce healthier foodstuffs as well. But Leonardo also recognized and respected the importance of a well-rounded lifestyle and meal choices.

In 1756, Voltaire compiled his literary criticism of religious doctrine of the 18th century, known as *Plato's Dream*. Asleep and dreaming, Plato interacts with Demogorgon about the formation of the world, and he tackles the difficult task of accepting both the perfection and faults that lie within humanity, the intricate balance of good and evil on earth. Following a healthy lifestyle that includes animal foods and products will always be seen as both good and evil, and a difficulty reconciling the two sides will accompany this consideration. Three years later, Voltaire created his literary masterpiece, *Candide;* he concluded this seminal work with a basic prescription remarkably reminiscent of both my grandfather John and my great-grandfather Leonardo: "Let us cultivate our garden." Let us not starve our gardens to avoid the growth of weeds, but instead provide deterrents by nurturing our healthy cells, stressing them when needed, and nourishing them in between.

EPILOGUE

We have covered a lot of material in this book, from the science of cancer and calorie restriction over the past hundred years to the philosophical undertones spanning millennia that are woven throughout our modern dietary recommendations. As I am sure you noticed, the material can be dense at times. What have we learned?

We have learned that the spartan-like activities of fasting, periods of low to minimal carbohydrates, heavy weightlifting exercises, and the consumption of bitter foods may be foreign concepts to our minds, but they are quite recognizable to our cells. In fact, they are so recognizable that upon application of these activities our cells engage in an array of mechanisms that help us to achieve optimal health, fight disease, and prune potential cancerous cells from within. Overloading our bodies with refined and simple carbohydrates, factory-produced fats, vegetable oils, and other "Frankenstein foods" that are unrecognizable to our cells leads to emergency cellular responses that, much like the small doses of radiation therapy I prescribe to my cancer patients, accumulate over time and take their toll.

Running counter to these acute spartan activities are the historic activities purposefully set out to elicit suffering and discipline. Intentional general calorie restriction, especially like that seen in the Minnesota Starvation Study, is a rare occurrence, albeit some religious or cultural ceremonies may purposefully channel its torturous aspects in display of sacrifice and discipline. Population-wide recommendations for calorie restriction ignore our bodies' ingrained mechanisms, eschew the macabre results of the Minnesota Starvation Study and the Biosphere 2 experience, and trample over millennia-old cultural traditions. Failure of these population-wide recommendations should come as no surprise. Should we connect with our food, or view it as a mild poison for which it is best left to minimize dosage? If you never leave the couch, you are unlikely to ever sprain an ankle, but even the most risk-averse orthopedic surgeon would be hard-pressed to recommend this as a healthy activity! Food is no different – if your cells are malnourished and barely surviving, they may be unlikely to form cancer, but is that a healthy strategy?

Outside of religious ceremonies, Leonardo never purposefully fasted; he never needed to, since his lifestyle often had him naturally going extended periods without food. When he did eat, his meals were comprised of nutrient-dense foods that provided him with adequate sustenance that satisfied his hunger, never leaving him at risk of excessive overeating. Dozens of randomized studies confirm this exact principle: when subjects can eat without limiting their calories but they instead opt to reduce appetite-stimulating foods like packaged and processed carbohydrates and thoughtfully increase fat consumption, they unanimously drop the amount of food they are eating due to their satisfied appetites. Furthermore, when subjects – regardless of whether adhering to a low-fat or low-carbohydrate diet – ignore calorie-counting, lower their overall consumption of processed foods and refined carbohydrates and grains, focus on wholesome foods like grass-fed beef and hearty vegetables, and change their relationship with food to view it as an important and normal part of daily life, lo and behold they also lose weight and end up healthier.[1] Interestingly, participants in this particular study were instructed to cook, eat with friends and family, avoid eating while driving or watching TV, and shop for food locally at farmers markets. In other words, they were asked to treat food much the same way that Leonardo Pesce and his family did.

Eating a well-rounded diet is not rocket science, and such a diet includes the most nutritious ingredients possible. Any discussion on which foods are "good" or "bad" for us usually becomes a nuanced, circular, and often subjective intermixing of science, religion, convenience, and cultural beliefs. All that said, most scientists and Average Joes alike would agree that any food that promotes uncontrolled overeating should be minimized. For many, this includes grains and simple carbohydrates – which often encourage overconsumption due to the blood sugar and insulin roller coaster that often follows – or even the ever so healthy nuts, which are kryptonite to some overeaters. Some solutions to avoid overeating are less subtle than others. It is not a coincidence that the avoidance of such addictive foods provides a metabolic benefit by fostering an anti-cancer cellular environment hospitable to our normal cells and unwelcoming to those budding cancer cells.

In what seems like a strictly Platonic move, population-wide dietary recommendations have ignored studies promoting the consumption of satiating, nutrient-dense foods and instead focused on promoting calorie counting, recommending anxious dieters to engage in the mind-numbing and oft-unsuccessful act of severe calorie restriction and consumption of low-fat, unsatisfying foods that make restricting anything nearly impossible. We are bombarded with messages touting a culture doomed to fail. How could this purposefully be accomplished? Did the dietary board members purposefully ignore the available studies? Were they unaware of them? Once again, there are inexplicable influences that could only have been manipulated by the undermining hidden hand of Plato and his refusal to view food and diet as anything more than a mechanism to test intestinal fortitude, as opposed to a source of fuel infusing the body with nutrients.

Furthermore, there are inalienable truths that surface when reviewing the cultural, historic, and scientific impact of our food and health. We need to reconnect with our food, and until we do, maximizing our health will remain out of reach for most of the population. These benefits go far beyond simply raising or lowering hormones like insulin or IGF-1 or normal processes that can be dangerous when in excess, such as our blood sugar levels. There are deep-rooted implications and physiologic responses that occur when we connect with our food, prepare meals, cook, and sit with family and friends over the dinner table. These undeniable benefits reveal that shortcuts to food provide shortcuts to sickness: we can count all the calories we want and continue to view food as poison, but until we take the long route and reconnect with our food, the rates of diabetes, obesity, and cancer will continue to rise.

Tannenbaum's mice grew fat and medically and metabolically morbid as they sat in their cage day after day, grazing on food around the clock. Such an experiment sounds all too familiar: modern humans have reached a woeful state where we must try harder to avoid living a life that resembles Tannenbaum's stuffed and sedentary mice miserably waiting around for their ultimate demise. His view of food as a currency and constant counting of calories – something we have all been told to do repeatedly as of late – only makes the experience that much more real. So, removing the ideologies, politics, religion, and multiple other external influences on what people recommend we eat, what makes up an anti-cancer diet and lifestyle?

To sell a successful diet book, authors are told to prescribe one simple eating strategy for everyone. Such an approach may be lucrative for authors and publishers, but certainly will not produce successful results for most of the population. Such an approach overlooks the point of food in the first place, its association with our cultural background, and the unique role it plays in our lives. Yet, several realities surface when attempting to prescribe an anti-cancer diet. Food is meant to nourish our bodies, and food that provides the most vitamins and nutrients is a good place to start. Along those lines, food and health are not valued or validated via a mathematical equation, so bread, grains, and other low-calorie but also low-nutrient foods are probably good foods to avoid, or at least not to be relied upon for nutritive reasons. I would be remiss if I did not at least provide a short prescription of an anti-cancer lifestyle, or at least some "tangible takeaways" (in the words of the health coach Roger Dickerman) based on what I personally do and what the famous researchers do:

1. Avoid grazing: Periods without food, fasting, intermittent fasting, or in whatever way you choose to quantify them as, trigger innate anti-cancer mechanisms, providing healthful benefits.

2. Engage in periods of low dietary carbohydrates: We experienced these periods extensively throughout our time on this earth during fasting and winter, engaging in ketosis, autophagy, and the pruning of superfluous and potentially dangerous energy sources and cellular components.

3. Avoid vegetable oils and sources of excess omega-6 fats: Aim to fight free radicals, not introduce external sources to our cells.

4. Stimulate indirect antioxidant production and sound the alarm on our defense systems: While direct antioxidant pills and vitamins have proven low-value thus far, mechanisms that indirectly increase our cellular production of antioxidants and cellular defense mechanisms to ward off cellular and DNA damage provide an array of anti-cancer benefits that enable our cells to battle disease and aging. Increase these mechanisms with numbers 1 and 2 above, along with intense exercise, heavy and muscle-stimulating lifting, spices, bitter vegetables, and even tannic wines.

5. Do what the researchers do: Kenyon eats a low-carbohydrate diet because she has seen so much research, including her own, supporting the health benefits of this path. She preaches what she practices, because she practices what she researches. Many diet gurus and armchair experts have a belief system first, then they preach a diet to back it up. Science

and data first, recommendations second. Who would you rather go to for the science, Kenyon and Ristow, or Plato and Pythagoras?

6. Remember cultural food habits and know why and where they come from. I am not suggesting we get our medical advice from a shepherd and an Italian grocery store owner, but if Leonardo were still alive today and were asked how best to remain healthy and avoid cancer, he would give simple advice like stay active and eat like your grandfather. This advice may not be newsworthy, but nevertheless it does parallel what is needed in our medical field.

I myself have published dozens of studies on cancer research, and my colleague Robert Weinberg has published many more which have rightfully earned him industry peer esteem, numerous international science awards, and millions of dollars in medical research funding grants. In the Ken Burns documentary based on Siddhartha Mukherjee's Pulitzer Prize winning novel *The Emperor of All Maladies*, Weinberg strongly voiced his views, opining:

"Without any doubt, that the greatest decreases in cancer-associated mortality will come from preventing the disease, rather than trying to treat it, as I try to do. The first major preventable cause of cancer is tobacco usage, and the second most important factor in causing cancer is, believe it or not, obesity. And if those two factors can be changed in our society, we are going to see decreases in cancer mortality, at least in the next decade or two, that dwarf anything I or my colleagues can produce in terms of new, miraculous cures."

To Weinberg, the entirety of science-based wellness research throughout history – from the dietary recommendations of Plato to the cutting-edge therapies of today – is far less important than the simple message of prevention through a healthy lifestyle.

I wholeheartedly concur.

REFERENCES

Chapter 2:

1. Davidovici, B. B. The role of diet in acne: facts and controversies. *Clin. Dermatol.* 2010.
2. Hu, F. B. et al. Dietary Fat Intake and the Risk of Coronary Heart Disease in Women. *N. Engl. J. Med.* 1997.
3. Kinlen, L. Sir Richard Doll, epidemiologist - a personal reminiscence with a selected bibliography. *Br. J. Cancer.* 2005.
4. Doll, R. & Hill, A. B. Smoking and carcinoma of the lung; preliminary report. *Br. Med. J.* 1950.
5. Doll, R. et al. Mortality in relation to smoking: 50 years' observations on male British doctors. *BMJ.* 2004.
6. Armstrong, B. & Doll, R. Environmental factors and cancer incidence and mortality in different countries, with special reference to dietary practices. *Int. J. Cancer.* 1975.
7. Willett, W. C. et al. Dietary fat and the risk of breast cancer. *N. Engl. J. Med.* 1987.
8. Schaefer, E. J. et al. Lack of efficacy of a food-frequency questionnaire in assessing dietary macronutrient intakes in subjects consuming diets of known composition. *Am. J. Clin. Nutr.* 2000.
9. Graham, S. et al. Diet in the Epidemiology of Breast Cancer. *Am. J. Epidemiol.* 1982.
10. Hunter, D. J. et al. Cohort Studies of Fat Intake and the Risk of Breast Cancer — A Pooled Analysis. *N. Engl. J. Med.* 1996.
11. Morganti, A. G. et al. Radioprotective Effect of Moderate Wine Consumption in Patients with Breast Carcinoma. *Int. J. Radiat. Oncol.* 2009.
12. Kristal, A. R., Peters, U. & Potter, J. D. Is It Time to Abandon the Food Frequency Questionnaire? *Cancer Epidemiol. Biomarkers Prev.* 2005.
13. Willett, W. C. et al. Dietary Fat and Fiber in Relation to Risk of Breast Cancer. *JAMA.* 1992.
14. Counsel on Scientific Affairs. Dietary Fiber and Health. *JAMA.* 1989.
15. Holmes, M. D. et al. Association of Dietary Intake of Fat and Fatty Acids with Risk of Breast Cancer. *JAMA.* 1999.
16. Schoenfeld, J. D. & Ioannidis, J. P. Is everything we eat associated with cancer? A systematic cookbook review. *Am. J. Clin. Nutr.* 2013.
17. Willett, W. C. Diet and cancer. *Oncologist.* 2000.
18. Willett, W. C. Diet and breast cancer. *J. Intern. Med.* 2001.

Chapter 3:

1. Bianchini, F. et al. Overweight, obesity, and cancer risk. *Lancet Oncol.* 2002.

2. Moreschi, C. Beziehungen zwischen Ernahrung und Tumorwachstum. Z. *Immunitatsforsch*. 1909.

3. Rous, P. The Influence of Diet on Transplanted and Spontaneous Mouse Tumors. *J. Exp. Med.* 1914.

4. Studies from the Rockefeller Institute for Medical Research, Volume 23. 1916.

5. Watson, A. F. & Mellanby, E. Tar Cancer in Mice. II. The Condition of the Skin, when Modified by External Treatment or Diet, as a Factor in Influencing the Cancerous Reaction. *Br. J. Exp. Pathol.* 1930.

6. Tannenbaum, A. The Dependence of Tumor Formation on the Composition of the Calorie-Restricted Diet as Well as on the Degree of Restriction. *Cancer Res.* 1945.

7. Van Alstyne, E. V. N. & Beebe, S. P. Diet studies in transplantable Tumors - I. The Effect of non-carbohydrate Diet upon the Growth of transplantable Sarcoma in Rats. *J Med Res.* 1913.

8. Beebe, S.P. The Autolysin Treatment for Cancer. *JAMA*. 1915.

9. Hursting, S. D. et al. Calories and carcinogenesis: lessons learned from 30 years of calorie restriction research. *Carcinogenesis*. 2010.

10. Bhatt, A. Evolution of clinical research: a history before and beyond james lind. *Perspect. Clin. Res.* 2010.

11. Proctor, R. N. The history of the discovery of the cigarette-lung cancer link: evidentiary traditions, corporate denial, global toll. *Tob. Control.* 2012.

12. Larsson, S. C. & Wolk, A. Red and processed meat consumption and risk of pancreatic cancer: meta-analysis of prospective studies. *Br. J. Cancer.* 2012.

13. Pancreatic cancer risk increases with every 2 strips of bacon you eat: Study - CBS News. Available at: https://www.cbsnews.com/news/pancreatic-cancer-risk-increases-with-every-2-strips-of-bacon-you-eat-study/. (Accessed: 29th January 2018)

14. Schoenfeld, J. D. & Ioannidis, J. P. Is everything we eat associated with cancer? A systematic cookbook review. *Am. J. Clin. Nutr.* 2013.

15. Stampfer, M. J. et al. A prospective study of postmenopausal estrogen therapy and coronary heart disease. *N. Engl. J. Med.* 1985.

16. Grady, D. et al. Cardiovascular disease outcomes during 6.8 years of hormone therapy: Heart and Estrogen/progestin Replacement Study follow-up (HERS II). *JAMA*. 2002.

17. Prasad V, et. al. Reversals of established medical practices: Evidence to abandon ship. *JAMA*. 2012.

18. Collaborative Group on Hormonal Factors in Breast Cancer. Breast cancer and hormone replacement therapy: collaborative reanalysis of data from 51 epidemiological studies of 52,705 women with breast cancer and 108,411 women without breast cancer. *Lancet*. 1997.

Chapter 4:

1. Life Under the Bubble | Discover Magazine. December 2010. Available at https://www.discovermagazine.com/environment/life-under-the-bubble
2. Poynter, J. The human experiment: two years and twenty minutes inside Biosphere 2. (Thunder's Mouth Press, 2006).
3. Walford, R. L. et al. Calorie restriction in biosphere 2: alterations in physiologic, hematologic, hormonal, and biochemical parameters in humans restricted for a 2-year period. *J. Gerontol. A. Biol. Sci. Med. Sci.* 2002.
4. Keys, A. et al. Experimental Starvation in Man. Defense Technical Information Center. 1945.
5. Walford, R. L. et al. The calorically restricted low-fat nutrient-dense diet in Biosphere 2 significantly lowers blood glucose, total leukocyte count, cholesterol, and blood pressure in humans. *Proc. Natl. Acad. Sci.* 1992.
6. Reider, R. Dreaming the Biosphere: The Theater of All Possibilities. (University of New Mexico Press, 2009).
7. Turner, C. CABINET // Ingestion / Planet in a Bottle. Cabinet Magazine (2011). Available at: http://www.cabinetmagazine.org/issues/41/turner.php. (Accessed: 26th November 2017)
8. The 100 Worst Ideas of The Century - TIME. Available at http://content.time.com/time/magazine/article/0,9171,991230,00.html. June 1999.
9. Lassinger, B. K. et al. Atypical parkinsonism and motor neuron syndrome in a Biosphere 2 participant: A possible complication of chronic hypoxia and carbon monoxide toxicity? *Mov. Disord.* 2004.
10. Patel, B. P. et al. Caloric Restriction Shortens Lifespan through an Increase in Lipid Peroxidation, Inflammation and Apoptosis in the G93A Mouse, an Animal Model of ALS. *PLoS One.* 2010.
11. Hanahan, D. Heritable formation of pancreatic β-cell tumours in transgenic mice expressing recombinant insulin/simian virus 40 oncogenes. *Nature.* 1985.
12. Hanahan, D. & Weinberg, R. A. The Hallmarks of Cancer. *Cell.* 2000.
13. Kritchevsky, D. et al. Influence of short-term heating on composition of edible fats. *J. Nutr.* 1962.
14. Kritchevsky, D. et al. Dietary Fat versus Caloric Content in Initiation and Promotion of 7,12-Dimethylbenz(a)anthracene-induced Mammary Tumorigenesis in Rats. *Cancer Res.* 1984.
15. Ip, M. et al. Prevention of mammary cancer with conjugated linoleic acid: role of the stroma and the epithelium. *J. Mammary Gland Biol. Neoplasia.* 2003.
16. Klurfeld, D. M. et al. Inhibition of dmba-induced mammary tumorigenesis by caloric restriction in rats fed high-fat diets. *Int. J. Cancer.* 1989.
17. Kritchevsky, I. D. The Quartercentenary Lecture Undernutrition and chronic disease: cancer. *Proc. Nutr. Soc.* 2017.

18. Quianzon, C. C. & Cheikh, I. The History of Insulin. *J Community Hosp Intern Med Perspect.* 2012

19. Heuson, J. C. & Legros, N. Influence of insulin deprivation on growth of the 7,12-dimethylbenz(a)anthracene-induced mammary carcinoma in rats subjected to alloxan diabetes and food restriction. *Cancer Res.* 1972.

20. Ruggeri, B. A. et al. Caloric restriction and 7,12-dimethylbenz(a)anthracene-induced mammary tumor growth in rats: alterations in circulating insulin, insulin-like growth factors I and II, and epidermal growth factor. *Cancer Res.* 1989.

21. Pekonen, F. et al. Receptors for epidermal growth factor and insulin-like growth factor I and their relation to steroid receptors in human breast cancer. *Cancer Res.* 1988.

22. Kritchevsky, D. Diet and cancer: what's next? *J. Nutr.* 2003.

Chapter 5:

1. Spiteller, G. The relation of lipid peroxidation processes with atherogenesis: a new theory on atherogenesis. *Mol. Nutr. Food Res.* 2005.

2. Gros, L. et al. Enzymology of the repair of free radicals-induced DNA damage. *Oncogene.* 2002.

3. Schulz, T. J. et al. Induction of Oxidative Metabolism by Mitochondrial Frataxin Inhibits Cancer Growth: Otto Warburg Revisited. *J. Biol. Chem.* 2006.

4. Schulz, T. J. et al. Activation of mitochondrial energy metabolism protects against cardiac failure. *Aging.* 2010.

5. Bjelakovic, G. et al. Mortality in randomized trials of antioxidant supplements for primary and secondary prevention: systematic review and meta-analysis. *JAMA.* 2007.

6. Bjelakovic, G. et al. Antioxidant supplements for prevention of mortality in healthy participants and patients with various diseases. *Cochrane Database Syst. Rev.* 2012.

7. Hanahan, D. et al. Hallmarks of cancer: the next generation. *Cell.* 2011.

8. Vander Heiden, M. G. et al. Understanding the Warburg Effect: The Metabolic Requirements of Cell Proliferation. *Science.* 2009.

9. Alegría-Torres, J. A. et al. Epigenetics and lifestyle. *Epigenomics.* 2011.

10. Warburg, O. On the origin of cancer cells. *Science.* 1956.

11. Weisz, G. M. Dr. Otto heinrich warburg-survivor of ethical storms. *Rambam Maimonides Med.* 2015.

12. Boland, M. L. et al. Mitochondrial dysfunction in cancer. *Front. Oncol.* 2013.

13. Mukherjee, P. et al. Dietary restriction reduces angiogenesis and growth in an orthotopic mouse brain tumour model. *Br J Cancer.* 2002.

14. Abdelwahab, M. G. et al. The Ketogenic Diet Is an Effective Adjuvant to Radiation Therapy for the Treatment of Malignant Glioma. *PLoS One.* 2012.

15. Kalaany, N. Y. & Sabatini, D. M. Tumours with PI3K activation are resistant to dietary restriction. *Nature.* 2009.

16. Champ, C. E. et al. Weight Gain, Metabolic Syndrome, and Breast Cancer Recurrence: Are Dietary Recommendations Supported by the Data? *Int. J. Breast Cancer.* 2012.

17. Bianchini, F. et al. Overweight, obesity, and cancer risk. *Lancet Oncol.* 2002.

18. Cao, Y. & Ma, J. Body Mass Index, Prostate Cancer-Specific Mortality, and Biochemical Recurrence: a Systematic Review and Meta-analysis. *Cancer Prev. Res.* 2011.

19. Gong, Z. et al. Obesity is associated with increased risks of prostate cancer metastasis and death after initial cancer diagnosis in middle-aged men. *Cancer.* 2007.

20. Meigs, J. B. et al. Body mass index, metabolic syndrome, and risk of type 2 diabetes or cardiovascular disease. *J. Clin. Endocrinol. Metab.* 2006.

21. Eckel, R. H. et al. The metabolic syndrome. *Lancet.* 2005.

22. Freedland, S. J. & Aronson, W. J. Examining the relationship between obesity and prostate cancer. *Rev. Urol.* 2004.

23. Heuson, J. C. & Legros, N. Influence of insulin deprivation on growth of the 7,12-dimethylbenz(a)anthracene-induced mammary carcinoma in rats subjected to alloxan diabetes and food restriction. *Cancer Res.* 1972.

24. Shuldiner, A. R. et al. Resistin, obesity and insulin resistance--the emerging role of the adipocyte as an endocrine organ. *N. Engl. J. Med.* 2001.

25. Mohamed-Ali, V. et al. Subcutaneous Adipose Tissue Releases Interleukin-6, But Not Tumor Necrosis Factor-α, in Vivo. *J. Clin. Endocrinol. Metab.* 1997.

26. Rivas, M. A. et al. TNF alpha acting on TNFR1 promotes breast cancer growth via p42/P44 MAPK, JNK, Akt and NF-kappa B-dependent pathways. *Exp. Cell Res.* 2008.

27. Michalaki, V. et al. Serum levels of IL-6 and TNF-α correlate with clinicopathological features and patient survival in patients with prostate cancer. *Br. J. Cancer.* 2004.

28. McArdle, P. A. et al. Systemic Inflammatory Response, Prostate-Specific Antigen and Survival in Patients with Metastatic Prostate Cancer. *Urol. Int.* 2006.

29. Steppan, C. M. et al. The hormone resistin links obesity to diabetes. *Nature.* 2001.

30. Boden, G. Role of fatty acids in the pathogenesis of insulin resistance and NIDDM. *Diabetes.* 1997.

31. Nam, S. Y. et al. Effect of obesity on total and free insulin-like growth factor (IGF)-1, and their relationship to IGF-binding protein (BP)-1, IGFBP-2, IGFBP-3, insulin, and growth hormone. *Int. J. Obes. Relat. Metab. Disord.* 1997.

32. Ludwig, D. Genetic Study Supports Carbohydrate-Insulin Model of Obesity. Medium (2018). Available at: https://medium.com/@davidludwigmd/genetic-study-supports-carbohydrate-insulin-model-of-obesity-327d84be6d2b. (Accessed: 3rd January 2018)

33. Banting, W. Letter on Corpulence, Addressed to the Public. *Obes. Res.* 1993.

34. Young, F. G. Claude Bernard and the discovery of glycogen; a century of retrospect. *Br. Med. J.* 1957.

35. Pawlak, D. B. et al. Effects of dietary glycaemic index on adiposity, glucose homoeostasis, and plasma lipids in animals. *Lancet.* 2004.

36. Leibel, R. L. et al. Changes in Energy Expenditure Resulting from Altered Body Weight. *N. Engl. J. Med.* 1995.

37. Miller, D. S. et al. Gluttony. 2. Thermogenesis in overeating man. *Am. J. Clin. Nutr.* 1967.

38. Saslow, L. R. et al. Twelve-month outcomes of a randomized trial of a moderate-carbohydrate versus very low-carbohydrate diet in overweight adults with type 2 diabetes mellitus or prediabetes. *Nutr. Diabetes.* 2017.

Chapter 6:

1. Kritchevsky, D. et al. Influence of short-term heating on composition of edible fats. *J. Nutr.* 1962.

2. Lavik, P. S. Dietary Fat and Tumor Formation. *Cancer Res.* 1941.

3. Kritchevsky, D. et al. Experimental atherosclerosis in rabbits fed cholesterol-free diets. *Atherosclerosis.* 1984.

4. Kritchevsky, D. & Tepper, S. A. Cholesterol vehicle in experimental atherosclerosis. Comparison of heated corn oil and heated olive oil. *J. Atheroscler. Res.* 1967.

5. Schulz, T. J. et al. Induction of Oxidative Metabolism by Mitochondrial Frataxin Inhibits Cancer Growth: Otto Warburg Revisited. *J. Biol. Chem.* 2006.

6. Siegel, R. L. et al. Cancer statistics, 2016. *CA. Cancer J. Clin.* 2016.

7. White, M. C. et al. Age and cancer risk: a potentially modifiable relationship. *Am. J. Prev. Med.* 2014.

8. Tomasetti, C. & Vogelstein, B. Variation in cancer risk among tissues can be explained by the number of stem cell divisions. *Science.* 2015.

9. 'Bad luck' of random mutations plays predominant role in cancer, study shows -- ScienceDaily. Available at: https://www.sciencedaily.com/releases/2015/01/150101142318.htm. (Accessed: 10th December 2015)

10. Siegel, R. et al. Cancer statistics, 2014. *CA. Cancer J. Clin.* 2014.

11. Champ, C. E. et al. Weight Gain, Metabolic Syndrome, and Breast Cancer Recurrence: Are Dietary Recommendations Supported by the Data? *Int. J. Breast Cancer* 2012.

12. Efstathiou, J. A. et al. Obesity and mortality in men with locally advanced prostate cancer: analysis of RTOG 85-31. *Cancer.* 2007.

13. Tomasetti, C. et al. Stem cell divisions, somatic mutations, cancer etiology, and cancer prevention. *Science.* 2017.

14. Zhu, L. et al. Multi-organ Mapping of Cancer Risk. *Cell.* 2016.

15. Berger, S. L. et al. An operational definition of epigenetics. *Genes Dev.* 2009.

16. El-Osta, A. et al. Transient high glucose causes persistent epigenetic changes and altered gene expression during subsequent normoglycemia. *J. Exp. Med.* 2008.

17. Riggs, M. G. et al. n-Butyrate causes histone modification in HeLa and Friend erythroleukaemia cells. *Nature.* 1977.

18. Dashwood, R. H. & Ho, E. Dietary histone deacetylase inhibitors: from cells to mice to man. *Semin. Cancer Biol.* 2007.

19. Donohoe, D. R. et al. The Warburg effect dictates the mechanism of butyrate-mediated histone acetylation and cell proliferation. *Mol. Cell.* 2012.

20. Bassett, S. A. & Barnett, M. P. The role of dietary histone deacetylases (HDACs) inhibitors in health and disease. *Nutrients.* 2014.

21. Couzin-Frankel, J. Debate reignites over the contributions of 'bad luck' mutations to cancer. *Science.* 2017

22. Dayton, S. et al. Controlled Trial of a Diet High in Unsaturated Fat for Prevention of Atherosclerotic Complications. *Lancet.* 1968.

23. Dayton, S. & Pearce, M. L. Diet and atherosclerosis. *Lancet.* 1970.

24. Lee Pearce, M. & Dayton, S. Incidence of Cancer in Men on a Diet High in Polyunsaturated Fat. *Lancet.* 1971.

25. Carroll, K. K. & Khor, H. T. Effects of level and type of dietary fat on incidence of mammary tumors induced in female sprague-dawley rats by 7,12-dimethylbenz(α) anthracene. *Lipids.* 1971.

26. Rose, G. A., Thomson, W. B. & Williams, R. T. Corn Oil in Treatment of Ischaemic Heart Disease. *Br. Med. J.* 1965.

27. Woodhill, J. M. et al. Low fat, low cholesterol diet in secondary prevention of coronary heart disease. *Adv. Exp. Med. Biol.* 1978.

28. Dayton, S. et al. Vitamin E Status of Humans During Prolonged Feeding of Unsaturated Fats. *J. Lab. Clin. Med.* 1965.

29. Harmon, E. M. et al. Relative rates of depletion of alpha-tocopherol and linoleic acid after feeding polyunsaturated fats. *Am. J. Clin. Nutr.* 1966.

30. Adkins, Y. & Kelley, D. S. Mechanisms underlying the cardioprotective effects of omega-3 polyunsaturated fatty acids. *J. Nutr. Biochem.* 2010.

31. Calder, P. C. Omega-3 polyunsaturated fatty acids and inflammatory processes: nutrition or pharmacology? *Br. J. Clin. Pharmacol.* 2013.

32. Oh, S. Y. et al. Eggs enriched in omega-3 fatty acids and alterations in lipid concentrations in plasma and lipoproteins and in blood pressure. *Am. J. Clin. Nutr.* 1991.

33. Rose, D. P. & Connolly, J. M. Omega-3 fatty acids as cancer chemopreventive agents. *Pharmacol. Ther.* 1999.

34. Rose, D. P. et al. Effect of omega-3 fatty acids on the progression of metastases after the surgical excision of human breast cancer cell solid tumors growing in nude mice. *Clin Can Res.*1996.

35. Masterjohn, C. AJCN Publishes A New PUFA Study That Should Make Us Long for the Old Days - The Weston A. Price Foundation. Available at: https://www.westonaprice.org/ajcn-publishes-a-new-pufa-study-that-should-make-us-long-for-the-old-days/. (Accessed: 29th August 2012)

36. Hibbeln, J. R. et al. Healthy intakes of n-3 and n-6 fatty acids: estimations considering worldwide diversity. *Am. J. Clin. Nutr.* 2006.

37. Meyer, B. & Groot, R. Effects of Omega-3 Long Chain Polyunsaturated Fatty Acid Supplementation on Cardiovascular Mortality: The Importance of the Dose of DHA. *Nutrients.* 2017.

38. Bradbury, J. Docosahexaenoic acid (DHA): an ancient nutrient for the modern human brain. *Nutrients.* 2011.

39. Martin, B. et al. "Control" laboratory rodents are metabolically morbid: why it matters. *Proc. Natl. Acad. Sci. U. S. A.* 2010.

40. Calle, E. E. et al. Overweight, obesity, and mortality from cancer in a prospectively studied cohort of U.S. adults. *N Engl J Med.* 2003.

41. Li, G. et al. Enriched Environment Inhibits Mouse Pancreatic Cancer Growth and Down-regulates the Expression of Mitochondria-related Genes in Cancer Cells. *Sci. Rep.* 2015.

42. Mattson, M. P. et al. Impact of intermittent fasting on health and disease processes. *Ageing Res. Rev.* 2017.

43. Shanks, N. et al. Are animal models predictive for humans? *Philos. Ethics. Humanit. Med.* 2009.

44. Sorge, R. E. et al. Olfactory exposure to males, including men, causes stress and related analgesia in rodents. *Nat. Methods.* 2014.

45. Masubuchi, Y. Metabolic and non-metabolic factors determining troglitazone hepatotoxicity: a review. *Drug Metab. Pharmacokinet.* 2006.

46. Harper, J. M. et al. Does caloric restriction extend life in wild mice? *Aging Cell.* 2006.

47. Klement, R. J. & Champ, C. E. Calories, carbohydrates, and cancer therapy with radiation: exploiting the five R's through dietary manipulation. *Cancer Metastasis Rev.* 2014.

48. Klement, R. J., Champ, C. E., Otto, C. & Kämmerer, U. Anti-Tumor Effects of Ketogenic Diets in Mice: A Meta-Analysis. *PLoS One.* 2016.

49. Catenacci, V. A. et al. A randomized pilot study comparing zero-calorie alternate-day fasting to daily caloric restriction in adults with obesity. *Obesity.* 2016.

50. Champ, C. E. et al. Nutrient Restriction and Radiation Therapy for Cancer Treatment: When Less Is More. *Oncologist*. 2013.

51. Simone, B. A. et al. Selectively starving cancer cells through dietary manipulation: methods and clinical implications. *Futur. Oncol.* 2013.

Chapter 7:

1. Bales, C. W. & Ritchie, C. S. Handbook of Clinical Nutrition and Aging. (Humana Press, 2009).

2. Koromila, K. Feasting with Archestratus. Available at: http://www.kathrynkoromilas.com/files/pdf/Feasting_With_Archestratus.pd f. (Accessed: 1st March 2019)

3. Cato, M. P. & Dalby, A. On farming: De agricultura. (Prospect Books, 1998).

4. Szymanski, I. F. The Significance of Food in Plato's Republic, Book I. *Food, Cult. Soc.* 2014.

5. Skiadas, P. & Lascaratos, J. Original Communication Dietetics in ancient Greek philosophy: Plato's concepts of healthy diet. *Eur Jour Clin Nut.* 2001.

6. Silvermintz, D. Plato and Food. in Encyclopedia of Food and Agricultural Ethics 1–7 (Springer Netherlands, 2014).

7. Center for Health Statistics. *National Health and Nutrition Examination Survey.* 2017.

8. Baserga, R. et al. The IGF-1 receptor in cancer biology. *Int. J. Cancer.* 2003.

9. Salmon, W. D. & Daughaday, W. H. A hormonally controlled serum factor which stimulates sulfate incorporation by cartilage in vitro. *J. Lab. Clin. Med.* 1957.

10. Caregaro, L. et al. Insulin-like growth factor 1 (IGF-1), a nutritional marker in patients with eating disorders. *Clin. Nutr.* 2001.

11. Chennaoui, M. et al. Sleep extension increases IGF-I concentrations before and during sleep deprivation in healthy young men. *Appl. Physiol. Nutr. Metab.* 2016.

12. Hedström, M. et al. Low IGF-I levels in hip fracture patients. A comparison of 20 coxarthrotic and 23 hip fracture patients. *Acta Orthop. Scand.* 1999.

13. Brugts, M. P. et al. Low Circulating Insulin-Like Growth Factor I Bioactivity in Elderly Men Is Associated with Increased Mortality. *J. Clin. Endocrinol. Metab.* 2008.

14. Rudman, D. et al. Effects of Human Growth Hormone in Men over 60 Years Old. *N. Engl. J. Med.* 1990.

15. Gelander, L. et al. Monthly Measurements of Insulin-Like Growth Factor I (IGF-I) and IGF-Binding Protein-3 in Healthy Prepubertal Children: Characterization and Relationship with Growth: The 1-Year Growth Study. *Pediatr. Res.* 1999.

16. Gunnell, D. Association of Insulin-like Growth Factor I and Insulin-like Growth Factor-Binding Protein-3 With Intelligence Quotient Among 8- to 9-Year-Old Children in the Avon Longitudinal Study of Parents and Children. *Pediatrics*. 2005.

17. Joseph D'Ercole, A. & Ye, P. Expanding the Mind: Insulin-Like Growth Factor I and Brain Development. *Endocrinology*. 2008.

18. Carro, E. et al. Serum insulin-like growth factor I regulates brain amyloid-β levels. *Nat. Med.* 2002.

19. Cittadini, A. et al. Insulin-like growth factor-1 protects from vascular stenosis and accelerates re-endothelialization in a rat model of carotid artery injury. *J. Thromb. Haemost.* 2009.

20. Jeschke, M. G. et al. Insulin-like growth factor I plus insulin-like growth factor binding protein 3 attenuates the proinflammatory acute phase response in severely burned children. *Ann. Surg.* 2000.

21. Brismar, K. et al. Effect of insulin on the hepatic production of insulin-like growth factor-binding protein-1 (IGFBP-1), IGFBP-3, and IGF-I in insulin-dependent diabetes. J. Clin. Endocrinol. *Metab.* 1994.

22. Sandhu, M. S. et al. Insulin, Insulin-Like Growth Factor-I (IGF-I), IGF Binding Proteins, Their Biologic Interactions, and Colorectal Cancer. *Cancer Spectrum Knowl. Environ.* 2002.

23. Fine, E. J. et al. An Evolutionary and Mechanistic Perspective on Dietary Carbohydrate Restriction in Cancer Prevention. *J. Evol. Heal.* 2016.

24. Serdula, M. K. et al. The association between fruit and vegetable intake and chronic disease risk factors. *Epidemiology*. 1996.

25. Mozaffarian, D. et al. Changes in Diet and Lifestyle and Long-Term Weight Gain in Women and Men. *N. Engl. J. Med.* 2011.

26. Wang, X. et al. Fruit and vegetable consumption and mortality from all causes, cardiovascular disease, and cancer: systematic review and dose-response meta-analysis of prospective cohort studies. *BMJ*. 2014.

27. Joshipura, K. J. et al. Fruit and Vegetable Intake in Relation to Risk of Ischemic Stroke. *JAMA*. 1999.

28. Hung, H.C. et al. Fruit and vegetable intake and risk of major chronic disease. *J. Natl. Cancer Inst*. 2004.

29. Boffetta, P. et al. Fruit and Vegetable Intake and Overall Cancer Risk in the European Prospective Investigation Into Cancer and Nutrition (EPIC). *J. Natl. Cancer Inst*. 2010.

30. Gandini, S. et al. Meta-analysis of studies on breast cancer risk and diet: the role of fruit and vegetable consumption and the intake of associated micronutrients. *Eur. J. Cancer*. 2000.

31. Freudenheim, J. L. et al. Premenopausal Breast Cancer Risk and Intake of Vegetables, Fruits, and Related Nutrients. *J. Natl. Cancer Inst*. 1996.

32. Giovannucci, E. et al. A prospective study of cruciferous vegetables and prostate cancer. *Cancer Epidemiol. Biomarkers Prev*. 2003.

33. Smith-Warner, S. A. et al. Intake of fruits and vegetables and risk of breast cancer: a pooled analysis of cohort studies. *JAMA.* 2001.

34. Farvid, M. S. et al. Fruit and vegetable consumption in adolescence and early adulthood and risk of breast cancer: population based cohort study. *BMJ.* 2016.

35. Blaut, M. Relationship of prebiotics and food to intestinal microflora. *Eur. J. Nutr.* 2002.

36. Maslowski, K. M. & Mackay, C. R. Diet, gut microbiota and immune responses. *Nat Immunol.* 2011.

37. Madara, J. Building an Intestine — Architectural Contributions of Commensal Bacteria. *N. Engl. J. Med.* 2004.

38. Claus, S. P. The gut microbiota: a major player in the toxicity of environmental pollutants? *Biofilms Microbiomes.* 2016.

39. Nakanishi, A. et al. Determination of the absolute configuration of a novel odour-active lactone, cis -3-methyl-4-decanolide, in wasabi (Wasabia japonica Matsum.). *Flavour Fragr.* 2014.

40. Williams, J. S. & Cooper, R. M. The oldest fungicide and newest phytoalexin - a reappraisal of the fungitoxicity of elemental sulphur. *Plant Pathol.* 2004.

41. Tsao, A. S. et al. Chemoprevention of cancer. *CA. Cancer J. Clin.* 2004

Chapter 8:

1. Kenyon, C. et al. C. elegans mutant that lives twice as long as wild type. *Nature.* 1993.

2. Mortality - Radiolab. (2007). Available at: http://www.radiolab.org/story/91562-mortality/. (Accessed: 20th November 2017)

3. Henderson, S. T. & Johnson, T. E. daf-16 integrates developmental and environmental inputs to mediate aging in the nematode Caenorhabditis elegans. *Curr. Biol.* 2001.

4. Lee, S. J. et al. Glucose shortens the life span of C. elegans by downregulating DAF-16/FOXO activity and aquaporin gene expression. *Cell Metab.* 2009.

5. Kenyon, C. The plasticity of aging: insights from long-lived mutants. *Cell.* 2005.

6. Pawlikowska, L. et al. Association of common genetic variation in the insulin/IGF1 signaling pathway with human longevity. *Aging Cell.* 2009.

7. Van Heemst, D. et al. Reduced insulin/IGF-1 signalling and human longevity. *Aging Cell.* 2005.

8. Bonafè, M. et al. Polymorphic Variants of Insulin-Like Growth Factor I (IGF-I) Receptor and Phosphoinositide 3-Kinase Genes Affect IGF-I Plasma Levels and Human Longevity: Cues for an Evolutionarily Conserved Mechanism of Life Span Control. *J. Clin. Endocrinol. Metab.* 2003.

9. Suh, Y. et al. Functionally significant insulin-like growth factor I receptor mutations in centenarians. *Proc. Natl. Acad. Sci.* 2008.

10. Vitale, G. et al. GH/IGF-I/insulin system in centenarians. *Mech. Ageing Dev.* 2016

11. Lee, R. Y. et al. Regulation of C. elegans DAF-16 and its human ortholog FKHRL1 by the daf-2 insulin-like signaling pathway. *Curr. Biol.* 2001.

12. Bluher, M. et al. Extended Longevity in Mice Lacking the Insulin Receptor in Adipose Tissue. *Science.* 2003.

13. Mair, W. et al. Calories Do Not Explain Extension of Life Span by Dietary Restriction in Drosophila. *PLoS Biol.* 2005.

14. Schulz, T. J. et al. Glucose restriction extends Caenorhabditis elegans life span by inducing mitochondrial respiration and increasing oxidative stress. *Cell Metab.* 2007.

15. Lin, S.-J. et al. Calorie restriction extends Saccharomyces cerevisiae lifespan by increasing respiration. *Nature.* 2002.

16. Emond, J. A. et al. Risk of Breast Cancer Recurrence Associated with Carbohydrate Intake and Tissue Expression of IGFI Receptor. Cancer Epidemiol. *Biomarkers Prev.* 2014.

17. Bitto, A. et al. Long-Term IGF-I Exposure Decreases Autophagy and Cell Viability. *PLoS One.* 2010.

18. Min, K.-J. & Tatar, M. Restriction of amino acids extends lifespan in Drosophila melanogaster. *Mechanisms of Ageing and Development.* 2006.

19. Klement, R. J. & Fink, M. K. Dietary and pharmacological modification of the insulin/IGF-1 system: exploiting the full repertoire against cancer. *Oncogenesis.* 2016.

20. Iwasaki, K. et al. Influence of the Restriction of Individual Dietary Components on Longevity and Age-Related Disease of Fischer Rats: The Fat Component and the Mineral Component. *J. Gerontol.* 1988.

21. Taguchi, A. et al. Brain IRS2 Signaling Coordinates Life Span and Nutrient Homeostasis. *Science.* 2007.

22. Yang, J. et al. Control of aging and longevity by IGF-I signaling. *Exp. Gerontol.* 2005.

23. Vance, M. L. Can Growth Hormone Prevent Aging? *N. Engl. J. Med.* 2003.

24. Howard, B. V. et al. Low-Fat Dietary Pattern and Risk of Cardiovascular Disease. *JAMA.* 2006.

25. Howard, B. V. et al. Low-Fat Dietary Pattern and Weight Change Over 7 Years. *JAMA.* 2006.

26. Prentice, R. L. et al. Low-Fat Dietary Pattern and Risk of Invasive Breast Cancer. *JAMA.* 2006.

27. Beresford, S. A. et al. Low-Fat Dietary Pattern and Risk of Colorectal Cancer. *JAMA.* 2006.

28. Lin, J. et al. Fat and Fatty Acids and Risk of Colorectal Cancer in Women. *Am. J. Epidemiol.* 2004.

29. Roth, J. A. et al. Economic return from the Women's Health Initiative estrogen plus progestin clinical trial: a modeling study. *Ann. Intern. Med.* 2014.

30. Pierce, J. P. et al. Influence of a Diet Very High in Vegetables, Fruit, and Fiber and Low in Fat on Prognosis Following Treatment for Breast Cancer. *JAMA.* 2007.

31. Champ, C. E. et al. Gain, Metabolic Syndrome, and Breast Cancer Recurrence: Are Dietary Recommendations Supported by the Data? *Int. J. Breast Cancer.* 2012.

32. Chlebowski, R. T. et al. Dietary Fat Reduction and Breast Cancer Outcome: Interim Efficacy Results from the Women's Intervention Nutrition Study. *J. Natl. Cancer Inst.* 2006.

33. Thiébaut, A. C. et al. Dietary Fat and Breast Cancer: Contributions from a Survival Trial. *J. Natl. Cancer Inst.* 2006.

34. Chlebowski, R. T. et al. Low-Fat Dietary Pattern and Breast Cancer Mortality in the Women's Health Initiative Randomized Controlled Trial. *J. Clin. Oncol.* 2017.

35. Brown, S. Shock, terror and controversy: how the media reacted to the Women's Health Initiative. *Climacteric.* 2012.

36. Champ, C. E. et al. Dietary Recommendations During and After Cancer Treatment: Consistently Inconsistent? *Nutr. Cancer.* 2013.

37. Houghton, C. A. et al. Sulforaphane: translational research from laboratory bench to clinic. *Nutr. Rev.* 2013.

38. Venugopal, R. & Jaiswal, A. K. Nrf1 and Nrf2 positively and c-Fos and Fra1 negatively regulate the human antioxidant response element-mediated expression of NAD(P)H:quinone oxidoreductase1 gene. *Proc. Natl. Acad. Sci.* 1996.

39. Zhang, Y. et al. Anticarcinogenic activities of sulforaphane and structurally related synthetic norbornyl isothiocyanates. *Proc. Natl. Acad. Sci.* 1994.

40. Cornblatt, B. S. et al. Preclinical and clinical evaluation of sulforaphane for chemoprevention in the breast. *Carcinogenesis.* 2007.

41. Belinsky, M. & Jaiswal, A. K. NAD(P)H:quinone oxidoreductase1 (DT-diaphorase) expression in normal and tumor tissues. *Cancer Metastasis Rev.* 1993.

42. Schulz, T. J. et al. Induction of Oxidative Metabolism by Mitochondrial Frataxin Inhibits Cancer Growth: Otto Warburg Revisited. *J. Biol. Chem.* 2006.

43. Zhang, Y. et al. Vegetable-derived isothiocyanates: anti-proliferative activity and mechanism of action. *Proceedings of the Nutrition Society.* 2017.

44. Ristow, M. et al. Antioxidants prevent health-promoting effects of physical exercise in humans. *Proc. Natl. Acad. Sci.* 2009.

45. International Agency for Research on Cancer. Glucosinolates, isothiocyanates and indoles. *IARC Publ.* 2004.

46. Nilius, B. & Appendino, G. Spices: The Savory and Beneficial Science of Pungency. *Reviews of physiology, biochemistry and pharmacology*. 2013.
47. Balstad, T. R. et al. Coffee, broccoli and spices are strong inducers of electrophile response element-dependent transcription in vitro and in vivo - Studies in electrophile response element transgenic mice. *Mol. Nutr. Food Res.* 2011.
48. Martínez-Huélamo, M. et al. Modulation of Nrf2 by Olive Oil and Wine Polyphenols and Neuroprotection. *Antioxidants*. 2017.
49. Champ, C. E. & Kundu-Champ, A. Maximizing Polyphenol Content to Uncork the Relationship Between Wine and Cancer. *Front. Nutr.* 2019.
50. Howard, L. R. et al. Antioxidant Capacity and Phenolic Content of Spinach as Affected by Genetics and Growing Season. *J. Agric. Food Chem.* 2002.
51. Young, J. E. et al. Phytochemical phenolics in organically grown vegetables. *Mol. Nutr. Food Res.* 2005.
52. Fahey, J. W. et al. Broccoli sprouts: An exceptionally rich source of inducers of enzymes that protect against chemical carcinogens. *Proc. Natl. Acad. Sci.* 1997.
53. McCaslin, T. Free radicals are not your enemy | An interview with Dr. Michael Ristow (part i). Geroscience (2018). Available at: http://geroscience.com/free-radicals-are-not-your-enemy-an-interview-with-dr-michael-ristow-part-i/. (Accessed: 8th February 2018)
54. Ristow, M. & Schmeisser, S. Extending life span by increasing oxidative stress. *Free Radic. Biol. Med.* 2011.
55. Ristow, M. et al. Frataxin activates mitochondrial energy conversion and oxidative phosphorylation. *Proc. Natl. Acad. Sci.* 2000.
56. Marmolino, D. et al. PGC-1alpha down-regulation affects the antioxidant response in Friedreich's ataxia. *PLoS One*. 2010.
57. Baserga, R. et al. The IGF-1 receptor in cancer biology. *Int. J. Cancer*. 2003.
58. Isley, W. L. et al. Dietary components that regulate serum somatomedin-C concentrations in humans. *J. Clin. Invest.* 1983.
59. Crowe, F. L. et al. The Association between Diet and Serum Concentrations of IGF-I, IGFBP-1, IGFBP-2, and IGFBP-3 in the European Prospective Investigation into Cancer and Nutrition. *Cancer Epidemiol. Biomarkers Prev.* 2009.
60. Maggio, M. et al. IGF-1, the cross road of the nutritional, inflammatory and hormonal pathways to frailty. *Nutrients*. 2013.
61. Rogers, I. et al. Milk as a food for growth? The insulin-like growth factors link. *Public Health Nutr.* 2006.
62. Allen, N. E. et al. Hormones and diet: low insulin-like growth factor-I but normal bioavailable androgens in vegan men. *Br. J. Cancer*. 2000.

63. Allen, N. E. et al. The Associations of Diet with Serum Insulin-like Growth Factor I and Its Main Binding Proteins in 292 Women Meat-Eaters, Vegetarians, and Vegans. *Cancer Epidemiol. Prev. Biomarkers*. 2002.

64. Wangen, K. E. et al. Effects of Soy Isoflavones on Markers of Bone Turnover in Premenopausal and Postmenopausal Women 1. *J. Clin. Endocrinol. Metab.* 2000.

65. Khalil, D. A. et al. Soy protein supplementation increases serum insulin-like growth factor-I in young and old men but does not affect markers of bone metabolism. *J. Nutr.* 2002.

66. Gann, P. H. et al. Sequential, randomized trial of a low-fat, high-fiber diet and soy supplementation: Effects on circulating IGF-I and its binding proteins in premenopausal women. *Int. J. Cancer*. 2005.

67. Report on Animal Welfare Aspects of the Use of Bovine Somatotrophin by the Scientific Committee on Animal Health and Animal Welfare. 1999.

Chapter 9:

1. O'Neill, B. In Methuselah's Mould. *PLoS Biol.* 2004.

2. Haddad, E. H. & Tanzman, J. S. What do vegetarians in the United States eat? *Am. J. Clin. Nutr.* 2003.

3. Orlich, M. J. et al. Vegetarian dietary patterns and mortality in Adventist Health Study 2. *JAMA Intern. Med.* 2013.

4. Kritchevsky, D. History of Recommendations to the Public about Dietary Fat. *J. Nutr.* 1998.

5. Cordain, L. et al. Origins and evolution of the Western diet: health implications for the 21st century. *Am. J. Clin. Nutr.* 2005.

6. Grotto, D. & Zied, E. The Standard American Diet and Its Relationship to the Health Status of Americans. *Nutr. Clin. Pract.* 2010.

7. U.S. Dept. of Agriculture. The Food Guide Pyramid. 1992.

8. Ferguson, K. The Music of Pythagoras: How an Ancient Brotherhood Cracked the Code of the Universe and Lit the Path from Antiquity to Outer Space. (Walker Books, 2008).

9. The Cult of Pythagoras | Classical Wisdom Weekly. Available at: https://classicalwisdom.com/philosophy/cult-of-pythagoras/. (Accessed: 4th March 2019)

10. Guthrie, K. S. & Fideler, D. R. The Pythagorean sourcebook and library: an anthology of ancient writings which relate to Pythagoras and Pythagorean philosophy. (Phanes Press, 1987).

11. Evans, J. Philosophy for life and other dangerous situations: ancient philosophy for modern problems. (New World Library, 2013).

12. Skiadas, P. & Lascaratos, J. Original Communication Dietetics in ancient Greek philosophy: Plato's concepts of healthy diet. *Eur Jour Clin Nut*. 2001

13. Lamb, W. Plato in Twelve Volumes, Vol. 9, Timaeus, section 89c. (Harvard University Press, 1925).

14. Standage, T. An edible history of humanity. (Walker & Co, 2010).
15. Diamond, J. The Worst Mistake in the History of the Human Race. Discov. Mag. 64–66 (1987).
16. Bowles, S. & Choi, J.K. Coevolution of farming and private property during the early Holocene. *Proc. Natl. Acad. Sci.* 2013.
17. Daley, C. et al. A review of fatty acid profiles and antioxidant content in grass-fed and grain-fed beef. *Nutr. J.* 2010.
18. Sofi, F. et al. Effects of a dairy product (pecorino cheese) naturally rich in cis-9, trans-11 conjugated linoleic acid on lipid, inflammatory and haemorheological variables: A dietary intervention study. *Nutr. Metab. Cardiovasc. Dis.* 2010.
19. Guadagni, F. et al. TNF/VEGF cross-talk in chronic inflammation-related cancer initiation and progression: an early target in anticancer therapeutic strategy. *In Vivo.* 2007.
20. Lehnen, T. E. et al. A review on effects of conjugated linoleic fatty acid (CLA) upon body composition and energetic metabolism. *J. Int. Soc. Sports Nutr.* 2015.
21. Kelley, N. S. et al. Conjugated Linoleic Acid Isomers and Cancer. *J. Nutr.* 2007.
22. Zhou, X.R. et al. Dietary conjugated linoleic acid increases PPARγ gene expression in adipose tissue of obese rat, and improves insulin resistance. *Growth Horm. IGF Res.* 2008.
23. Cho, K. et al. Conjugated linoleic acid supplementation enhances insulin sensitivity and peroxisome proliferator-activated receptor gamma and glucose transporter type 4 protein expression in the skeletal muscles of rats during endurance exercise. *Iran. J. Basic Med. Sci.* 2016.
24. Aubert, J. et al. Up-Regulation of UCP-2 Gene Expression by PPAR Agonists in Preadipose and Adipose Cells. *Biochem. Biophys. Res. Commun.* 1997.
25. Heinze, V. M. & Actis, A. B. Dietary conjugated linoleic acid and long-chain n -3 fatty acids in mammary and prostate cancer protection: a review. *Int. J. Food Sci. Nutr.* 2012.
26. Chajès, V. et al. Conjugated Linoleic Acid Content in Breast Adipose Tissue of Breast Cancer Patients and the Risk of Metastasis. *Nutr. Cancer.* 2003.
27. Hubbard, N. E. et al. Effect of separate conjugated linoleic acid isomers on murine mammary tumorigenesis. *Cancer Lett.* 2003.
28. Aro, A. et al. Inverse association between dietary and serum conjugated linoleic acid and risk of breast cancer in postmenopausal women. *Nutr. Cancer.* 2000.
29. Larsson, S. C. et al. High-fat dairy food and conjugated linoleic acid intakes in relation to colorectal cancer incidence in the Swedish Mammography Cohort. *Am. J. Clin. Nutr.* 2005.

30. Larsson, S. C. et al. Conjugated linoleic acid intake and breast cancer risk in a prospective cohort of Swedish women. *Am. J. Clin. Nutr.* 2009.

31. Jouanna, J. Greek Medicine from Hippocrates to Galen: Selected Papers. (Brill, 2012).

32. Settanni, L. & Moschetti, G. Non-starter lactic acid bacteria used to improve cheese quality and provide health benefits. *Food Microbiol.* 2010.

33. Scharlau, D. et al. Mechanisms of primary cancer prevention by butyrate and other products formed during gut flora-mediated fermentation of dietary fibre. *Mutat. Res. Mutat. Res.* 2009.

34. Wong, J. M. et al. Colonic health: fermentation and short chain fatty acids. *J. Clin. Gastroenterol.* 2006.

35. Zheng, H. et al. Metabolomics Investigation to Shed Light on Cheese as a Possible Piece in the French Paradox Puzzle. *J. Agric. Food Chem.* 2015.

36. Khosrova, E. Butter: A Rich History. (Algonquin Books of Chapel Hill).

37. Martin, C. K. et al. Change in food cravings, food preferences, and appetite during a low-carbohydrate and low-fat diet. *Obesity.* 2011.

38. Kindstedt, P. Cheese and culture: a history of cheese and its place in western civilization. (Chelsea Green Pub, 2012).

39. Keys, A. Mediterranean diet and public health: personal reflections. *Am. J. Clin. Nutr.* 1995.

40. St-Onge, M. P. & Jones, P. J. Physiological Effects of Medium-Chain Triglycerides: Potential Agents in the Prevention of Obesity. *J. Nutr.* 2002.

41. Mozaffarian, D. et al. Trans-palmitoleic acid, metabolic risk factors, and new-onset diabetes in U.S. adults: a cohort study. *Ann. Intern. Med.* 2010.

42. Huffington Post Canada. Harvard Milk Study: It Doesn't Do A Body Good. (2013). Available at: http://www.huffingtonpost.ca/2013/07/05/harvard-milk-study_n_3550063.html. (Accessed: 23rd March 2018)

43. Ludwid, D. 3 Foods That Are Surprisingly Good for You. David Ludwig MD PHD (2016). Available at: https://www.drdavidludwig.com/3-foods-that-are-surprisingly-good-for-you-2/. (Accessed: 23rd March 2018)

44. Scharf, R. J. et al. Longitudinal evaluation of milk type consumed and weight status in preschoolers. *Arch. Dis. Child.* 2013.

45. Kratz, M. et al. The relationship between high-fat dairy consumption and obesity, cardiovascular, and metabolic disease. *Eur. J. Nutr.* 2013.

46. Ericson, U. et al. Food sources of fat may clarify the inconsistent role of dietary fat intake for incidence of type 2 diabetes. *Am. J. Clin. Nutr.* 2015.

47. Arcidiacono, B. et al. Insulin resistance and cancer risk: an overview of the pathogenetic mechanisms. *Exp. Diabetes Res.* 2012.

48. Warensjö, E. et al. Biomarkers of milk fat and the risk of myocardial infarction in men and women: a prospective, matched case-control study. *Am. J. Clin. Nutr.* 2010.

49. Kirschner, B. S. & Sutton, M. M. Somatomedin-C levels in growth-impaired children and adolescents with chronic inflammatory bowel disease. *Gastroenterology.* 1986.

50. Lecornu, M. et al. Low serum somatomedin activity in celiac disease. A misleading aspect in growth failure from asymptomatic celiac disease. *Helv. Paediatr. Acta.* 1978.

51. Fontana, L. et al. Long-term effects of calorie or protein restriction on serum IGF-1 and IGFBP-3 concentration in humans. *Aging Cell.* 2008.

52. McCarty, M. F. et al. The low-methionine content of vegan diets may make methionine restriction feasible as a life extension strategy. *Med. Hypotheses.* 2009.

53. Fontana, L. et al. Long-term low-protein, low-calorie diet and endurance exercise modulate metabolic factors associated with cancer risk. *Am. J. Clin. Nutr.* 2006.

54. Sucher, S. et al. Comparison of the effects of diets high in animal or plant protein on metabolic and cardiovascular markers in type 2 diabetes: A randomized clinical trial. Diabetes, *Obes. Metab.* 2017.

55. Viguiliouk, E. et al. Effect of Replacing Animal Protein with Plant Protein on Glycemic Control in Diabetes: A Systematic Review and Meta-Analysis of Randomized Controlled Trials. *Nutrients.* 2015.

56. Roberts, I. F. et al. Malnutrition in infants receiving cult diets: a form of child abuse. *Br Med J.* 1979.

57. Kühne, T. et al. Maternal vegan diet causing a serious infantile neurological disorder due to vitamin B12 deficiency. *Eur. J. Pediatr.* 1991.

58. Ingenbleek, Y. & McCully, K. S. Vegetarianism produces subclinical malnutrition, hyperhomocysteinemia and atherogenesis. *Nutrition.* 2012.

59. Perry, C. L. et al. Characteristics of vegetarian adolescents in a multiethnic urban population. *J. Adolesc. Health.* 2001.

60. Baines, S. et al. How does the health and well-being of young Australian vegetarian and semi-vegetarian women compare with non-vegetarians? *Public Health Nutr.* 2007.

61. Jacobi, F. et al. Prevalence, co-morbidity and correlates of mental disorders in the general population: results from the German Health Interview and Examination Survey (GHS). *Psychol. Med.* 2004.

62. Larsson, C. L. et al. Lifestyle-related characteristics of young low-meat consumers and omnivores in Sweden and Norway. *J. Adolesc. Health.* 2002.

63. Robinson-O'Brien, R. et al. Adolescent and Young Adult Vegetarianism: Better Dietary Intake and Weight Outcomes but Increased Risk of Disordered Eating Behaviors. *J. Am. Diet. Assoc.* 2009.

64. Burkert, N. T. et al. Nutrition and Health – The Association between Eating Behavior and Various Health Parameters: A Matched Sample Study. *PLoS One.* 2014.

65. Maggio, M. et al. IGF-1, the cross road of the nutritional, inflammatory and hormonal pathways to frailty. *Nutrients.* 2013.

66. Lee, C. et al. Reduced Levels of IGF-I Mediate Differential Protection of Normal and Cancer Cells in Response to Fasting and Improve Chemotherapeutic Index. *Cancer Res.* 2010.

67. Clemmons, D. R. et al. Reduction of Plasma Immunoreactive Somatomedin C during Fasting in Humans. *J. Clin. Endocrinol. Metab.* 1981.

68. Mattson, M. P. et al. Impact of intermittent fasting on health and disease processes. *Ageing Res. Rev.* 2017.

69. Young, L. R. et al. Low-fat diet with omega-3 fatty acids increases plasma insulin-like growth factor concentration in healthy postmenopausal women. *Nutr. Res.* 2013.

70. Fulgoni, V. L. Current protein intake in America: analysis of the National Health and Nutrition Examination Survey, 2003-2004. *Am. J. Clin. Nutr.* 2008.

71. Zhu, K. et al. The effects of a two-year randomized, controlled trial of whey protein supplementation on bone structure, IGF-1, and urinary calcium excretion in older postmenopausal women. *J. Bone Miner. Res.* 2011.

72. Klement, R. J. & Fink, M. K. Dietary and pharmacological modification of the insulin/IGF-1 system: exploiting the full repertoire against cancer. *Oncogenesis.* 2016.

73. Herzog, H. & Railsback, B. Motivations for Meat Consumption Among Ex-Vegetarians. in National Council on Undergraduate Research. 2009

74. Rozin, P. et al. Moralization and Becoming a Vegetarian: The Transformation of Preferences into Values and the Recruitment of Disgust. *Psychological Science.* 1997

Chapter 10:

1. Scientists 'find key to longevity' in Italian village where one in 10 people live beyond 100 years | The Independent. Available at: https://www.independent.co.uk/life-style/health-and-families/health-news/scientists-key-to-longevity-italy-acciaroli-centenarian-mediterranean-diet-a7230956.html. (Accessed: 8th September 2016)

2. Rockhill, B. et al. A Prospective Study of Recreational Physical Activity and Breast Cancer Risk. *Arch. Intern. Med.* 1999.

3. Miller, W. C. et al. A meta-analysis of the past 25 years of weight loss research using diet, exercise or diet plus exercise intervention. *Int. J. Obes. Relat. Metab. Disord.* 1997.

4. Curioni, C. C. & Lourenço, P. M. Long-term weight loss after diet and exercise: a systematic review. *Int. J. Obes.* 2005.

5. McGill, S. Core training: Evidence translating to better performance and injury prevention. *Strength Cond. J.* 2010.

6. Romijn, J. A. et al. Regulation of endogenous fat and carbohydrate metabolism in relation to exercise intensity and duration. *Am J Physiol Endocrinol Metab.* 1993.

7. Bonn, S. E. et al. Physical activity and survival among men diagnosed with prostate cancer. *Cancer Epidemiol. Biomarkers Prev.* 2015.

8. Devlin, J. T. & Horton, E. S. Effects of Prior High-Intensity Exercise on Glucose Metabolism in Normal and Insulin-resistant Men. *Diabetes.* 1985.

9. Newsom, S. A. et al. A single session of low-intensity exercise is sufficient to enhance insulin sensitivity into the next day in obese adults. *Diabetes Care.* 2013.

10. Kritchevsky, D. The effect of over- and undernutrition on cancer. *Eur. J. Cancer Prev.* 1995.

11. Tannenbaum, A. & Silverstone, H. Effect of low environmental temperature, dinitrophenol, or sodium fluoride on the formation of tumors in mice. *Cancer Res.* 1949.

12. Champ, C. E. et al. Fortifying the Treatment of Prostate Cancer with Physical Activity. *Prostate Cancer.* 2016.

13. Gao, N. et al. Role of PI3K/AKT/mTOR signaling in the cell cycle progression of human prostate cancer. *Biochem. Biophys. Res. Commun.* 2003.

14. O'Reilly, K. E. et al. mTOR inhibition induces upstream receptor tyrosine kinase signaling and activates Akt. *Cancer Res.* 2006.

15. Freburger, J. K. et al. The rising prevalence of chronic low back pain. *Arch. Intern. Med.* 2009.

16. Merry, T. L. & Ristow, M. Do antioxidant supplements interfere with skeletal muscle adaptation to exercise training? *J. Physiol.* 2016.

17. Adams, G. R. & Haddad, F. The relationships among IGF-1, DNA content, and protein accumulation during skeletal muscle hypertrophy. *J. Appl. Physiol.* 1996.

18. Rainsford, K. D. et al. Anti-Inflammatory Drugs in the 21st Century Inflammation in the Pathogenesis of Chronic Diseases. in (eds. Harris, R. E. et al.) (Springer Netherlands, 2007).

19. Hanahan, D. et al. Hallmarks of cancer: the next generation. *Cell.* 2011.

20. Ekbom, A. et al. Ulcerative Colitis and Colorectal Cancer. *N. Engl. J. Med.* 1990.

21. Eaden, J. A. et al. The risk of colorectal cancer in ulcerative colitis: a meta-analysis. *Gut.* 2001.

22. Lowenfels, A. B. et al. Pancreatitis and the Risk of Pancreatic Cancer. *N. Engl. J. Med.* 1993.

23. Brody, J. S. & Spira, A. State of the Art. Chronic Obstructive Pulmonary Disease, Inflammation, and Lung Cancer. *Proc. Am. Thorac. Soc.* 2006.

24. Barber, M. D. et al. Relationship of serum levels of interleukin-6, soluble interleukin-6 receptor and tumour necrosis factor receptors to the acute-phase protein response in advanced pancreatic cancer. *Clin. Sci.* 1999.

25. Wang, C. S. & Sun, C. F. C-reactive protein and malignancy: clinico-pathological association and therapeutic implication. *Chang Gung Med. J.* 2009.

26. Hall, G. van et al. Interleukin-6 Stimulates Lipolysis and Fat Oxidation in Humans. *The Journal of Clinical Endocrinology & Metabolism.* 2013.

27. Plomgaard, P. et al. Tumor necrosis factor-alpha induces skeletal muscle insulin resistance in healthy human subjects via inhibition of Akt substrate 160 phosphorylation. *Diabetes.* 2005.

28. Shackelford, D. B. & Shaw, R. J. The LKB1-AMPK pathway: metabolism and growth control in tumour suppression. Nat Rev Cancer 9, 563–575 (2009).

29. Crawley, D. J. et al. Serum glucose and risk of cancer: a meta-analysis. BMC Cancer 14, 985 (2014).

30. Goodwin, M. L. Blood glucose regulation during prolonged, submaximal, continuous exercise: a guide for clinicians. *J. Diabetes Sci. Technol.* 2010.

31. Adams, O. P. The impact of brief high-intensity exercise on blood glucose levels. Diabetes. *Metab. Syndr. Obes.* 2013.

32. Pedersen, B. K. et al. Muscle-derived interleukin-6: lipolytic, anti-inflammatory and immune regulatory effects. *Arch. Eur. J. Physiol.* 2003.

33. Keller, P. et al. Interleukin-6 production by contracting human skeletal muscle: autocrine regulation by IL-6. *Biochem. Biophys. Res. Commun.* 2003.

34. Pedersen, B. K. & Febbraio, M. A. Muscle as an Endocrine Organ: Focus on Muscle-Derived Interleukin-6. *Physiol. Rev.* 2008.

35. Febbraio, M. A. et al. Glucose ingestion attenuates interleukin-6 release from contracting skeletal muscle in humans. *J. Physiol.* 2003.

36. Starkie, R. et al. Exercise and IL-6 infusion inhibit endotoxin-induced TNF-alpha production in humans. *FASEB J.* 2003.

37. Lira, F. S. et al. Endotoxin levels correlate positively with a sedentary lifestyle and negatively with highly trained subjects. *Lipids Health Dis.* 2010.

38. Gratas-Delamarche, A. et al. Physical inactivity, insulin resistance, and the oxidative-inflammatory loop. *Free Radic. Res.* 2014.

39. Oberley, T. D. Oxidative damage and cancer. *Am. J. Pathol.* 2002.

40. García-López, D. et al. Effects of strength and endurance training on antioxidant enzyme gene expression and activity in middle-aged men. Scand. *J. Med. Sci. Sports.* 2007.

41. Green, A. S. et al. The LKB1/AMPK signaling pathway has tumor suppressor activity in acute myeloid leukemia through the repression of mTOR-dependent oncogenic mRNA translation. *Blood.* 2010.

42. Champ, C. E. et al. Nutrient Restriction and Radiation Therapy for Cancer Treatment: When Less Is More. *Oncologist.* 2013.

43. Faubert, B. et al. AMPK is a negative regulator of the Warburg effect and suppresses tumor growth in vivo. *Cell Metab.* 2013.

44. Vavvas, D. et al. Contraction-induced changes in acetyl-CoA carboxylase and 5'-AMP-activated kinase in skeletal muscle. *J. Biol. Chem.* 1997.

45. Winder, W. W. & Hardie, D. G. Inactivation of acetyl-CoA carboxylase and activation of AMP-activated protein kinase in muscle during exercise. *Am. J. Physiol.* 1996.

46. Rasmussen, B. B. & Winder, W. W. Effect of exercise intensity on skeletal muscle malonyl-CoA and acetyl-CoA carboxylase. *J. Appl. Physiol.* 1997.

47. Draznin, B. et al. Effect of Dietary Macronutrient Composition on AMPK and SIRT1 Expression and Activity in Human Skeletal Muscle. *Horm Metab Res.* 2012.

48. Cantó, C. et al. Interdependence of AMPK and SIRT1 for metabolic adaptation to fasting and exercise in skeletal muscle. *Cell Metab.* 2010.

49. Bae, H. R. et al. B-Hydroxybutyrate suppresses inflammasome formation by ameliorating endoplasmic reticulum stress via AMPK activation. *Oncotarget.* 2016.

50. Hardie, D. G. Sensing of energy and nutrients by AMP-activated protein kinase. *Am J Clin Nutr.* 2011.

51. Hamrick, M. W. A role for myokines in muscle-bone interactions. *Exerc. Sport Sci. Rev.* 2011.

52. Layne, J. E. & Nelson, M. E. The effects of progressive resistance training on bone density: a review. *Med. Sci. Sports Exerc.* 1999.

53. Coleman, M. E. et al. Myogenic vector expression of insulin-like growth factor I stimulates muscle cell differentiation and myofiber hypertrophy in transgenic mice. *J. Biol. Chem.* 1995.

54. Kraemer, W. J. et al. Effects of exercise and alkalosis on serum insulin-like growth factor I and IGF-binding protein-3. *Can. J. Appl. Physiol.* 2000.

55. Rojas Vega, S. et al. Effect of Resistance Exercise on Serum Levels of Growth Factors in Humans. *Horm. Metab. Res.* 2010.

56. Brahm, H. et al. Net fluxes over working thigh of hormones, growth factors and biomarkers of bone metabolism during short lasting dynamic exercise. *Calcif. Tissue Int.* 1997.

57. Schiffer, T. et al. Effects of Strength and Endurance Training on Brain-derived Neurotrophic Factor and Insulin-like Growth Factor 1 in Humans. *Horm. Metab. Res.* 2009.

58. Suikkari, A. M. et al. Prolonged Exercise Increases Serum Insulin-Like Growth Factor-Binding Protein Concentrations. *J. Clin. Endocrinol. Metab.* 1989.

59. Cappon, J. et al. Effect of brief exercise on circulating insulin-like growth factor I. *J. Appl. Physiol.* 1994.

60. Berg, U. & Bang, P. Exercise and circulating insulin-like growth factor I. *Horm. Res.* 2004.

61. Carro, E. et al. Circulating insulin-like growth factor I mediates effects of exercise on the brain. *J. Neurosci.* 2000.

62. Carro, E. et al. Circulating insulin-like growth factor I mediates the protective effects of physical exercise against brain insults of different etiology and anatomy. *J. Neurosci.* 2001.

63. Tsai, C. L. et al. The effects of long-term resistance exercise on the relationship between neurocognitive performance and GH, IGF-1, and homocysteine levels in the elderly. Front. *Behav. Neurosci.* 2015.

64. Levine, M. E. et al. Low protein intake is associated with a major reduction in IGF-1, cancer, and overall mortality in the 65 and younger but not older population. *Cell Metab.* 2014.

65. Church, D. D. et al. l -Leucine Increases Skeletal Muscle IGF-1 but Does Not Differentially Increase Akt/mTORC1 Signaling and Serum IGF-1 Compared to Ursolic Acid in Response to Resistance Exercise in Resistance-Trained Men. *J. Am. Coll. Nutr.* 2016.

66. Ahlborg, G. et al. Substrate Turnover during Prolonged Exercise in Man. *J. Clin. Invest.* 1974.

67. D'Antona, G. et al. Branched-Chain Amino Acid Supplementation Promotes Survival and Supports Cardiac and Skeletal Muscle Mitochondrial Biogenesis in Middle-Aged Mice. *Cell Metab.* 2010.

68. Sjödin, B. et al. Biochemical Mechanisms for Oxygen Free Radical Formation During Exercise. *Sport. Med.* 1990.

69. Austin, S. & St-Pierre, J. PGC1$^{\alpha}$ and mitochondrial metabolism - emerging concepts and relevance in ageing and neurodegenerative disorders. *J. Cell Sci.* 2012.

70. Ristow, M. et al. Antioxidants prevent health-promoting effects of physical exercise in humans. *Proc. Natl. Acad. Sci.* 2009.

71. Moskalev, A. A. et al. Genetics and epigenetics of aging and longevity. *Cell Cycle.* 2014.

72. Cao, L. et al. Environmental and Genetic Activation of a Brain-Adipocyte BDNF/Leptin Axis Causes Cancer Remission and Inhibition. *Cell.* 2010.

Chapter 11:

1. Willett, W. C. Diet and breast cancer. *J. Intern. Med.* 2001.

2. Dreyfuss, E. Want to Make a Lie Seem True? Say It Again. And Again. And Again | WIRED. Wired (2017). Available at: https://www.wired.com/2017/02/dont-believe-lies-just-people-repeat/. (Accessed: 5th April 2018)

3. Willett, W. C. Diet and cancer. *Oncologist.* 2000.

4. Daley, C. et al. A review of fatty acid profiles and antioxidant content in grass-fed and grain-fed beef. *Nutr. J.* 2010.

5. Realini, C. E. et al. Effect of pasture vs. concentrate feeding with or without antioxidants on carcass characteristics, fatty acid composition, and quality of Uruguayan beef. *Meat Sci.* 2004)

6. Haskins, C. P. et al. Meat, eggs, full-fat dairy, and nutritional boogeymen: Does the way in which animals are raised affect health differently in humans? *Crit. Rev. Food Sci. Nutr.* 2018.

7. O'Dea, K., Deakin U. Kangaroo meat - polyunsaturated and low in fat: ideal for cholesterol-lowering diets. *Aust. Zool.* 1988.

8. Arya, F. et al. Differences in postprandial inflammatory responses to a 'modern' v. traditional meat meal: a preliminary study. *Br. J. Nutr.* 2010.

9. Chan, D. S. M. et al. Red and processed meat and colorectal cancer incidence: meta-analysis of prospective studies. *PLoS One.* 2011.

10. Koeth, R. A. et al. Intestinal microbiota metabolism of L-carnitine, a nutrient in red meat, promotes atherosclerosis. *Nat. Med.* 2013.

11. Bae, S. et al. Plasma choline metabolites and colorectal cancer risk in the Women's Health Initiative Observational Study. *Cancer Res.* 2014.

12. Zhang, A. Q. et al. Dietary precursors of trimethylamine in man: a pilot study. *Food Chem. Toxicol.* 1999.

13. Zheng, H. et al. Metabolomics Investigation To Shed Light on Cheese as a Possible Piece in the French Paradox Puzzle. *J. Agric. Food Chem.* 2015.

14. Micha, R. et al. Red and processed meat consumption and risk of incident coronary heart disease, stroke, and diabetes mellitus: a systematic review and meta-analysis. *Circulation.* 2010.

15. Key, T. J. et al. Cancer incidence in vegetarians: results from the European Prospective Investigation into Cancer and Nutrition (EPIC-Oxford). *Am. J. Clin. Nutr.* 2009.

16. Institute of Medicine et al. Dietary reference intakes for vitamin A, vitamin K, arsenic, boron, chromium, copper, iodine, iron, manganese, molybdenum, nickel, silicon, vanadium, and zinc. A Report of the Panel on Micronutrients (National Academies Press, 2001).

17. Sawa, T. et al. Lipid peroxyl radicals from oxidized oils and heme-iron: implication of a high-fat diet in colon carcinogenesis. Cancer Epidemiol. *Biomarkers Prev.* 1998.

18. Vipperla, K. & O'Keefe, S. J. The microbiota and its metabolites in colonic mucosal health and cancer risk. *Nutr. Clin. Pract.* 2012.

19. Guarner, F. & Malagelada, J.-R. Gut flora in health and disease. *Lancet.* 2003.

20. Curing Ground Meat: Soppressata | Ruhlman. Available at: https://ruhlman.com/2011/10/18/soppressata-recipe/. (Accessed: 7th May 2016)

21. Virk-Baker, M. K. et al. Dietary acrylamide and human cancer: a systematic review of literature. *Nutr. Cancer.* 2014.

22. Alomirah, H. et al. Concentrations and dietary exposure to polycyclic aromatic hydrocarbons (PAHs) from grilled and smoked foods. *Food Control.* 2011.

23. Lijinsky, W. The formation and occurrence of polynuclear aromatic hydrocarbons associated with food. *Mutat. Res. Toxicol.* 1991.

24. Phillips, D. H. Polycyclic aromatic hydrocarbons in the diet. Mutat. Res. Toxicol. Environ. *Mutagen.* 1999.

25. Stołyhwo, A. & Sikorski, Z. E. Polycyclic aromatic hydrocarbons in smoked fish – a critical review. Food Chem. 91, 303–311 (2005).

26. Tfouni, S. A. et al. Polycyclic aromatic hydrocarbons in coffee brew: Influence of roasting and brewing procedures in two Coffea cultivars. *Food Sci. Technol.* 2013.

27. Poole, R. et al. Coffee consumption and health: umbrella review of meta-analyses of multiple health outcomes. *BMJ.* 2017.

28. Sinha, R. et al. Pan-Fried Meat Containing High Levels of Heterocyclic Aromatic Amines but Low Levels of Polycyclic Aromatic Hydrocarbons Induces Cytochrome P4501A2 Activity in Humans. *Cancer Res.* 1994.

29. Grainger, S. Cooking Apicius: Roman recipes for today. (Prospect Books, 2006).

30. Gibis, M. Effect of Oil Marinades with Garlic, Onion, and Lemon Juice on the Formation of Heterocyclic Aromatic Amines in Fried Beef Patties. *J. Agric. Food Chem.* 2007.

31. Farhadian, A. et al. Effects of marinating on the formation of polycyclic aromatic hydrocarbons (benzo[a]pyrene, benzo[b]fluoranthene and fluoranthene) in grilled beef meat. *Food Control.* 2012.

32. Tkacz, K. et al. Influence of Marinades on the Level of PAHS in Grilled Meat Products. *Ital. J. Food Sci.* 2012.

33. Joosen, A. M. et al. Effect of processed and red meat on endogenous nitrosation and DNA damage. *Carcinogenesis.* 2009.

34. Murray, S. Effect of cruciferous vegetable consumption on heterocyclic aromatic amine metabolism in man. *Carcinogenesis.* 2001.

35. Herman, K. M. et al. Outbreaks attributed to fresh leafy vegetables, United States, 1973-2012. *Epidemiol. Infect.* 2015.

36. Mirvish, S. S. et al. Nitrate and nitrite concentrations in human saliva for men and women at different ages and times of the day and their consistency over time. *Eur. J. Cancer Prev.* 2000.

37. Kapil, V. et al. Physiological role for nitrate-reducing oral bacteria in blood pressure control. *Free Radic. Biol. Med.* 2013.

38. Tiso, M. & Schechter, A. N. Nitrate Reduction to Nitrite, Nitric Oxide and Ammonia by Gut Bacteria under Physiological Conditions. *PLoS One.* 2015.

39. Rowland, I. R. & Grasso, P. Degradation of N-nitrosamines by intestinal bacteria. *Appl. Microbiol.* 1975.

40. Horne, B. D. et al. Usefulness of Routine Periodic Fasting to Lower Risk of Coronary Artery Disease in Patients Undergoing Coronary Angiography. *Am. J. Cardiol.* 2008.

41. Varady, K. A. & Hellerstein, M. K. Alternate-day fasting and chronic disease prevention: a review of human and animal trials. *Am J Clin Nutr.* 2007.

42. Mattson, M. P. & Wan, R. Beneficial effects of intermittent fasting and caloric restriction on the cardiovascular and cerebrovascular systems. *J Nutr Biochem.* 2005.

43. Safdie, F. et al. Fasting enhances the response of glioma to chemo- and radiotherapy. *PLoS One.* 2012.

44. Harvie, M. & Howell, A. Energy restriction and the prevention of breast cancer. *Proc Nutr Soc.* 2012.

45. Bjelakovic, G. et al. Mortality in randomized trials of antioxidant supplements for primary and secondary prevention: systematic review and meta-anal sis. *JAMA.* 2007.

46. Hakooz, N. & Hamdan, I. Effects of Dietary Broccoli on Human in Vivo Caffeine Metabolism: A Pilot Study on a Group of Jordanian Volunteers. *Curr. Drug Metab.* 2007.

47. Bansal, S. S. et al. Curcumin Implants, Not Curcumin Diet, Inhibit Estrogen-Induced Mammary Carcinogenesis in ACI Rats. *Cancer Prev. Res.* 2014.

48. Thapliyal, R. & Maru, G. Inhibition of cytochrome P450 isozymes by curcumins in vitro and in vivo. *Food Chem. Toxicol.* 2001.

49. Boyanapalli, S. S. et al. Nrf2 Knockout Attenuates the Anti-Inflammatory Effects of Phenethyl Isothiocyanate and Curcumin. *Chem. Res. Toxicol.* 2014.

50. McWalter, G. K. et al. Transcription factor Nrf2 is essential for induction of NAD(P)H:quinone oxidoreductase 1, glutathione S-transferases, and glutamate cysteine ligase by broccoli seeds and isothiocyanates. *J. Nutr.* 2004.

51. Guyonnet, D. et al. Modulation of Phase II Enzymes by Organosulfur Compounds from Allium Vegetables in Rat Tissues. *Toxicol. Appl. Pharmacol.* 1999.

52. Dinkova-Kostova, A. T. et al. Potency of Michael reaction acceptors as inducers of enzymes that protect against carcinogenesis depends on their reactivity with sulfhydryl groups. *Proc. Natl. Acad. Sci.* 2001.

53. Concerted action of antioxidant enzymes and curtailed growth under zinc toxicity in Brassica juncea. *Environ. Exp. Bot.* 1999.

54. Wu, X. et al. Are isothiocyanates potential anti-cancer drugs? *Acta Pharmacol.* 2009.

55. Hecht, S. S. et al. Effects of watercress consumption on metabolism of a tobacco-specific lung carcinogen in smokers. *Cancer Epidemiol. Biomarkers Prev.* 1995.

56. Chung, F. L. et al. Inhibition of tobacco-specific nitrosamine-induced lung tumorigenesis by compounds derived from cruciferous vegetables and green tea. *Ann. N. Y. Acad. Sci.* 1993.

57. Stoner, G. D. & Morse, M. A. Isothiocyanates and plant polyphenols as inhibitors of lung and esophageal cancer. *Cancer Lett.* 1997.

58. International Agency for Research on Cancer. Glucosinolates, isothiocyanates and indoles. *IARC Publ.* 2004.

59. Xu, M. et al. Effect of carcinogen dose fractionation, diet and source of F344 rat on the induction of colonic aberrant crypts by 2-amino-3-methylimidazo[4,5-f]quinoline. *Carcinogenesis.* 1999.

60. Kassie, F. et al. Chemoprevention of 2-amino-3-methylimidazo[4,5-f]quinoline (IQ)-induced colonic and hepatic preneoplastic lesions in the F344 rat by cruciferous vegetables administered simultaneously with the carcinogen. *Carcinogenesis.* 2003.

61. Kassie, F. et al. Chemoprotective effects of garden cress (Lepidium sativum) and its constituents towards 2-amino-3-methyl-imidazo[4,5-f]quinoline (IQ)-induced genotoxic effects and colonic preneoplastic lesions. *Carcinogenesis.* 2002.

62. Liew, C. et al. Protection of conjugated linoleic acids against 2-amino-3-methylimidazo[4,5-f]quinoline-induced colon carcinogenesis in the F344 rat: a study of inhibitory mechanisms. *Carcinogenesis.* 1995.

63. Nowak, A. & Libudzisz, Z. Ability of probiotic Lactobacillus casei DN 114001 to bind or/and metabolise heterocyclic aromatic amines in vitro. *Eur. J. Nutr.* 2009.

64. Balstad, T. R. et al. Coffee, broccoli and spices are strong inducers of electrophile response element-dependent transcription in vitro and in vivo - Studies in electrophile response element transgenic mice. *Mol. Nutr. Food Res.* 2011.

65. Chih-Chung Wu, et al. Differential Effects of Garlic Oil and Its Three Major Organosulfur Components on the Hepatic Detoxification System in Rats. *J. Agric. Food Chem.* 2001.

66. Shi, L. et al. Alliin, a garlic organosulfur compound, ameliorates gut inflammation through MAPK-NF-κB/AP-1/STAT-1 inactivation and PPAR-γ activation. *Mol. Nutr. Food Res.* 2017.

67. Shibata, T. et al. Toll-like receptors as a target of food-derived anti-inflammatory compounds. *JBC. 2014.*

68. Sarvan, I. et al. Sulforaphane formation and bioaccessibility are more affected by steaming time than meal composition during in vitro digestion of broccoli. *Food Chem.* 2017.

69. Saha, S. et al. Isothiocyanate concentrations and interconversion of sulforaphane to erucin in human subjects after consumption of commercial frozen broccoli compared to fresh broccoli. *Mol. Nutr. Food Res.* 2012.

70. Wang, G. C. et al. Impact of Thermal Processing on Sulforaphane Yield from Broccoli (Brassica oleracea L. ssp. italica). *J. Agric. Food Chem.* 2012.

71. Ghawi, S. K. et al. The potential to intensify sulforaphane formation in cooked broccoli (Brassica oleracea var. italica) using mustard seeds (Sinapis alba). *Food Chem.* 2013.

72. Mahn, A. & Pérez, C. Optimization of an incubation step to maximize sulforaphane content in pre-processed broccoli. *J. Food Sci. Technol.* 2016.

73. Song, K. & Milner, J. A. The influence of heating on the anticancer properties of garlic. *J. Nutr.* 2001.
74. Liu, X. et al. Dietary Broccoli Alters Rat Cecal Microbiota to Improve Glucoraphanin Hydrolysis to Bioactive Isothiocyanates. *Nutrients.* 2017.
75. Oberley, T. D. Oxidative damage and cancer. *Am. J. Pathol.* 2002.
76. García-López, D. et al. Effects of strength and endurance training on antioxidant enzyme gene expression and activity in middle-aged men. *Scand. J. Med. Sci. Sports.* 2007.

INDEX

Made in the USA
Monee, IL
19 September 2020